Yog-Ethos

A simple compilation of personal experiences and contemporary information for conducting a successful and meaningful yoga session detailing yoga choreography.

Yog-Ethos

A Handbook for Aspiring Yoga Teachers and Students

Geeta Rao

ALLIED PUBLISHERS PVT. LTD.

New Delhi • Mumbai • Kolkata • Lucknow • Chennai
Nagpur • Bangalore • Hyderabad • Ahmedabad

ALLIED PUBLISHERS PRIVATE LIMITED

Regd. Off. : 15 J.N. Heredia Marg, Ballard Estate, Mumbai–400001, Ph.: 022-22626476
E-mail: mumbai.books@alliedpublishers.com

12 Prem Nagar, Ashok Marg, Opp. Indira Bhawan, Lucknow–226001, Ph.: 0522-2614253
E-mail: appltdlko@sify.com

Prarthna Flats (2nd Floor), Navrangpura, Ahmedabad–380009, Ph.: 079-26465916
E-mail: ahmbd.books@alliedpublishers.com

3-2-844/6 & 7 Kachiguda Station Road, Hyderabad–500027, Ph.: 040-24619079
E-mail: hyd.books@alliedpublishers.com

5th Main Road, Gandhinagar, Bangalore–560009, Ph.: 080-22262081
E-mail: bngl.books@alliedpublishers.com

1/13-14 Asaf Ali Road, New Delhi–110002, Ph.: 011-23239001
E-mail: delhi.books@alliedpublishers.com

17 Chittaranjan Avenue, Kolkata–700072, Ph.: 033-22129618
E-mail: cal.books@alliedpublishers.com

81 Hill Road, Ramnagar, Nagpur–440033, Ph.: 0712-2521122
E-mail: ngp.books@alliedpublishers.com

751 Anna Salai, Chennai–600002, Ph.: 044-28523938
E-mail: chennai.books@alliedpublishers.com

Website: www.alliedpublishers.com

ISBN : 978-81-8424-447-2

Published by Sunil Sachdev and printed by Ravi Sachdev at Allied Publishers Pvt. Ltd.
(Printing Division), A-104 Mayapuri Phase II, New Delhi-110064

Acknowledgements

The book would not have been possible without the pillar of my strength—my beloved husband, Mohan. His unrelenting encouragement at every step of the way has been inspirational. My daughter, Ritika Paul and her loving support, innovative ideas and constant inputs has meant a lot. I am proud that she lights up the pages of the entire book with her perfect yoga poses. My spiritual mentor and my son, Rishab's invaluable assistance has been motivating. My family has been extremely supportive, shoring up my endeavour with their positive energy and insight. I am eternally grateful to the Almighty for showering His Divine Grace and all my Gurus for their inspiration and guidance in helping me complete this book. Most importantly I offer my sincere salutations to all my yoga students who have played a major role in this blissful journey of my spiritual transformation.

Preface

At the outset I would like to thank you for taking the time off to read this book. The contents will walk you through from the start to the finish of each yoga session.

Today you have taken the initiative to improve your life along with those of others by promoting a new lease of hope for so many yoga practitioners. I assure you that I will not let you down and will not let you regret your decision of touching many lives through the medium of yoga. To get an idea of the individual flexibility levels, let us start with some simple and easy stretches.

Once you get the gist of it, we will carry on with more specific and complex postures.

Every session will include six parts:
1. The warm-up—these are preparatory poses
2. The standing postures
3. The sitting postures
4. The lying down on the floor postures (supine and prone position)
5. The breath workout
6. The pose of tranquillity (Shavasan).

So what *exactly* are we doing in our yoga practice?

If you recommend yoga to anyone, the most common response is "Oh God! Yoga makes my whole body ache…." The truth is that just as the theromometer reads the body temperature, yoga postures are scientifically designed to detect stiffness in the body. When you realise that it is *only through yoga* that certain aspects of the 'self' namely, the physical (stiffness), mental (rigidity) and spiritual (ignorance) can be detected, it makes yoga all the more interesting to ponder over and practice.

Yoga comprises three main features: Postures (Asanas), Deep Breathing (Pranayama) and Meditation (Dhyana) which help in uniting the *Body, Mind and Spirit.*

Yoga Postures

The primary function of yoga postures is to make the person *mentally aware* of one's *physical state*. In other words, yoga diverts one's attention to the *union* or the connection between the mind and the body which may not be possible when one is busy walking, talking or working. Thus when you are busy or stressed, you are not aware of certain aspects of yourself but when you start performing a posture, you become aware of the aches, pains, stiffness or discomfort in certain areas. In other words, these postures give you a good chance to peer into your body's stiff or problematic areas because they are 'scientifically designed' to identify stiffness or discomfort. By allowing you to become aware of your physical state, they create what is known as *Increased Awareness*.

Any pain or stiffness signifies a blockage in the energy system of the body and these yoga postures help in removing these blockages. With the regular practice of yoga, the energy system gets balanced, and as renewed energy begins to flow freely and evenly throughout the body, you begin to feel supple, flexible and physically better without the pains and aches.

Deep Breathing

As you continue the practice of yoga, the body begins to feel totally relaxed and devoid of pains and aches. This condition allows you to focus on your mind, setting you thinking about your thoughts, actions and emotions. You begin to scan your mental 'innerscape' to understand your behaviour and check whether it needs any change, correction or improvement. Here, the deep breathing practices of yoga called '*Pranayam*' help you to remove *mental irregularities* such as unwanted thoughts, negative emotions, etc. Deep breathing connects you to your mind and you begin to feel mentally aware and clear. When you become conscious of this mental clarity, there is a union between your conscious and subconscious levels which is known as *Higher Awareness*.

Meditation

Your journey does not stop here. From easing the body through the postures and the mind through the deep breathing techniques, you travel further through meditation to still the mind to block the flow of thoughts which cause anxiety, depression or unhappiness. You not only look within but begin to look beyond yourself and your surroundings.

In yoga, meditation unfolds to you that you are the outcome and a replica of the universal consciouness. Therefore, you do not limit yourself to 'increased awareness' or the 'higher awareness' but flow further towards what is known as 'Spiritual Awareness' or 'Awakening'. This leads you to understand the true purpose and the meaning of your very existence on earth and the ultimate union between you and the creator. This is the ultimate awareness for any human being. This kind of awareness is extremely rejuvenating for your own self or spirit. In such a state of attainment, your spirituality radiates around you, uplifting the spirits of others as well and you become spiritual in the true sense. So through yoga, what started out with physical awareness ends in peace and spiritual bliss.

Therefore yoga is a journey to ease the body, mind and spirit through physical, mental and spiritual experiences to finally unite with the Ultimate. It is a journey to evolve from one level to the next. Some people will accomplish the physical level, some will achieve the mental level, and yet others will master the spiritual level in which case they will be truly enlightened souls.

Every human being is potentially divine and yoga gives you the opportunity to ultimately unite with the Ultimate Bliss or Divinity. This is the main objective of yoga.

Total Postures at a Glance

Number of Warm-up Postures	30
Number of Standing Postures	34
Number of Sitting Postures	37
Number of Lying Down Postures (Floor Postures)	34
Deep Breathing Techniques and Others	25
Total	**160**

These specially chosen 160 postures/techniques will keep you fit all through the year.

Contents

SECTION–I

Introduction

SECTION–II

Sukshma Vyaayam (Warm-up)

Section—III

Standing Postures

Section–IV

Sitting Postures

xiv

The Lying Down Postures

SECTION–VI

Various Yogic Techniques

Appendices

SECTION–I
Introduction

Sarve Bhavantu Sukhinaha
Sarve Bhavantu Niraamayaha
Sarve Bhadrani Pashantu
Maa Kaschid Dukh Bhaag Bhave !

May all beings be happy
May all beings be healthy
May all beings receive strength
From the Almighty to perceive
Happiness and unhappiness alike !

Namaste to You All

Namaste is an Indian traditional greeting signifying a salute, a farewell or a gesture of humility based on the belief that there is divine energy in every human being. Yoga has a humble way of expressing this traditional greeting. It is done with affection, utmost respect or total gratitude. It is performed by placing the hands/palms together as in the 'prayer pose', bowing the head slightly as a sign of modesty or humility and verbalising the word 'Namaste', to acknowledge its essence.

There are three energy *chakra* sites for presenting Namaste, namely:

The Heart or Anahata Chakra: The most common form of greeting is by placing the joined palms close to the heart. This represents affection and fond regards, and is expressed generally to greet all human beings, elders or youngsters.

The Third Eye (Bhrumadhya—in between the eyebrows) or Ajna Chakra: The same gesture with the joined palms placed near the third eye indicates a sign of devotion and deep respect and proffered generally to the elders and gurus.

The Crown (of the head) or Sahasrara Chakra: Finally, the same gesture with the joined palms placed on the head signifies eternal gratitude and total surrender or submission in front of the Almighty.

There are three ways of presenting this gesture, denoting three different sentiments.

Namaste—Meaning and Importance

The word is split into: nama+as+te; 'nama' = bowing, 'as' = I, 'te' = you.

The divine spirit in me bows to the divine spirit in you.

The Light in me salutes the Light in you.

I honour the Universal Spirit in you.

With respect, I bow my head with folded hands and palms together in front of the divine energy of your soul.

Namaskar—Meaning and Importance

This is another way of paying one's respect to one's elders, Guru and God.

The word splits into nama+as+kar, that is, 'nama'= bowing, 'as' = I, 'kar' = hands/action. In this expression of reverence, a younger person kneels down at the feet of an older person, placing his/her right hand on the right foot and the left hand on the left foot of the older person who, in return, places his/her right or both hands on the younger person's head. In this form of salutation, an energy circuit is created between them, in the form of an electro-magnetic current which serves as a catalyst in increasing the receptivity of the younger person for absorbing positive energy from the elder. This pure and positive energy comes in the form of an assurance or a blessing from the elder to the younger person, boosting the latter's self-confidence, self-reliance, self-esteem, self-awareness and self-healing.

The ultimate demonstration of devotion is displayed through Saashtanga Namaskar (This is used in the Sun Salutations as in Step 6).

Saashtanga Namaskar—Meaning and importance

This is yet another way of paying one's respect to one's elders, Guru and God. The word splits into sa+ashta+anga, that is, 'sa' = with, 'ashta' = eight, 'anga' = limbs, parts or eight points of the body: the forehead (bhrumadhya), the chest (heart), two palms, two knees and the two sets of toes which come in contact with the earth.

When performed in front of a Guru, God or the Sun (as in the Sun Salutation) it is in the form of prostration which depicts total surrender, faith and humility—the main factors for mental clarity and sanity. This gesture of reverence helps in unburdening one's woes and worries, trials and tribulations, physical ailments or mental pressures at the feet of a Guru or in front of God or the Sun. Many people have experienced solace and a feeling of divine energy being bestowed especially when one feels victimised, frustrated or depressed. Done as a routine practice, the human ego gets dissolved, opening new dimensions to one's personality, leading them towards wisdom. Generally, people get drawn to this pose with ease as there is some sort of hidden symmetry or inexplicable attraction attached to this pose which appeals to the subconscious mind. It teaches the most profound form of alignment with reality and is believed to have something to do with gravity, solemnity and the human instinct. The belief is that when one's personal will does not have any power to change a despairing situation on its own, one turns to the Higher Power or the Almighty and that triggers a sense of serenity, contentment and new hope that creates a very calming effect and a feeling of security.

My Personal Experience in the Field of Yoga

When I began teaching yoga a few decades ago, I faced several practical difficulties like what exactly to teach, when, to whom and why. Although there were plenty of yoga books available, not a single book seemed describable as a guide for yoga teachers. Those days in the early '70s, yoga was not as popular as it is today. Also, there were hardly any good teachers around to explain the correct definition of yoga, the purpose of the postures and the importance of deep breathing. The yoga classes were pretty boring and tedious as one was expected to perform postures and that too perfectly, without understanding why. I found some yoga teachers who were excellent 'picture-perfect, posture performers' but they too did not seem to understand or explain yoga from the students' point of view. At that time I often felt that *yoga is not a performing art but a transforming art.* If I had some guidelines then on sensible choreography, I would have saved my time on the energy-consuming and time-intensive task of structuring and sequencing the postures in a well balanced manner. I could then have paid attention to something more important like the students' expectations and concerns. This is how I was compelled to attend yoga classes conducted by several different teachers to learn various teaching techniques. I absorbed several influences and compiled all the skills. Several books on yoga and 'Yoga Journal' magazine were also key inspirations. I kept records of what I taught and also made notes of certain sessions which became popular and those which proved boring and ultimately decided to combine all the necessary features required to make a yoga class successful.

At this juncture I decided to share my experiences in the form of simple guidelines for the upcoming yoga teachers to make them self-reliant and also prevent them from groping in the dark regarding the uncertainty of what to teach and why. With the help of these leads they would conduct a flawless class keeping the practitioners' interest and safety intact.

It is my mission to offer this simple guide for those yoga teachers who wish to impart their knowledge to their students' satisfaction, become truly accomplished in conducting a successful yoga class and also make teaching a gratifying experience.

Balancing all the factors to make a session successful may become a tight rope walk when 10–15 students with different levels of accomplishment may come at one time. This can become pretty demanding as each one comes with their individual expectation and it is necessary to make sure that everyone is safe and satisfied with their yoga practice.

The secret of a **successful formula** for conducting a good class is through the practical and convincing explanation of the meaning of yoga and its physical, psychological and spiritual benefits as well as the **structuring** and **sequencing** of the yoga postures i.e., '**yoga choreography**'. Apart from all this, incorporating **synchronised breathing** is equally important.

Structuring

Structuring of the yoga postures is a science and an art. As a science it underscores two important aspects that are **selection of postures proportionately** and **which ones**. The first aspect is to select an equal number of postures from each section of 'Warm-up, Standing, Sitting and Lying-Down postures. The other aspect is to ensure a proper blend by clubbing of the complementary postures. For instance, after performing a 'forward bend' posture, it should be followed by a 'backward bend' posture.

As an art, it requires conducting the class at a graceful and flowing pace. Simultaneously, the teacher's positive energy, creativity and spontaneity should reflect in the journey of yoga that can be savoured by the teacher along with the students.

Sequencing

Sequencing is basically designing the entire section on postures keeping in mind and targeting the usual problems of the practitioners. This can be done by selecting postures that work on the stiff joints or weak muscles, sluggish internal organs which usually take the brunt of the daily stress and strain, mental restlessness and lack of concentration.

Mindfulness and the presence of mind have prime importance in observing and taking several decisions on the spot. The yoga postures should be arranged in a very well-balanced manner at a professional level. All this has to be executed at the same time without forgetting the level of flexibility of the practitioners. These postures will work gently on the areas such as the neck, shoulders, lungs, spine, the spinal-discs, their connective tissues and the limbs. This will make a difference especially when these postures are performed in the sequence mentioned in the guide since they are hand-picked postures blended with effective stretches to soothe and strengthen the body simultaneously. While performing these postures, the main aim is to make the most targeted areas respond favourably by easing their stiffness and strengthening the weak spots in order to receive nutrients through life-force or *prana* energy and an oxygenated blood supply.

Breathing

Breathing is another vital aspect of yoga and different from normal breathing. Each inhalation and exhalation is slower and retained for approximately 4 seconds each.

Synchronising each move of the posture with the specific action of either inhalation or exhalation results in a bonus of 'improved breathing' simultaneously. This enhances the performance of a posture and as a result optimises the benefits accrued from the posture.

Yog Ethos

One of the facts that teachers must keep in mind is that they would be assessed by the students who need to be convinced of the calibre and capability of the teacher in order to accept them. At the beginning of the session, never assume that students know nothing about yoga. Some may not know as much as the teacher but may have read, discussed and practised a lot. Whereas, others do not wish to show their ignorance and this happens invariably in a class comprising beginners and non-beginners. This situation may stymie the teacher in deciding how and at what level of yoga to begin with. Therefore, the best bet is to be subtle in the introduction to yoga and to elaborate on the understanding of the true meaning of yoga. This helps to dissolve differences and bring the whole class on a common wavelength.

The word "Yoga" comes from the ancient Indian language, Sanskrit. "Yuj", which means to yoke, bind, blend, attach or bridge. The question is, what is it that needs to be joined or bound and why is the medium of yoga needed to yoke or bind?

The answer is—it is our body, mind and spirit which ought to be united ultimately in our journey of life. These three parts correspond with the three aspects of yoga. The postures (Asanas) correspond with the body, the deep breathing (Pranayam) corresponds with the mind and the meditation (Dhyan) corresponds with the spirit. Linking these three aspects is done through our breath. Breathing bridges the body, mind and spirit and is the main aspect of yoga.

Amongst the various types of yoga, we will be practising the most popular form of yoga known as *Hatha Yoga.* The word Hatha is derived from Sanskrit and lays emphasis on the two sides of the body. 'Ha' embodies the properties of the sun which denotes heat, light, warmth, creativity, activity, passion and positive energy (male energy) and is represented by the right side of the body. 'Tha' reflects the properties of the moon which denotes coolness, receptivity and negative energy (female energy) and is represented by the left side of the body. The terms 'positive' and 'negative' energy refer to the electro-chemical charge of the body and have nothing to do with 'higher' or 'lower' in terms of the quality. The right side is positively charged and the left side is negatively charged and both have equal importance.

Our biological clock ticks throughout the day and night and our physical energy alternates between the solar and the lunar forces. Both warmth and coolness, provided by the solar and lunar energies to the body, are necessary and should be in balance to create harmony in the body. Through Hatha Yoga, the postures, deep breathing and meditation make this happen almost immediately.

The mind also has its own polarities and our thought process often moves from one extreme to the other without our realising it. This is quite natural due to our habitual thinking, daily experiences, preconceived ideas and a wide range of set opinions and assumptions. However, this oscillation most often becomes the cause of our daily anxiety and strife resulting in stress or confusion of the mind.

The ultimate goal of yoga is for the mind to remain in the centre of this polarity range. Yogic practice makes it simple and easy through postures, deep breathing and meditation. Through postures, the body is trained to be steady for an extended period of time. Through deep breathing, the mind is trained to be still and devoid of thoughts for a while and through meditation, the spirit or conscious is prepared to be silent for introspection. Soon we learn to look beyond ourselves, develop the ability to identify with the other person and understand true empathy which leads to compassion which is the first sign of an accomplished yoga practitioner.

However, when one begins to be compassionate, there are situations when one tends to go overboard with altruistic emotions and once again this can also result in emotional imbalance. When altruistic emotions sway fully towards others or egotistical emotions swing totally towards self, it becomes a weakness either way and in that case it is time for introspection. So, you soon learn a new concept that is *moderation* and *balance* which are the key words where compassion or other extreme emotions like self-centredness are concerned.

This is the best time to be in touch with one's conscience and only then will the true answers emerge restoring balance. Through the regular practice of yoga one does not feel the strain of remaining in balance or in controlling one's excesses. One learns to become realistic and practical whenever required. There is no need to 'control' one's 'weaknesses' as one learns to 'overcome' it as yoga takes one to a higher level of understanding to know the difference between 'controlling' and 'conquering'.

Apart from Hatha Yoga, there are various kinds of yoga, for instance, karma (action) yoga, bhakti (devotion) yoga, kriya or shatkarma (detox) yoga, kundalini (meditational) yoga, Jnyan (knowledge) yoga, etc., which ultimately have a common goal and that is to unite oneself with the higher consciousness. Equally fascinating is Ashtang Vinyasa Yoga which is also a part of Hatha yoga but has a much deeper connotation. In Sanskrit, 'Ashta' means eight, 'Anga' means limbs and 'Vinyasa' means step by step, breath synchronised movements. The breath is the reference, like a scale of measure. The eight fold path or the eight commandments comprise a scientific way of living. 1. Yama—Don'ts, 2. Niyama—Do's, 3. Asanas—Postures, 4. Pranayam—Controlled Breathing, 5. Pratyahara—Practice of controlling senses, 6. Dharana—Focusing on any object, 7. Dhyana—Meditation with full concentration, and 8. Samadhi— Super-consciousness and perfect harmony.

EIGHT FOLD PATH—ASHTANG VINYASA YOGA		
1. Yama	–	moral conduct
2. Niyama	–	religious observances
3. Asanas	–	right postures
4. Pranayam	–	control of prana, subtle life currents
5. Pratyahara	–	withdrawal of senses from external objects
6. Dharana	–	concentration
7. Dhyana	–	meditation
8. Samadhi	–	super-consciousness experience

Some Special Features of Yoga Postures

- In traditional yoga, there are some postures named after birds, beasts or reptiles since these are designed based on their characteristics. Similarly, in this book you may find that some of the postures have unfamiliar names which have been maintained for the sake of convenience and where the literal translation (transliteration) is used to help associate the English names with those in Sanskrit.

- One point requires particular mention. Some people tend to wrongly associate yoga with the Hindu religion. In fact, Hinduism has adopted yogic principles in their rituals after having realised their values in maintaining balance and harmony in life. The way karate cannot be equated with Buddhism, yoga, too, cannot be associated with Hinduism. Therefore, yoga is not a religion although one should practice yoga religiously just as we eat, rest, shop or entertain ourselves with great interest. Yoga is a way of life and an art of living.

- Yoga is practised barefoot since our feet have tiny receptors in the form of acupressure points which make the right contact between the feet and the floor and serve like an earthing connection. Earthing improves the inner awareness and develops balance between the left and the right hemispheres of the brain. It also promotes balance between the body (physical actions) and the mind (emotions).

- Remember to come to class on an empty stomach. Any meal should be taken at least 2–3 hours before yoga practice. If you feel thirsty, you may sip water in between your practice but do not gulp water. The spleen chakra is the major entry point of oxygen. The practice of yoga brings about an ample oxygenation of the blood supply to your system. Gulping water results in an excess flow of liquid which interferes with the oxygen exchange and makes the stomach ache.

- Do not be tense about your practice as the slightest tension blocks the energy flow. Practising yoga is a healing process and it is not about getting the poses 'picture-perfect'. It is about being sensitive to your own body and getting connected to your true self—your conscience.

- Do not compete with the other practitioners as their levels differ from yours. If you wish to compete with anyone it should be with yourself by comparing your progress from the previous week to this week.

- Turning off your cellphone is a good idea in order to be quiet enough to hear your own inner voice.

- You can always express your queries and concerns either before beginning the class or at the end of the class.

Yoga Choreography

The basic principle of Hatha Yoga embodies postures performed with synchronised yogic breathing, within a specified time frame. Each move of the posture is synchronised with the specific action of either inhalation or exhalation. This breathing is different from the normal breathing as each inhalation and exhalation is stretched to a comfortable pace of 4 seconds each. This is again different from Deep Yogic Breathing where each breath is stretched to its full capacity.

Postures

Generally each posture has three parts:
  A. The first part is *going into the posture.*
  B. The second part is *remaining in the posture.*
  C. The third part is *coming out of the posture.*

Breathing

Each breath comprises two parts—inhalation and exhalation:
  • Each inhalation takes 4 seconds and there is a pause of 1 second.
  • Each exhalation takes 4 seconds and there is a pause of 1 second.

This means each breath takes about 10 seconds.

Posture and Breathing

Now synchronise postures with breathing as follows:
  1. The first part—going into the posture involves *two breaths*:
     This becomes one sequence of 20 seconds.
  2. The second part—remaining in the posture involves *four breaths*:
     This becomes one sequence of 40 seconds.
  3. The third part—coming out of the posture, just like the way you go into the posture, once again involves *two breaths*:
     This becomes one sequence of 20 seconds.

At the end of each posture, *one supplementary breath* is required to bring the breathing back to normal. This supplementary breathing sequence takes an additional 10 seconds.

Therefore, one posture takes about 20 + 40 + 20 + 10 seconds = 90 seconds.

So each posture takes about one and a half minutes using one side of the body. Then you repeat the same posture using the other side of the body which takes another one and a half minutes which means that each posture (using both sides) takes about 3 minutes.

A standard yoga session can be conducted for either 60 minutes or 90 minutes.

The 60 Minutes Yoga Session

When you perform 4 postures, you will take precisely 12 minutes. In a yoga session, the postures comprise 4 sections viz: warm-up, standing, sitting and lying down postures and each section comprises 4 postures. Since 12 minutes are taken up by each section of 4 postures, a total of 48 minutes are required for 4 sections consisting of 16 postures. After the postures, it is necessary to add 2 more sections of 12 minutes viz: Deep Breathing and Shavasan which would add at least a further 10 minutes for deep breathing practice and the remaining 2 minutes for Shavasan. This 6 section format is ideal for the 60 minutes yoga session.

If you adhere to the above time format of 60 minutes, the yoga session will look somewhat like this:
1. 12 minutes—warm-up/preparatory section comprising 4 gentle exercises
2. 12 minutes—4 standing postures
3. 12 minutes—4 sitting postures
4. 12 minutes—4 lying down postures
5. 10 minutes—3 deep breathing techniques
6. 2 minutes—Shavasan for total relaxation at the end of the session.

The 90 Minutes Yoga Session

For the 90 minutes session, the 60 minutes format can be extended proportionately for the extra 30 minutes.

When you conduct the 90 minutes session, you can begin with 5 minutes of gentle breathing, 60 minutes for the postures, 20 minutes for deep breathing and 5 minutes for Shavasan.

At the outset it is important to relax and settle down the class by asking the students to breathe gently for 5 minutes and to make them focus their attention inward. This also gives some 'late comers' a chance to join the class without disturbing others.

The 60 minutes will be spread equally over 20 postures i.e. 5 postures in each of the 4 sections (warm-up, standing, sitting and lying down postures) instead of 16 postures i.e. 4 postures in each of the 4 sections of the 60 minutes session. With the extra 5th posture of 3 minutes each in each section, a total of extra 4 postures and 15 minutes are required. These can be reserved for instance for Neck Circles or Self-Blessing from the warm-up section; any easy pose like the Mountain Pose in the standing postures; the Child Pose in the sitting postures and the Crocodile Pose in the lying down postures.

In the warm-up section you may pick any exercise. For the remaining 3 sections of postures i.e. standing, sitting and lying down, you may refer to the Index for structured postures and pick any 2 odd numbered and 2 even numbered postures.

Now you can avail of the remaining 25 minutes by allotting 20 minutes for deep breathing practice and 5 minutes for Shavasan at the end.

Of the 20 minutes for deep breathing techniques, you can take the breathing practice either in the beginning or at the end of the session, but remember that breathing practice is as important if not, even more important than performing postures.

Finally you may reserve the last 5 minutes to unwind, through meditation or through Shavasan where you focus your attention only on your breathing. Apart from this there is no other mental activity like thinking, counting or getting distracted by any outside factor.

Every yoga teacher is free to experiment with this choreography through one's own approach and perspective. This format which has been evolved through several years of teaching and research is meant to help understand the holistic nature of a yoga session and how to conduct it effectively within the given time frames and simultaneously incorporating various important aspects like safety, degree of flexibility, level of exposure and understanding, etc.

If you adhere to the above format, your 90 minutes' yoga session will look somewhat like this:

The session will consist of seven sections:
  1. 5 minutes—gentle and easy breathing to feel settled
  2. 15 minutes—warm up/preparatory poses comprising 5 gentle exercises

14

3. 15 minutes—standing postures comprising 4 postures + 1 of any easy pose
4. 15 minutes—sitting postures comprising 4 postures + 1 of any easy pose
5. 15 minutes—lying-down postures comprising 4 postures + 1 of any easy pose
6. 20 minutes—deep breathing comprising 3 breathing techniques
7. 5 minutes—total relaxation at the end with Shavasan.

General Instructions

Sometimes a variation in the number of postures can be done. Repeating the same posture twice provides a better insight into each posture. Performing it for the second time may help in improving their performance and quality in the posture giving them enough time to go deeper into the pose and absorb the benefits. In this case the students will perform only 2 postures out of the 4 in one section. This is left to the teacher's discretion and the energy level of the students.

In the 60 minutes session, perform 16 main yoga postures from the 4 sections: warm-up, standing, sitting and lying down postures. Once you have grasped the concept of time management for each posture, in the 90 minutes session, you can decide which postures should be repeated and which ones can be done just once depending on the practitioners' level of achievement. For example in sitting postures, certain difficult ones such as the Camel Pose (Ushtrasan), Cow-head (Gomukhasan), the Royal Dove (Raj Kapotasan) and Complete Spine Twist (Poorna Matsyendrasan) need to be repeated to achieve better performance.

Similarly, there are difficult ones in standing and lying down postures which may need to be repeated.

You will journey through each yoga posture following a route over 9 headings or key elements. This gives a complete summary of each posture. Apart from that, look for easy clues given in the numbers i.e. all the odd numbered postures are complemented by the even numbered postures. You will notice that the odd numbered postures are mostly for the upper body and the even numbered postures are mostly for the lower body. Also, the odd numbered postures involve stretching upward or bending forward whereas the even numbered postures involve stretching downward or bending backward. In addition to this, when postures are done with the right and left side of the body, they too become complementary to each other.

After this systematic practice one will realise that yoga is a beautiful tool that *toughens* the body, *strengthens* the mind, *sharpens* the focus, *heightens* the will-power and finally *evokes* the spirit in transforming one into feeling self-reliant and content for the rest of one's life.

Special Clues for the Class

While in the posture, it is a good idea to tell your students to channelise their mental energy to a particular part of the body by saying 'send your energy to your legs or arms or your abdomen' depending on which part of the body is involved. By sending their 'Thought Energy' to different parts of the body, your students become aware of their physical being. This will make them practice yoga with more awareness and involvement rather than practising it absent-mindedly or mechanically. With regular practice they begin to feel the stillness of the body and mind. Synchronising each individual move precisely with either inhalation or exhalation is very important. Each sequence will allow them to settle down in each posture and absorb all the benefits. It is important to take care to stay *within the natural limits of their flexibility*. Side by side their focus on correct breathing will help them release blockages in their energy flow and also relieve them from petty mindedness and unwanted mental clutter. Apart from this, the postures have a profound effect at a cellular level and on your emotional energy which will erase certain painful memories or unwanted emotional scars. The entire effect will result in regulating their subtle energy to heal themselves from within, feel connected with their inner pristine energy and awaken their true spirit which they will soon realise is full of unconditional love, understanding, peace, care and compassion.

In case they experience certain negative thought patterns, regular yoga practice will convert those into new forms of inspiration and confidence for them. When their flexibility level improves, you can lead them to the more advanced postures. Although certain postures may challenge them initially, they may find them gratifying ultimately as they will love to take up challenges in their yoga practice as well as in real life situations. Similarly, in the beginning their sense of balance and coordination may feel threatened but by giving sufficient time they will understand the concept behind each and every posture. Balancing postures boost their concentration and soon they will begin to love them. Yoga postures cannot be understood in one attempt. Only repeated practice of the postures which is called 'sadhana' will allow them to realise that yoga is not acrobatics or mere athletics but an inner awakening of their body, mind and spirit.

While practising warm-up exercises in the form of sukshma vyaayam, yoga postures, deep breathing or meditation, it is customary to close the eyes.

Students can close their eyes once they have learnt to perform and do not need to look at the teacher for guidance. Teachers need to be trained to be articulate in giving instructions immaculately in such a way that even when the students are blind folded, they should be able to understand the teacher's verbal instructions perfectly well. Closing one's eyes has a special significance. It is believed in yoga that we have two physical eyes and a third unseen eye, known as the spiritual eye, located in between and slightly above the physical eyes. When our physical eyes are closed, our spiritual eye opens up. It opens from the inside and absorbs all the sensory stimuli from your surroundings like a magnet. When our third eye is open, you cannot miss any sight, sound, smell, touch or even the taste in your mouth. We become acutely aware of our senses which lead us to *increased awareness*. This increased awareness is related to our bodily or physical consciousness. Once we are familiar with this response, we reach a higher level where our mind awakens and leads us to a *higher awareness*. This higher awareness is related to our subconscious or super conscious level. When we experience this level, it is like an inner mirror introducing us to our true self. Ultimately we are supposed to reach at a level where we see ourselves in the utmost clarity. With this experience one remains honest with one's inner self. We realise what is right and what is wrong and avoid 'wrong' in order to keep ourselves sane and happy, pure and enlightened. This is the essence of yoga.

Selection of Postures

Select postures which need to work on the following areas.

1. *The Neck and Shoulder Area*—Perform postures mostly involving your upper body including the torso and the spine, along with the neck and shoulders which will help stretch your spine in all directions: forward, backward, upward and downward. You will perform postures involving twisting or partial rotation of your spine for suppleness which will help in loosening up and unblocking the energy in the upper body.
2. *The Limbs*—You will use your limbs in most postures and also work on them by stretching, twisting and bringing your own body weight to bear on them. Working on your limbs will strengthen and prepare you for further postures.
3. *The Lower Body*—You will be working on your waist, abdomen, hip-joint and the internal soft tissue organs which will either be energised or stabilised depending on their energy level.

4. *The Entire Body*—Some of the postures will strengthen the energy centres by working on your entire body and boosting all the systems including the skeletal, muscular, respiratory, circulatory, digestive, nervous, reproductive and endocrine or the glandular systems. The glandular system is important as the hormones that are secreted regulate and influence your entire being. You should be aware of some important glands in your body. They are as follows:

(a) Gonads—Reproductive Gland
(b) The Pancreas Gland
(c) The Adrenal Gland
(d) The Thymus Gland
(e) The Thyroid/Para Thyroid Gland
(f) The Pineal Gland
(g) The Pituitary Gland.

When you work on them through several, appropriate yoga postures, the effect will be manifold in strengthening and balancing of the entire hormonal system.

5. *The Balancing Postures*—You will perform certain balancing postures that will make you aware of and improve your physical strength and balance and also train you to learn the techniques to make your body and mind still. Initially, the balancing postures make you wobbly, requiring an effort to steady the body. To achieve steadiness, the mind has to take charge of the situation in order to command the body. This can only be done if the mind is still and not wavering. Becoming aware of the stillness of the body and mind is very important to realise that imbalance is the root cause of all your turmoil.

At the physical level, the moment you achieve balance of the body, you begin to experience steadiness and strength.

At the mental level, you will overcome anxiety, chaos or confusion, experiencing renewed confidence, concentration and creative thought patterns along with contentment.

At the emotional level, each yoga posture communicates its own unique message to the brain and you will have your own interesting interpretation through the body and mind mechanism.

At the creative level, the balancing postures will elicit and utilise the untapped energy from both hemispheres of the brain and bring out your latent talents and positive energy.

6. *The Mind and Body*—You will be working on your breathing pattern to either increase or decrease and balance your energy level in the body. The deep breathing techniques will have an overall cleansing effect of your body and mind.

7. *At the End of your yoga practice*—You will be focusing your attention on the simplest of processes like your own breathing. When you meditate, you can tap into your inner resources which will have a refreshing effect on your body and mind.

8. *The Time to Wind* up—To conclude your yoga practice, lie in the Pose of Tranquillity or Shavasan to remove any strain which has occurred from any posture or deep breathing.

In most postures, bending, twisting and stretching are common, being integral parts of yoga but you should bear in mind that *stretching within the natural limits of your flexibility is good* and when it starts hurting at any given point, you should stop there, since pain indicates 'Negative Stretching' which is harmful and can lead to overheating of the body. Overheating creates tremendous energy which may often result in sleeplessness or restlessness.

There are different causes leading to overheating of the body *generally applicable to beginners*. The accomplished yoga practitioners with years' of practice may not experience the same overheating effect.

Causes and Reasons of Overheating

1. *Overheating Due to the Extended Period of Time in One Posture*: Remember, stretching is an integral part of yoga to ensure an oxygenated blood supply to the spine. To remain stretched for an extended period of time, say for four breaths in any posture, is a good interval to hydrate the spinal discs and its connective tissues with a flow of freshly oxygenated blood and prana energy. However, continuous stretching for more than four breaths begins to overheat the body.

2. *Overheating Due to the Continuous and Consecutive Vigorous Postures*: This happens if you continue with energy charging postures one after the other, without a break, as in the 'Vinyasa—Step by step' style.

3. *Overheating Due to Overstretching*: Most postures involve the limbs and there are certain postures such as the Heart Openers or the Hip Openers which exert extra pressure on the upper and lower limbs respectively. The heart openers involve mostly the upper body including the neck, shoulders,

19

arms and torso. Similarly, the hip openers involve mostly the lower body i.e. legs, sacrum and pelvis. When you perform such postures, the stretch is not limited only to the limbs but designed to exert pressure through a range of stretching motions extending to the vital organs as well, uniformly energising and stabilising them. This range is sometimes prone to over extension and therefore care should be taken.

Therefore the art of sequencing is given prime importance in a good yoga class to avoid overstretching which may lead to overheating of the body. Overheating leads to hyperactivity of the body and restlessness of the mind which defeats the whole purpose of practising yoga.

Hence, as an additional safeguard, the 'cool-down' poses are added to ensure a stabilising effect. This also results in inducing sound sleep at night without any interference in your normal sleep pattern.

Before you wrap up the session, you practice various breathing techniques which serve as the most effective methods ever devised for saturating the blood with anti-oxidants and balancing the biochemistry of the entire body. You will unfold many major secrets of anti-ageing; enlightenment and contentment, peace and bliss.

Some Popular Styles of Hatha Yoga and their Description

Iyengar Yoga

This type of yoga is said to use traditional hatha techniques (physical aspect) in fluid and dance-like, graceful sequences. This is one of the oldest and most authentic types of yoga which stresses on physical form, alignment of the body and precision in poses. The postures can be tailored to specific needs and abilities. Each posture is held for longer periods of time than in other types of hatha yoga, but it's not as physically demanding. It uses props such as belts, chairs, blocks, cushions, pillows and blankets to accommodate anyone with injuries or special needs.

Kundalini Yoga

This yoga is believed to mainly concentrate on awakening the energy at the base of the spine and drawing it upward through chakras or the energy wheels. A typical class includes chanting, meditation, postures and breathing exercises.

Kripalu Yoga

This yoga has been described as 'Meditation in Motion'. It allows you to focus on a flowing sequence of postures whilst achieving a meditative state. It is perfect for beginners. This yoga focuses on self-empowerment and self-improvement. Students focus on their bodies and their psychological reactions to the poses.

Viniyoga

This gentle form of yoga is tailored to each person's body type and requirements which also serve beginners well. This is based on your dominant 'Dosha' (mind-body type). Choosing the right poses and the type of practice are determined as per your type.

Ananda Yoga

This form of yoga focuses on simple postures that move the psychic energy up to the brain and prepare the body for meditation. This lays emphasis on proper body alignment and breathing.

Bikram Yoga

This is supposed to be 'hot-yoga' which is done in a sauna-style room that is heated to over 100 degrees Fahrenheit. The theory behind the heat is to warm the muscles so that they stretch farther and postures become easier.

Jivamukti Yoga

This type is said to be both physically challenging and highly meditative. This is mostly for advanced students. Beginner classes emphasise several continuous, standing poses with forward and backward bends. It sometimes includes chanting and meditation.

Kriya Yoga or Shatkarma

This includes various cleansing rituals of traditional yoga therapies. There are 'Dhauti' and 'Neiti' techniques which are detoxifying, healing and rejuvenating. They should be done under supervision and in a proper environment with facilities like a vomitorium. A lot of warm water is consumed and then thrown out to bring about the right pH in the body which is considered to bring harmony.

The Seven Energy Wheels (Chakra)

In yogic philosophy it is believed that there are seven energy centres in our body which are located vertically starting right from the base of the spine up to the crown of the head. These are referred to as Energy Wheels or *chakras* because of their continuous whirling energy. Each *chakra* is like a concentrated energy hub which radiates subtle life energy and although not visible to the eyes, one can zero in on them in order to assess one's physical, mental, emotional and spiritual status. As long as the *chakras* are active and in balance, individually and collectively, the subtle life energy moves throughout the body freely and evenly, bringing harmony. But at times, due to several factors, one or more *chakras* may become inactive, underactive or overactive and cause imbalance which is manifested in the physical, mental, emotional or spiritual malfunction. It is interesting to know that each *chakra* is associated with a specific colour corresponding to the 7 colours of the rainbow in the same order. Also, there are five natural elements which are associated with the five *chakras* starting from the base upwards.

1. **Mooladhara Chakra** (*The Base or Root Wheel*): It is located at the base of the spine or more precisely at the perineum, between the anus and the genitals. It is the foundation of the *chakra* system. Its element is the **earth** and it is symbolised by the colour red. When this *chakra* is in balance, one feels happy, relaxed, safe and grounded in the surroundings, experiencing calm. There is a normal tendency to be logical or realistic and a willingness to go at an easy pace in life or at times even allowing oneself to let go of certain impractical situations. Surrendering to the Almighty comes easily and naturally. But when the *chakra* is not in balance, it is manifested in physical malfunctions like aches and pains in the feet, legs or bones, disorders of the stomach like constipation, indigestion or diarrhoea. The psychological disorders include, having very low self-esteem, lack of confidence, procrastination, failing to take simple commitments, being unemotional, feeling threatened or seeming to be in a survival crisis, constant agitated mind, being unrealistic and unable to let go of any issue. Such people will also face constant problems relating to the earthy issues like family, business and property, etc.

The balance can be restored by certain postures and some of them are: The Wind Release Pose, Lying Spine-Twist, Reclining Buddha, Child Pose and the Pose of Tranquillity.

2. **Swadhishthan Chakra** (*The Sacrum Wheel or the Pelvis Plexus*): It is located at the lower abdomen or pelvis. Its element is **water** and it is symbolised by the colour orange. When this *chakra* is in balance, one is able to enjoy life with harmony, adaptability, receptivity, capacity to love and enjoy all sensual pleasures. But when the *chakra* is not in balance it is manifested in physical malfunctions like lower back pain particularly pain in the tail bone or sciatica, rigidity in the hip bones, various ailments concerning genitals, womb, bladder and kidneys. Besides, water being its element, there are constant problems with fluids of the body like urination, blood circulation, saliva, tears, ejaculation, menstruation and orgasms. The psychological disorders can be manifested in sexual obsession, inability to express deep emotions or enjoy any sensual pleasure, suffering from mental unrest and loneliness.

The balance can be restored through certain postures that bring healthy pressure on the hip bone and allow free movement in the pelvis. These are known as the **hip-openers,** for instance, the Cow-head Pose, Seated Forward Bends, Pigeon Pose or the Royal Dove Pose, Butterfly Pose, the Seated Angle Pose, Air Douche and Seated Warrior Pose.

3. **Manipur Chakra** (*The Solar Plexus Wheel*): It is located near the navel. Its element is **fire** and it is symbolised by the colour yellow. When the *chakra* is in balance it governs the digestive fire in the body by promoting good digestion, healthy metabolism, self-confidence, an assertive attitude, bright and courageous personality, the willingness to help others and an altruistic approach. But when the *chakra* is not in balance, it is manifested in physical malfunctions related to the stomach like indigestion, sluggish metabolism and various types of eating disorders. The psychological disorders include feelings of guilt or hate, mood-swings, emotional meltdowns, persecution complex, a constant need for reassurance from near and dear ones, being a perfectionist, craving for supremacy or material things, wanting to be rich and famous, etc. The balance can be restored by certain postures which are: The Palm Tree Pose, The Warrior Pose I, II and III, Sun Salutation, Tree Pose, Boat Pose, Half-boat Pose, Back bends, Spinal twist.

Deep breathing exercises like Kapalbhati and Ujjayi help a lot.

4. **Anahata Chakra** (*The Heart Wheel or Cardiac Plexus*): It is located at the heart radiating energy to the lungs, thymus gland, upper chest and back, shoulders, arms and hands. Its element is **air** and it is symbolised by the colour green. It is interesting to note that this is the fourth *chakra* either from the bottom or from the top since it is in the middle of the *chakra* system and joins the upper

three *chakras* with the lower three. When this *chakra* is in balance, it is manifested by tremendous positive energy, feeling of love and compassion, caring and sharing attitude, understanding and appreciating others, sacrificing and bringing harmony wherever it is possible. But when the *chakra* is not in balance, it is manifested in physical malfunctions like irregular breathing, breathlessness, palpitation, listlessness, lung disease or asthma, etc. The psychological disorders are manifested in feelings of acute insecurity, dejection, timidness, loneliness, lack of self-confidence or esteem, lack of empathy and an inability to 'forget and forgive'. The balance can be restored by certain postures known as **chest openers** like the Standing Bridge Pose, the Camel Pose and Backbends and Cow Head Pose, etc. Once the chest is opened and expanded, the heart chakra is activated which drives away fear, doubt and insecurity. Particularly, the High Shoulder Stand and the Head Stand Pose reverse the usual position of the heart by bringing the heart above the head as opposed to the usual position where the head is always above the heart. By reversing the usual position a great deal of emotional shuffling takes place and the mind ceases its dominant role. The heart then takes over the dominant role bringing about a miraculous trans-formation in the usual pattern of thinking or emotions. In addition, the Forward Bend Poses, either standing or sitting, are also recommended as they teach grounding, introspection and surrender to the cosmic power.

Also, Deep Breathing exercises which help in activating the higher *chakras* are particularly helpful for balancing this *chakra* as its element is air.

5. **Vishuddhi Chakra** (*The Throat Wheel*): It is located in the cavity formed by the throat, neck, jaws and mouth. Its element is **space** and it is symbolised by the colour blue. This *chakra* is associated with vibration or rhythm. When this *chakra* is in balance, people are interested in self development through skillful communication, articulation, personal progress, purification of the body and mind through a proper diet, yoga and meditation, as the fifth chakra focuses on spiritual development. But when the *chakra* is not in balance, it is manifested in physical malfunctions like stiffness in the neck and shoulders, tension in the upper back or in the jaw, various throat ailments particularly hypo (under-active) or hyper (over-active) thyroid problems. The psychological disorders can be fear of expressing or speaking or sometimes speech problems like stammering, stuttering or perhaps excessive talking and an inability to listen to others, hearing difficulties, etc. The balance can be restored by certain postures and they are: Neck Circles like Brahma Mudra, Shoulder openers like the Camel Pose, the Bridge Pose, the Cart Wheel, High Shoulder Stand and Plough Pose.

Deep Breathing exercises like Udgeet Pranayam with Omkar chanting, Bhraamari or Bumble Bee Sound vibrations help a lot. Any sound like singing or giving a speech, mock-news reading or reciting poems aloud, create vibrations in this *chakra* that help in bringing balance to the *chakra*.

6. **Ajna/Adnya Chakra** (*The Command Wheel*): It is located between the eyebrows. This is known as the third *eye* or the spiritual *eye*. Its element is ***perception*** and it is symbolised by the colour indigo. This serves like a sensor or the control panel of the body commanding all the sensory stimuli. The two *eyes* are meant for viewing this material world whereas the third *eye* viusalises the spiritual aspect and perceives beyond the physical entity. When this *chakra* is in balance, it helps in interpreting dreams, subliminal messages or decoding imagination or intuition. Since it involves perception, one can develop the art of telepathy and clairvoyance which have a powerful impact in one's spiritual journey. When the *chakra* is not in balance, it is manifested in physical malfunctions like *eye* problems, headaches, migraines, inability to concentrate, loss of immediate memory. The psychological disorders are having nightmares or hallucinations, being sceptical or cynical and having a negative or distorted view of the world.

The balance can be restored by certain postures comprising the *eye* exercises like covering the *eyes* with an *eye* mask to activate the third *eye* and to bring a fresh perspective in life, palming exercise to bring the necessary energy to the third *eye*, etc. The Seated Forward Bend, the Simplified Fish Pose, Child's Pose, Lotus Pose also help. Pressing the palms and the fingertips on the floor help stimulate the area around the third *eye* as our body's weight and pressure on the palms create positive images and boost imagination and creativity. It induces positive thinking and an assertive approach.

7. **Sahasrara Chakra** (*The Crown Wheel*): It is located at the crown of the head and serves as the crown of the *chakra* system. Its element is ***thought*** and it is symbolised by the colour violet. Sahasra in Sanskrit means thousand. In this case it is assumed to be the invisible lotus that has a thousand petals. These thousand petals represent one thousand nerve centres in the brain. This is believed to be the origin of our thought process, faith or belief system. With yogic practice like regular meditation the mental levels can be elevated to lead to a higher state of spirituality. Purifying and cleansing of the conscience becomes easy. Touching base with the true self or being honest with one's conscience is the primary state of enlightenment. Purity and spirituality can be seen through one's actions and can be felt at the spiritual level. When such enlightened

26

people are around they uplift others' spirits who begin to feel energetic and content. When this *chakra* is not in balance, it is manifested in physical malfunctions like difficulty in coherent thinking, indifference towards oneself and the surroundings, general lack of interest and a feeling of mental inertia. The psychological disorders include scepticism, cynicism, pessimism, suspicion and a craving for materialism through a religious medium, displaying pedanticism, spiritual arrogance, ego and sycophancy. The balance can be restored through certain postures and they are: Simple meditation focusing on one's breath which serves like mental cleansing. This chakra energy helps us to open to the Divine energy through simple humility. All types of meditation practices allow the mind to become more clear and insightful.

Yawn and Yoga

Some yoga practitioners begin to yawn the moment they enter a yoga class but the teacher should not feel offended. Although a yawn is somtimes a symbol of the body's protest against an action perceived as a boring activity, it has a different connotation while practising yoga. Some yoga teachers may find the act of yawning in their class pretty strange and may construe that something must be wrong with their style of conducting the class. Even if efforts are taken to make the classes more interesting, you may notice some more yawns. However, the verbal instructions or the soothing voice of the teacher is not making them feel bored or drowsy and instead of wondering about this natural or mostly nocturnal phenomenon, here is a little observation on this subject of 'yawning' and its interesting connection with yoga. This will help you understand some interesting facts and make you guilt-free about your proficiency.

Many people yawn in anticipation of stretching the body. 'Yawning' and 'Stretching' go together. The human mind has a deeper understanding than we think and yawning and stretching prepares the body for sudden stretching without the risk of injury. Injury occurs from a combination of an enthusiastic mind with an unprepared body. In other words, at times, if the mind is ready to perform the yoga poses but the body is a bit lethargic, an unhealthy resistance is created. A yawn can fix that situation in seconds by preparing the body for stretching and hence deal with unaccustomed stretches. Stretching in yoga is like an enlarged version of yawning.

Create Your Own Spiritual Sanctuary—
Yoga Utopia

When you cannot go on a vacation to recharge your spirit, you can unwind and rejuvenate in the comforts of your own home. The following regimen will give you some ideas on how to boost your spirit and feel joy and peace. Set aside a day and follow these tools and techniques.

Early Morning

To fill your mind with soothing thoughts, you need to create a spiritual sanctuary.

- *Early Morning Super Splash*: As you wake up, wash your face, ears and neck with cool or warm water depending on your need and the weather. Hold cool water in your palms and dip your eyes in it while keeping the mouth filled with water. When the water in your palms becomes warm, it indicates that it has absorbed the heat from your eyes. Also, when the water in your mouth becomes warm, spit it out.
- Perform the yogic style 'Sun Gazing' at the rising Sun when it is in its pinkish-red tinge by simply gazing at it and slowly rotating the eyes along its circumference clockwise and counter clockwise for two to three minutes.
- Kick-start your day with a 'Daily Detox'. A great beverage would be a glass of warm water with a few drops of freshly squeezed lemon and a few drops of honey that will stimulate your digestive fire to eliminate toxins from the body.
- Locate the energy spot in your house where you experience joy and hope. Spend a few moments there soaking this energy in.
- Keep some fresh flowers in a vase.
- Light a mild incense stick or an aromatic candle.
- Play some soft music and diffuse light by drawing the curtains.
- Adjust the temperature of the room as per your requirement.
- Chant your own name, your beloved's name or chant 'OM' or 'OM SHANTI'.
- Have breakfast consisting of fresh organic fruit, plain yogurt and muesli.
- Massage your skin with orange peel dipped in milk cream. Brushing removes impurities and dead skin cells and stimulates the lymphatic system and blood circulation. You can also use 'loofah' making small brisk circular movements.

- Massage your body with a few drops of your favourite essential oil mixed in almond oil and take a hot shower. It will vaporise and cover you in a cloud of fragrant steam. Revel in the sensation.
- Begin your daily meditation. Meditate by sitting on a cushion, cross your legs and keep your back straight. Set an alarm to go off 30 minutes later, then close your eyes and concentrate on your breathing. When your mind starts to wander off, bring it back to focus on your breathing. This will put you in touch with the 'come alive' feeling.

Mid Morning

- *Moving Meditation can also be a part of meditation*—Play some music of your choice depending on your mood at that point of time. Stand still and focus on your physical self. The music will guide you into making movements that will come naturally to you.

Have you tried dancing or swirling like a 'Sufi Whirling Dervish'? Open and raise the right palm to the skies as if ready to receive the Almighty's Grace. The left arm is stretched down with palm facing the earth in a gesture of bestowal. Log on to your own inner rhythm and begin revolving slowly. You will feel some connection through the cosmic energy from above which enters through the right palm, passes through the body and through the left palm into the earth. Make 3–4 whirls. This mystical experience leads to abundant positive energy, tolerance, clarity and charity, compassion, faith and awareness. The whirling of Dervishes represents a spiritual journey with the seekers turning towards the Almighty or simply inward. Dervish literally means 'doorway' 'Dar' (door) 'Vesh' (threshold) and is thought to be a door from this material world to the spiritual world. This is believed to help transcend all differences or prejudices and unifies one and all.

- Take a blank sheet of paper and a pen. Start drawing or painting whatever comes to your mind. If not, write words, images, thoughts, sensations or feelings. Take a few minutes to reflect on what you have written or drawn.
- Glance at these words everyday. List them as per their importance to you. You will be surprised to discover that your priorities will change from time to time. Today's sequence may not remain the same after six months. These words sink into your subconscious and remain imprinted helping you transform. This is your evolving journey through this life.
- *The Words:* Focus, Fulfilment, Peace, Relaxation, Energy, Hope, Confidence, Healing, Faith, Trust, Commitment, Honesty, Balance, Ethics, Integrity, Awareness, Clarity, Charity.

- *The Emotions:* Passion, Compassion, Love, Patience, Tolerance or any other emotion you think of intensely.
- *Ask yourself*—which frame of mind am I in today: Aesthetic, Spiritual, Moral, Social, Personal, Emotional, Intellectual, Mental or Heavenly or it could be a combination of two or more.
- Chant your *mantra* on prayer beads. Write a *japa* (mental repetition of a sacred word or name).

Lunch Time

- Try a tofu sandwich and some steamed vegetables for lunch. Feel the taste of each mouthful and be aware of the sensations as you swallow.

Evening Ritual

- Take a walk in the evening after eating and resting, leaving the sanctuary for half an hour. Start walking at a brisk but sustainable pace. As you walk, be aware of your surroundings. Notice the trees or buildings as you pass because you will be seeing things with a more meditative frame of mind.
- Sit in front of the window and watch the Sun Set. Observe how the colours around the setting sun change and finally blend in one tone. Wait for the moment when the sun actually sinks below the horizon. As the light fades, take a few minutes to enjoy your sense of calm and peace. You may feel the skyline transporting you into a different world.
- Have a cup of your favourite herbal tea like lemon-ginger or honey-vanilla.
- Prepare for a soothing bath by adding a few drops of your favourite essential oil. Then light candles, place them around the bathroom and play some Gregorian chant, any spa music or a 'New Age' tune. This simple ritual can turn into a meaningful and soothing experience.
- Lie back in the bath and remain aware of the water swirling around your body. Slowly pour a stream of water over your head. This form of ritual ablution is traditionally used to cleanse the aura and will help you disperse any troubled thoughts that may have surfaced during the day. Simply enjoy the sensation of the warm water and the therapeutic effect of the oils.
- Have a *Sattvic* (an Ayurvedic diet system) dinner with sprouts, fruits, nuts, vegetables and cow's milk.
- Select a prayer and start chanting at a pace that suits your natural inner rhythm. Continue the prayer for half an hour.

- Perform Kapalbhati, Agnisar, Anuloma-Viloma, Bhastrika, Ujjayi, Bhraamari, Udgeet Pranayam with chanting of OM for about half an hour.
- Climb into bed and take a moment to dwell on everything you have achieved today. Retire with Peace.

Going through this experience will transform your emotions and moods into feelings of contentment and serenity that will easily allow you to enter your inner landscape. Soon you will feel connected to your supreme self. This state of mind will lead you beyond yourself and beyond this worldly strife giving you a broader perspective of life and making you feel cleansed and purified. You will begin to float in your sacred, spiritual sanctuary where you will fulfil your dreams and desires and also accomplish your ambitions and aspirations. Later on you will begin to motivate others to fulfil their dreams and desires as well and people too will look up to you as their spiritual mentor.

SECTION–II
Sukshma Vyaayam (Warm-up)

Warm-up is to limber up the body before beginning any sort of exercise. This applies to yoga too. There are subtle physical exercises known as 'Sukshma Vyaayam' in Sanskrit which have a positive effect on the body, mind and the spirit. These exercises are as follows:

1. The Neck Circles
2. Finger Rotation
3. Five Fingers Technique
4. Sunflowers Bloom
5. Breathing through a Ten Petals Lotus
6. Blessing Oneself for Purification
7. The Dynamic Arms Twist
8. Five Sensory Point Massage
9. The Divine Triangle
10. Yoga for Energy Wave Balance
11. Chakra Meditation
12. Palming
13. The Wrist-joint Rotations
14. The Big Zero with the Elbows and the Shoulders
15. Ankle Circles
16. Knee Press
17. Rolls—Side to Side in Sitting Position
18. Knee Crank
19. Extended Stretch in Lying Down Position
20. Leg Scissors
21. The Breath Coordination
22. Sixteen Point Upper Body Stretch
23. Sixteen Point Lower Body Stretch
24. Knee Press (Front)
25. Knee Press (Back)
26. The Yogic Sit-ups
27. Leg Kicking I
28. Dynamic Stretch and Swing
29. Arm Scissors
30. Leg Kicking II

1

Brahma Mudra or Greeva Sanchalan (The Neck Circles)

Aim—To feel relaxed at the beginning of your practice. This also helps to stave off workplace injuries and to stretch the neck muscles which help release stored tension from the neck area and around the shoulders.

Time Span—Two to three minutes.

Technique—Sitting in any comfortable pose, preferably in the Easy Pose. This can also be done in the Diamond, Adept Pose or any Easy Pose of your choice. Breathe gently. Inhale and turn your head to the right, remain in this position and exhale. Once again inhale, exhale and return to the centre. Inhale and exhale. In the same way, inhale and turn your head to the left, remain in this position and exhale. Once again inhale, exhale and come back to the centre. Inhale and exhale. Inhale and raise the head upward towards the ceiling, exhale. Inhale, keeping the head up, stretch your neck comfortably. Exhale and bring it back to the centre. Inhale and stay in the centre. Exhale and drop the head downward, chin touching the breastbone. Inhale and exhale.

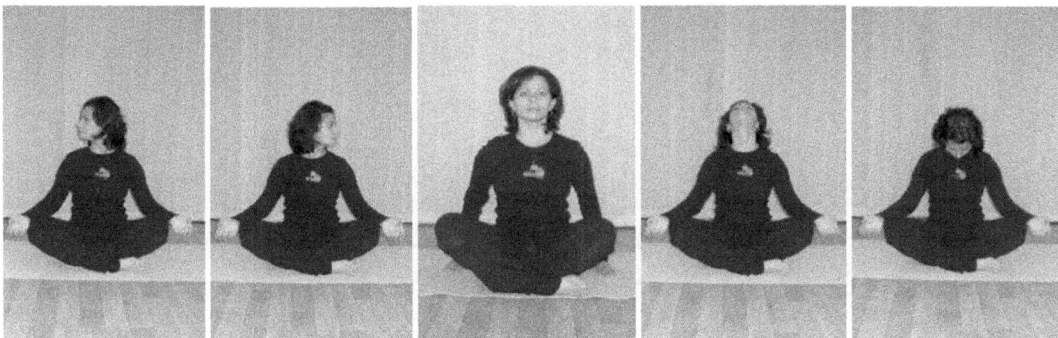

Coming Out of the Pose—Inhale and gently lift the head to bring it back to the centre, in the normal position. Exhale and stay in the centre. Inhale and exhale gently.

Focus—Should be on the breathing and the stretching of the muscles.

Breathing Pattern—During the posture, each inhalation and each exhalation should last for approximately four seconds.

Physical Benefits—All the nerves connecting the different organs and limbs of the body pass through the neck. Therefore, the muscles of the neck and shoulders accumulate tension. This 'Sukshma Vyaayam' releases tension, heaviness and stiffness in the head, neck and the shoulder region.

Psychological Benefits—Looking into all directions serves like opening the windows to all sides of the mind which teaches you to have an overall view of any situation without having a one track mind. This broadens the horizon of the mind and offers a deeper dimension of the situation.

Spiritual Benefits—With gentle breathing, these neck movements activate the higher chakras and allow free and unobstructed thinking.

Contraindications—Those suffering from cervical spondylosis, low or very high blood pressure and elderly and weak people should avoid this exercise.

Value Addition—While doing the neck circles, you are looking to the right, left, up and down. How many directions are you looking at?

The answer is five (right, left, centre (in front), up and down).

Thought for the Day

The Buddhist philosophy says that we cannot escape old age, illness or death; we cannot escape separation from our loved ones or disappointment from our dear ones. The only thing that stays with us is our action and we cannot escape from the consequences of our actions. Therefore our actions must always be righteous.

2

Angulika Chakra
(Finger Rotation)

Aim—To develop single or one-pointedness using finger rotation technique.

Time Span—Five minutes.

Technique—Extend your arms in front at the shoulder level. Open your palms facing outward, keeping them vertical and stretch your fingers wide. Start rotating the little fingers of both hands clockwise and counter-clockwise, five times. Repeat the same with other corresponding fingers individually.

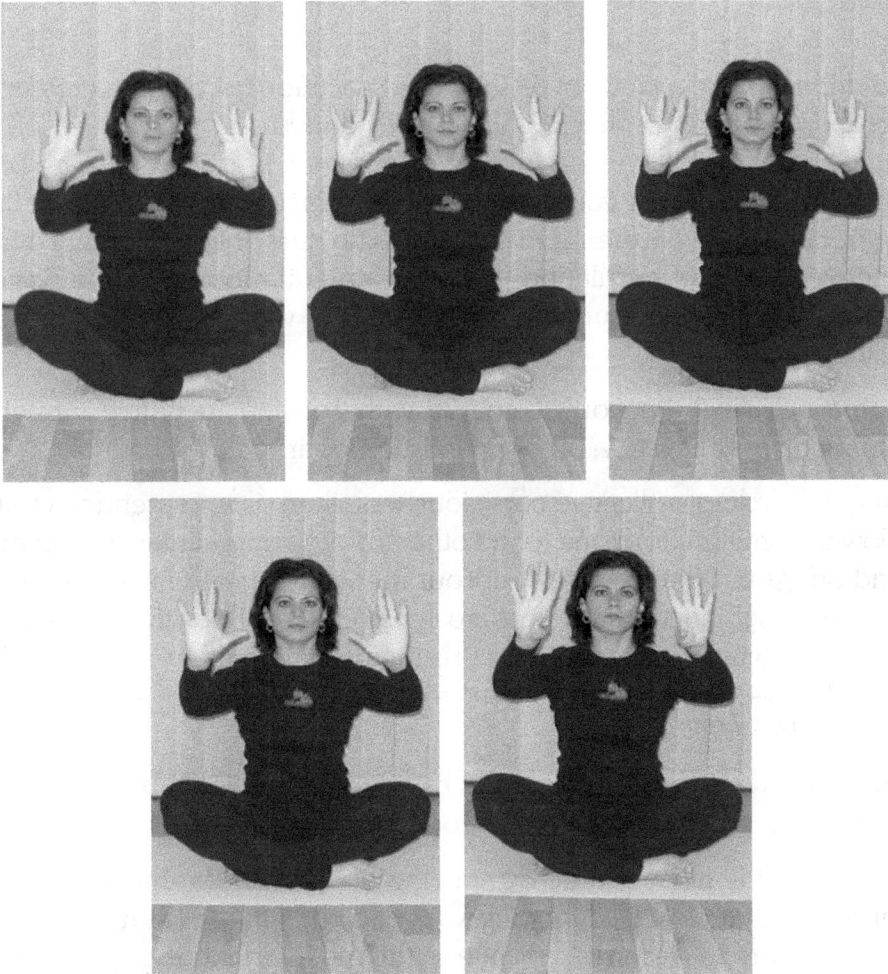

Focus—On the coordination and rotation of each finger of both hands clockwise and counter-clockwise five times.

Breathing Pattern—Normal and easy.

Physical Benefits—Develops steadiness and physical coordination. This training leads you to a heightened awareness.

Psychological Benefits—Improves mental concentration and reflexes.

Contraindications—Do not do this if you have severe arthritis of the finger joints.

Value Addition—Make a circle of all the yoga practitioners. Sit with crossed legs. Ask all of them to open both the palms. Each one has to place their left palm (facing upward) on their left side partner's right knee and your left side partner will place her right palm on your left palm. Now place the right palm on the left palm of your right side partner. If this is confusing, just hold each other's hands. This synergy helps in circulating the built-up, vibrant energy among the practitioners soon after the yoga session. Make a wish or a silent prayer for peace. It works.

When some people drain you of energy with constant negative thoughts or threats, try to balance it with a bit of optimistic vigour.

By making the circle of collective consciousness, there is a tremendous uplifting energy flow transmitted from one to the other through the cellular contact of your palms and brings out the best in you. Your mental connections will be stronger and emotions heightened when you are surrounded by positive energy which also allows you to tune into your own pristine positive energy.

Thought for the Day

Coordination awakens the awareness of your body. Use this awareness to observe the movement of the chest through your breathing.

Even if you decide to be physically still, the body cannot remain totally still. You will notice that your body moves with each breath and that is absolutely normal. You learn to become sensitive to the inner workings of your body.

3

Shun Mukhi Mudra
(Five Fingers Technique)

Aim—To protect the eight gates* of the sense organs from any negativity or excess stimulation. It is a powerful practice for withdrawing the mind from all association with sensory objects or external stimuli which functions like 'Pratyahara'—the fifth limb from Ashtang Yoga.

Time Span—Five minutes.

Technique—Using both hands, place the corresponding finger of each hand on each of your five senses, your index fingers on the forehead i.e. on your main sensor, your middle fingers on your eyes, the ring fingers close to your nostrils, the little fingers close to your mouth and your thumbs gently on your ears. Inhale and exhale gently. On each inhalation, imagine that your fingertips are injecting divine energy into your senses. On each exhalation, imagine that your senses are expelling negative energy absorbed from any of your surroundings.

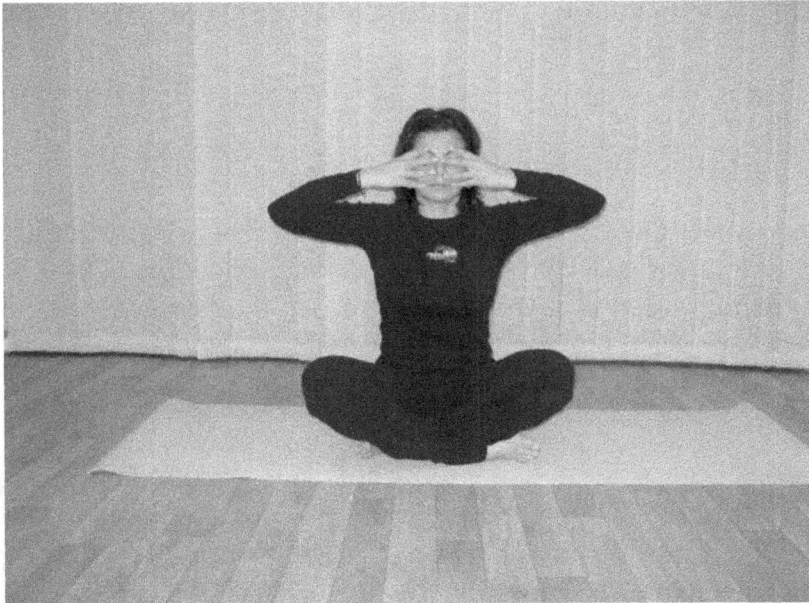

---

* Eight Gates are—Bhrumadhya or the third eye area, two eyes, two nostrils, two ears and the mouth.

Focus—Should be on each sense organ. Concentrate on the inner sounds and visions of a divine and psychic nature.

Breathing Pattern—Gentle and easy.

Physical Benefits—It balances the internal and external awareness.

Psychological Benefits—Awakens psychic sensitivity and induces the state of 'Pratyahara' or the withdrawal of excessive stimuli absorbed by the senses.

Contraindications—People suffering from acute depression should avoid this.

Value Addition—Before you begin this exercise, join and connect all the five fingertips of your right hand with the corresponding fingertips of your left hand. Push and expand, vibrating them. This increases the positive energy of your acupressure points which are connected to various internal organs.

Thought for the Day

As your senses keep absorbing energy from your surroundings, sometimes unwittingly you absorb negative energy. By placing each finger on each of your senses, you expel negativity from your senses. Your fingertips/acupressure points inject fresh flow of energy to the corresponding area of the sense which brings positive energy and stability to the senses and also clarity to the mind. You also create a strong, protective shield around your senses whereby you are not affected by any negativity for quite sometime.

4

Prasaarita Pushpasan (Suryamukhi)
(Sunflowers Bloom)

Aim—To stretch the finger joints and to open and activate the mini/minor chakras of the palms.

Time Span—Five minutes.

Technique—Make tight fists of both hands with the thumbs inside, keeping them at the shoulder level, with fists facing outside. Imagining the bloom of sunflowers, open the fists very slowly with resistance, till all the fingers stretch backward. Widen the palm and feel the stretch. Breathe normally. Make a circular movement of your arms as if you are running your hands over the periphery of two huge sunflowers and visualise the bright yellow colour of your imaginary sunflowers.

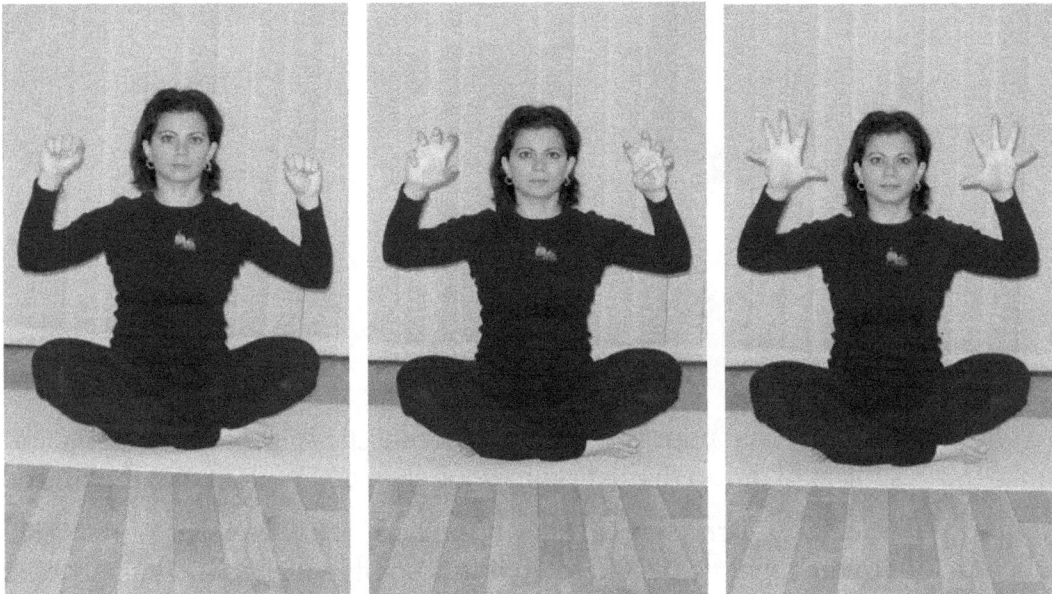

Focus—Should be on the stretching of the fingers and the palms.

Breathing Pattern—Normal.

Physical Benefits—Protects the finger joints from arthritis and improves your grip. The knuckles become flexible and strong.

Psychological Benefits—It brings brightness to your mood when you imagine a bright yellow colour. It improves your visualisation and coordination.

Contraindications—Do not do this if you have severe arthritis of the finger joints.

Value Addition—Find out your views on a 'Minimalistic Approach' to living and make this a subject of group discussion in your class when you have the time.

A group discussion often serves like a guided tour to your inner self, subconscious mind, inner voice and to your true spirit as well as a preview of the outside world. You come to know yourself a little better and the society at large, each time you participate in group discussions.

Thought for the Day

He who finds fault with others cannot see his own.

---

5 | Dasha-Bhuja Padma
(Breathing through a Ten Petals Lotus)

Aim—To feel calm, composed and centred.

Time Span—Five minutes.

Technique—Connect the index finger and thumb of both hands. Outlining the inner and outer perimeters of a lotus petal through two semicircles, inhale and raise your hands in a semicircular movement joining them above your head and exhale and lower your hands joining them near your heart. Then connect the middle finger and the thumb of both hands. Inhale and raise your hands, exhale and lower your hands, again forming a second lotus petal. Repeat the same with the ring fingers, the little fingers and finally with all five fingers together to complete all ten petals. Check the picture of this pose.

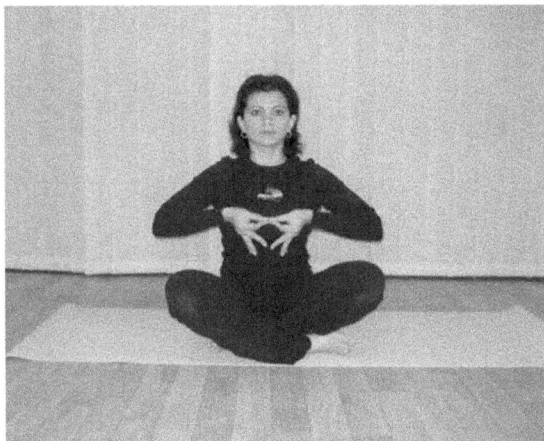

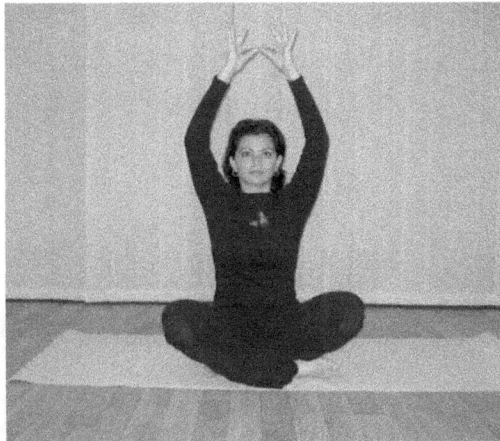

Focus—Form an imaginary lotus by joining the thumb and each finger; synchronising your breath and the hand movement to make each petal.

Breathing Pattern—Inhale as you raise your arms and exhale as you bring your arms down. Each inhalation and exhalation should last for four seconds.

Physical Benefits—It improves steadiness of your hands and coordination.

Psychological Benefits—This helps particularly during emotional stress which leads to unhealthy behaviour like overeating, working too hard, absentmindedness and constriction of the arteries, etc. It also promotes rhythmic breathing and a regulated thought process and teaches mindfulness and improves communication skills. This is the first lesson in visualisation and imagination.

Contraindications—Nil.

Value Addition—Imagine a rainbow in front of your mental screen. Now draw it on a piece of paper and colour it, using all the rainbow colours.

Thought for the Day

A common man cannot do uncommon deeds.

| 6 | **Shubha Aashish or Kundalini Jagriti
(Blessing Oneself for Purification)** |

Aim—To capture the universal energy on the palms and direct it inwards through your head. This is to cleanse and purify the aura by dispelling any negative energy or obstructions.

Time Span—Two minutes.

Technique—Sit in Easy Pose and stretch your arms out sideways, palms facing upward. Inhale, raise your arms overhead and bring your palms together. Exhale, separate your palms and gently place them on your head. Breathe four times slowly. Check how you feel. Inhale and get ready to come out of the pose. Exhale and lower your arms to the normal position. Breathe gently.

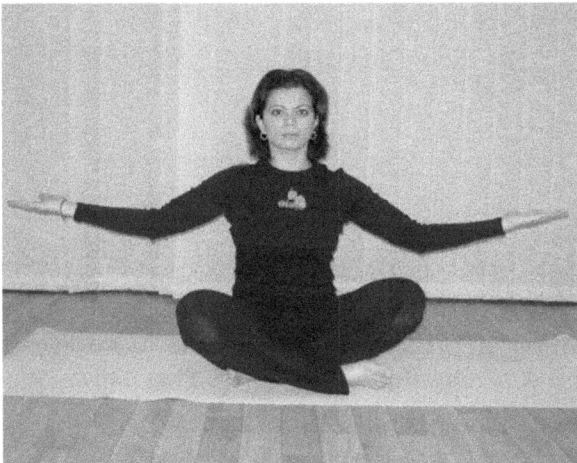

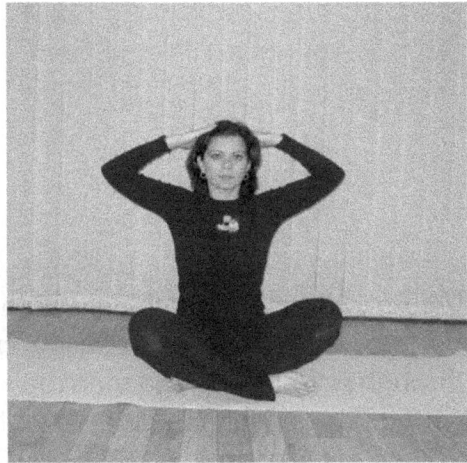

Focus—Around yourself or from the top of your head all the way down to the base chakra (Mulaadhar chakra) or still further down to your toes.

Breathing Pattern—Inhale while raising the arms. Breathe four times while in the posture. Exhale while lowering the arms. If you wish to get the best calming effect, repeat two or three times.

Physical Benefits—Steadies the nerves and brings overall stability to all the seven chakras. It balances the chakra energies of the head and heart. Raising the arms over the head and gently placing the palms on the head especially activates the higher centres of the brain through the pineal gland.

Psychological Benefits—You bless yourself with universal energy which has a soothing effect and you become aware of the protective energy field around yourself. With regular practice it awakens the Kundalini Shakti.*

Contraindications—Nil. It is safe for anyone.

Value Addition—If anything is bothering you, draw a swastika the opposite way. Perform the above exercise by creating a protective shield over your head through self-blessing and then draw the swastika the correct way. This will set the wrong things right to a great extent by instilling positive energy in you.

Thought for the Day

The path of truth is as narrow as it is straight.

---

* Kundalini comes from the Sanskrit word *kundal* which has several meanings, but the most appropriate connotation here is a sleeping serpent, synonymous with the vital force or the primal energy, coiled at the base of the spine. Uncoiling of this energy awakens the unlimited potential already existing in every human leading to higher awareness and enlightenment.

Jagriti means awakening.

7   Gatyatmak Bhuja Vakrasan (The Dynamic Arms Twist)

Aim—To loosen up the upper body muscles.

Time Span—Five minutes.

Technique—Sit on the floor with both legs outstretched in front of you. Do not bend the knees. Stretch the arms forward at the shoulder level, parallel to your legs. Inhale and keep the arms straight. Exhale and twist to the right, stretching the right arm behind as much as possible. Turn the head and gaze at the outstretched right hand. Inhale and bring the right arm in front. Exhale and stretch the left arm behind just like the right arm. Repeat four rounds, alternating each arm.

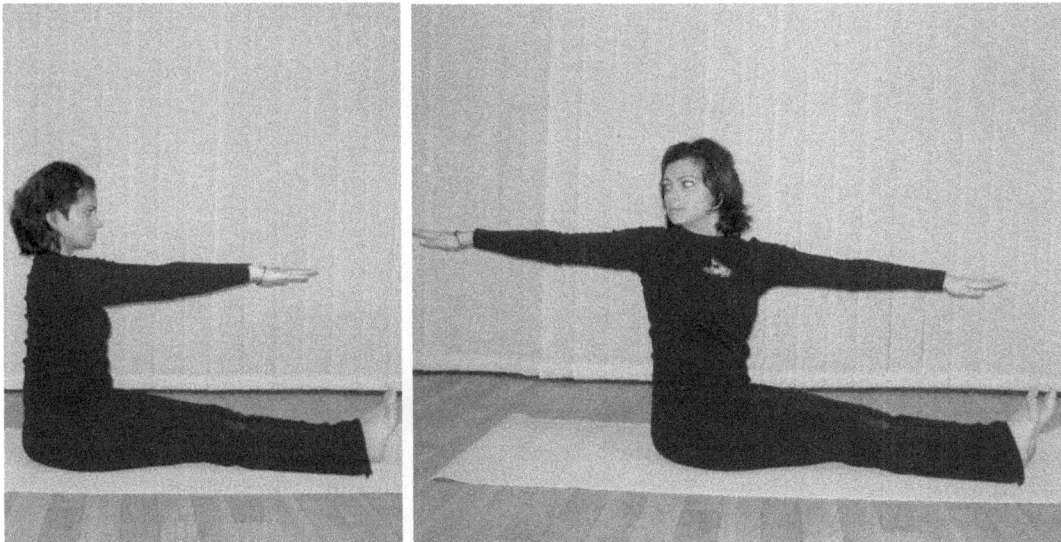

Focus—Applying maximum pressure on the abdomen, exhale while twisting and inhale while returning back to the normal position.

Breathing Pattern—As described in the 'Technique'.

Physical Benefits—This loosens up the vertebrae and removes stiffness of the back. Exaggerate the twist and the shoulders and arms respond remarkably.

Psychological Benefits—Allows you to forget the past painful or unpleasant memories and encourages you to march ahead confidently.

Contraindications—If you are suffering from a frozen shoulder.

Value Addition—How will you know that you are an accomplished yoga practitioner? Find out through the changes in your daily perception.

Ans: You will know that you are an accomplished yoga practitioner when you begin to create a utopia around yourself and the world around you. Wherever you go, you go with ease and peace. Yoga rewards you with an integrated energy in abundance and you share it freely with others.

Thought for the Day

Empathy is the golden key that unlocks the 'blocked' heart.

8

Pancha Marma Bindu
(Five Sensory Point Massage)

The third eye centre (the third eye centre is in between the two eyes/eyebrows), the temples, the flare of the nostrils, behind the earlobes and the back of the head (behind the third eye point where the spine begins)

Aim—To direct the energy within to travel and heal all the sense organs.

Time Span—Five minutes.

Technique—Massage with your middle finger by pressing and releasing the pressure on the third eye point (where the Indian women apply a dot on the forehead). Feel the sensation. Similarly, press and release the temples with your index and the middle fingers; press and release the flare of the nostrils with your middle fingers; press and release behind the earlobes with the index and the middle fingers and finally with the same fingers, press and release at the back of your head (behind the third eye point where the spine begins).

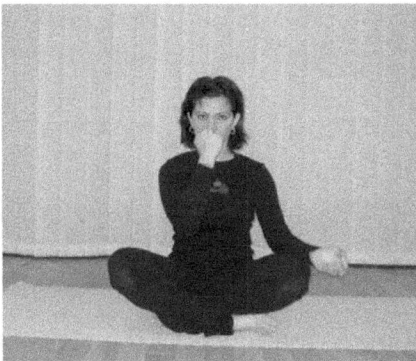

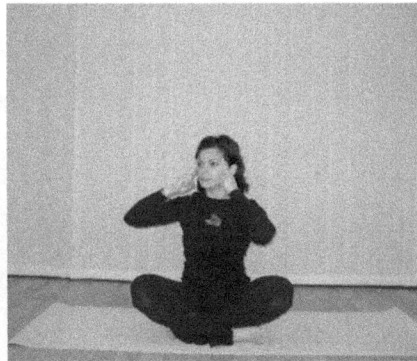

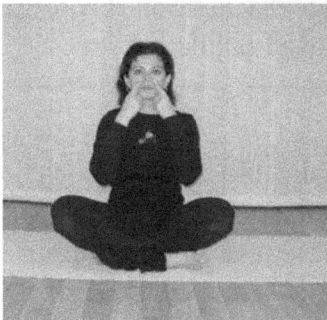

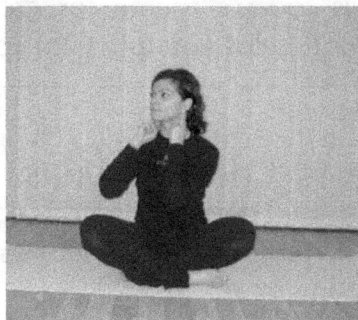

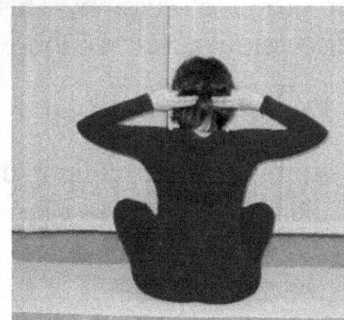

Focus—On each sensory organ. Try to locate the right spot where you feel the maximum relaxing sensation.

Breathing Pattern—Normal.

Physical Benefits—Senses begin to function better. You become aware of the innate capacity of your sight, hearing, smell, taste and touch.

Psychological Benefits—Brings relief by ridding you of negative stimuli. This also helps in cultivating empathy, compassion, forgiveness and altruism.

Contraindications—Nil.

Value Addition—Discuss about the 'Law of Impermanence' in the class as a part of group discussion. This is today's theme for group discussion. A group discussion is like free therapy. It helps you to invent yourself a little better.

Thought for the Day

Nothing is permanent except 'CHANGE'. Do not take life *too* seriously. Ultimately your decisions should depend on your conscience. Do not try to change the world. Always be judicious wherever possible and leave the final justice in the hands of the Almighty.

9

Divya Trikone
(The Divine Triangle)

Aim—To log on to your inner energy which gives a fresh perspective to the postures and their healing qualities.

Time Span—Five minutes.

Technique—Sit in the Diamond Pose and bend forward, lifting your buttocks. Make your hand position like an *eye mask* by joining your index finger and the thumb together and place your hands on the floor. Close your eyes, rest your forehead on the floor and place your eyes inside the eye mask which you have formed with your fingers. Breathe gently.

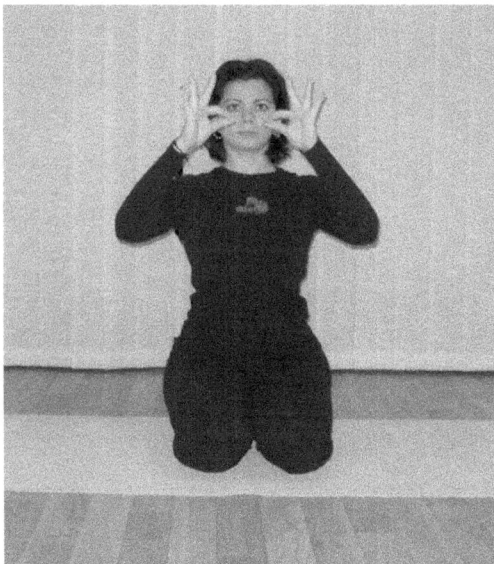

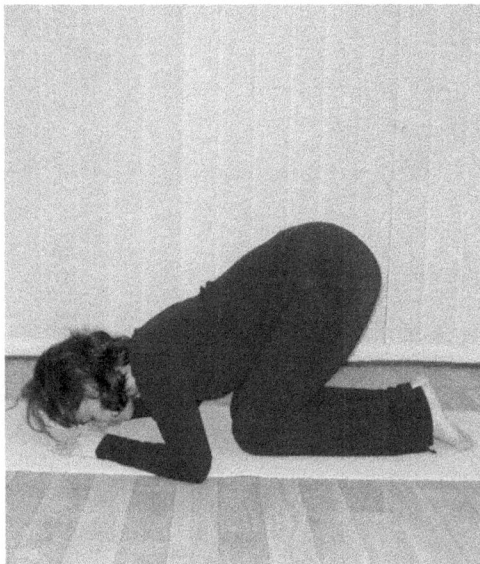

Focus—On gentle breathing and resting the forehead on the floor and on your third eye centre. The third eye centre is in between the two eyes/eyebrows.

Breathing Pattern—Slow and gentle.

Physical Benefits—Strengthens the back muscles. This is a journey of consciousness which travels and balances the energy from the conscious to the subconscious level into your inner world. Also, from the lower chakras, gross energy or primal energy moves upward to the higher chakras.

Psychological Benefits—The energy starts ascending towards the subtle chakras which awakens your third/spiritual eye or the 6th energy centre. This improves your perception. You learn to take initiative and responsibilities in new assignments.

Contraindications—High blood pressure, weak knees or any neck injury.

Value Addition—A group discussion on 'Telepathy'.

Thought for the Day

The 'Third Eye' is the inner window of your mind and this is the home of intuition, visions, dreams and imagination. When this energy is awakened, it improves your memory, telepathy, creativity and ESP.

If this 6th chakra is in imbalance, we see certain symptoms; for instance, if it is overactive, you may experience difficulty in concentration because it is loaded with various stimuli. This interferes with the normal functioning and is manifested in headaches, hallucinations, bad dreams, etc. If the 6th chakra is underactive, the mind is blank, forgetful or dull with hazy thoughts.

10　Laya Yoga
(Yoga for Energy Wave Balance)

Aim—To transform the gross energy into subtle energy and expand the capacity for developing the finer qualities. A prolonged pressure on the base of your spine, specifically on the muscles of the perineum, causes the flow of gross energy located at the root chakra to ascend upward in the form of subtle energy to the other higher chakras. This has a stabilising and calming effect on the mind and body which promotes concentration and steadiness. This pose is almost addictive as it has a beautiful soothing effect on the body and mind. We all have gross energy which is the primal force for our basic survival but since only survival is not enough for humans, we practice yoga. We develop the finer qualities like increased and higher awareness understanding of self and going beyond 'Me' 'Myself' and 'I' with regard to understanding and empathy for others.

Time Span—Ten minutes.

Technique—Squat or sit on the Medicine Ball in the Diamond Pose. If the medicine ball is not available, any football will do. Feel the base of the spine where the Mooladhar Chakra is located. Feel it getting gently pressed. Breathe slowly for five or ten minutes. Within moments, the energy starts flowing upward and you will feel very relaxed. This energy balances all the upper and lower chakras equally bringing harmony.

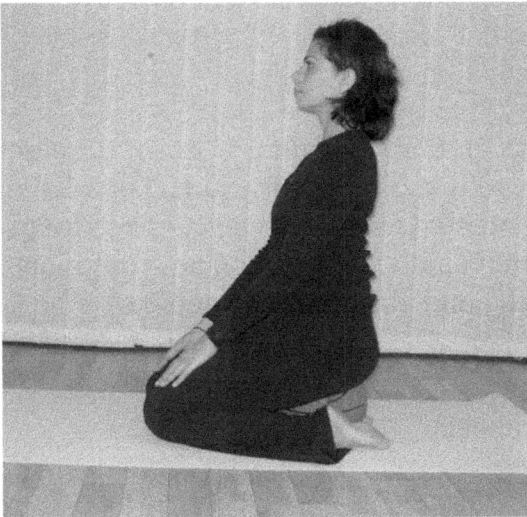

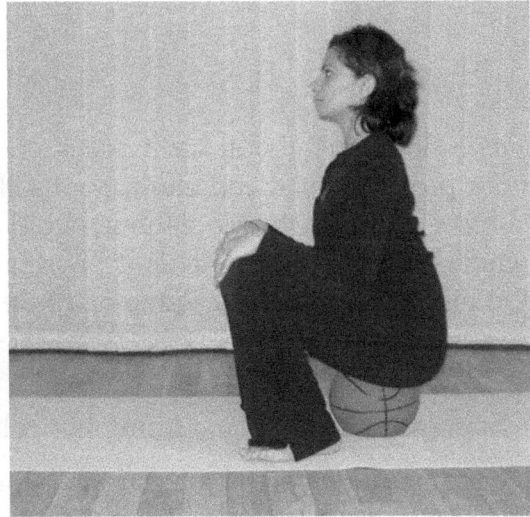

Focus—Perineum or the Mooladhar Chakra.

Breathing Pattern—Steady and normal.

Physical Benefits—Strengthens the spine, helps digestion.

Psychological Benefits—You will feel the 'Energy Flow' in the spine, spiralling upward, giving you harmony and an extremely divine feeling. It improves concentration, awareness and understanding about self and others.

Contraindications—If you have weak or sore knees.

Value Addition—If you have deficit energy in the Mooladhar Chakra, increase your protein intake and earthy foods like root vegetables. If you feel you have surplus energy in the Mooladhar, avoid processed foods. Eat organic fresh fruits, whole grains and increase your physical movement by spending time outdoors. Go bike riding, power walking or gardening and absorb earthy energy.

Thought for the Day
Strength does not come from physical capacity.
Greatness lies not in being strong but in the right use of strength.

11 Chakra Dhyana
(Chakra Meditation or Wave of Breath)

Aim—To balance chakras with optimum energy.

Time Span—Five minutes.

Technique—You can perform this either by sitting in any comfortable pose or lying down in a supine (face up) position. Place your left hand on your heart and the right hand on your diaphragm. If you are lying down, make sure your elbows rest on the floor to feel comfortable. Inhale slowly but deeply and check that your right hand is rising like the swell of a wave of water. Exhale from your abdomen and make sure your right hand descends. Your breathing creates a wave as if the breath is a wave of flowing water. As you inhale it travels from the ocean of your abdomen/diaphragm towards the shore of your heart and as you exhale it moves from your heart towards your abdomen/diaphragm.

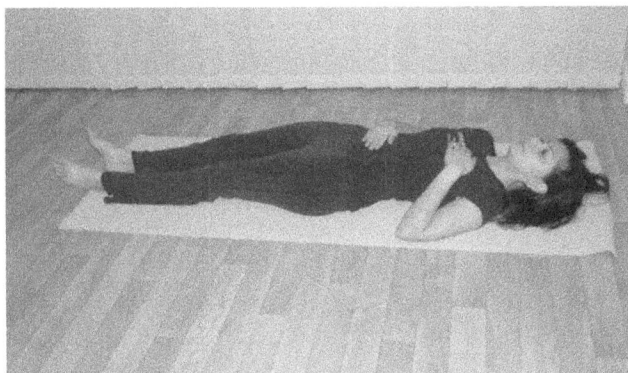

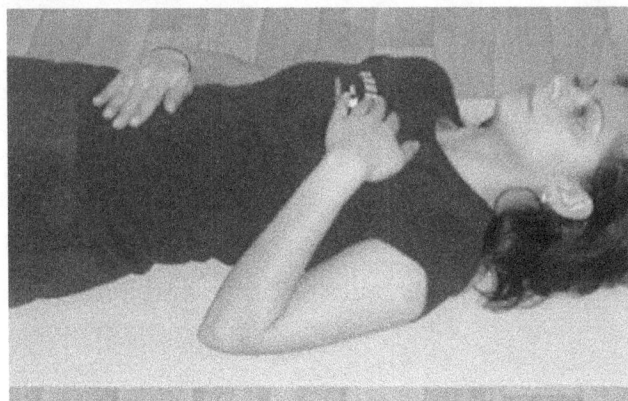

Focus—On slow and deep breathing.

Breathing Pattern—Slow, steady, regular breathing.

Physical Benefits—All the seven systems (respiratory, circulatory, digestive, immune, nervous, reproductive and endocrine) function harmoniously.

Psychological Benefits—When each system functions well, your relationship with the world improves and you experience life filled with joy.

Contraindications—Nil.

Value Addition—Check how many times you need people in your daily routine. How you feel when you need others for your own requirements? Now find out how many times people need you for their requirements and how you react to that.

Thought for the Day

Yoga teaches self reliance which is independence and that is a great virtue but do you know that yoga also teaches inter-dependence which is an even greater virtue.

12

Hasta Mudra
(Palming)

Aim—To bathe the eyes in soothing darkness until the heat from the hands has been absorbed by the eyes.

Time Span—Three to four minutes.

Technique—Sit in any comfortable pose. Close your eyes. Stretch your arms over the head and join your palms in your aura or the energy field of the Sahasrara Chakra (Crown Centre). Rub your palms until they become warm and place them gently over the eyelids without any pressure. Breathe normally for three to four minutes.

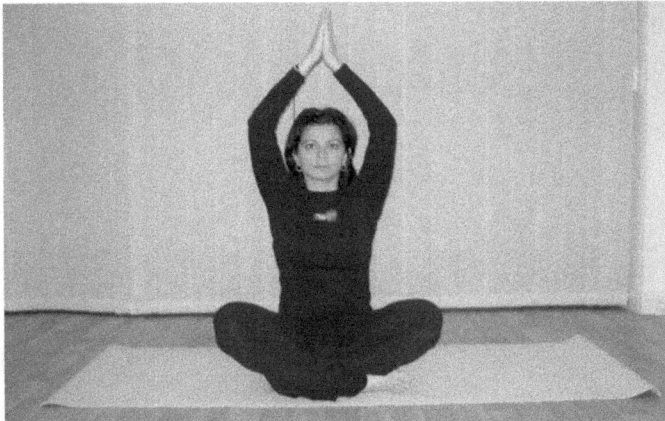

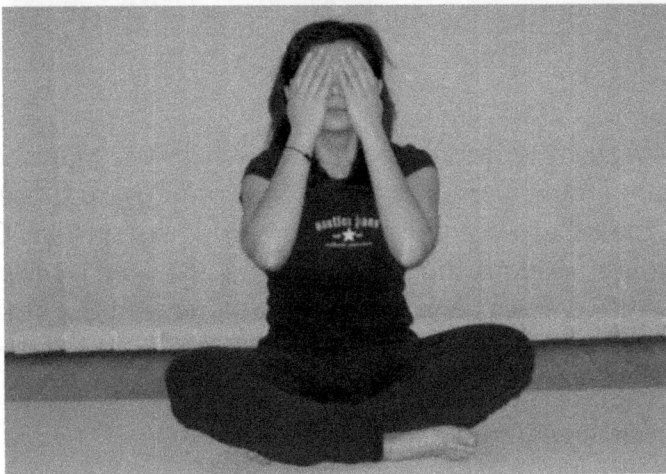

Focus—Feel the warmth and energy being transmitted from the hands into the eyes and the optic muscles.

Breathing Pattern—Normal.

Physical Benefits—Palming relaxes and revitalises the optic muscles and stimulates the circulation of the aqueous humour, the liquid that runs between the cornea and the lens of the eye, helping in the correction of defective vision.

Psychological Benefits—Palming allows you to look inward at your mental screen which helps in meditation.

Contraindications—Those suffering from major eye diseases or disorders like glaucoma, trachoma, cataract, retinal detachment, conjunctivitis, etc.

Value Addition—Watch the rising sun when it is still in its pinkish, reddish hue. Let your eyes bathe in the warmth and the light of the sun. Close one eye and looking through the other eye, put an imaginary cross on top, below and on each side of the sun. Rotate the pupil around the sun clockwise and then counter-clockwise three times each. Repeat the same with the other eye.

Thought for the Day

Yoga lightens your stress and enlightens your spirit.

13

Mushtika Chakra
(The Wrist-joint Rotations)

Aim—To relieve tension from the wrist joints.

Time Span—Two minutes.

Technique—Sitting in any comfortable position, extend your arms in front at shoulder level. Make fists with the thumb inside. Slowly rotate the fists. The arms and elbows should remain perfectly straight and still. Practice it ten times clockwise and ten times counter-clockwise. Exaggerate the movement for better effect.

Focus—On the breath, mental counting up to ten counts; movement of the wrist joints and stretching of the forearm muscles.

Breathing Pattern—Normal.

Physical Benefits—Beneficial for arthritis of the finger-joints, wrist-joints. Releases tension caused by prolonged writing, typing and so on.

Psychological Benefits—Teaches mindfulness and concentration.

Contraindications—Nil.

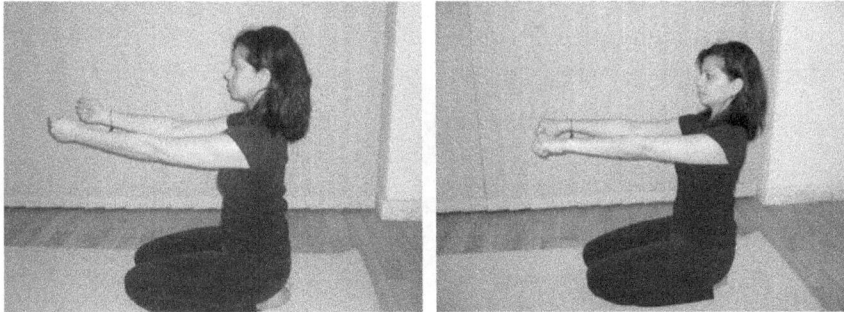

Value Addition—Try a hot tub bath at home or if available a 'Moroccan Bath' at your favourite spa.

Thought for the Day
Being indecisive or non-committal is a mental weakness.

14 | Skanda Chakra
(The Big Zero with the Elbows and the Shoulders)

Aim—To relieve tension and strain from the shoulders due to driving, office/desk work, etc.

Time Span—Two minutes.

Technique—Keeping your fingertips on the shoulders, fully rotate both elbows at the same time in a large circle as if you are making a big zero. Try to touch the elbows in front of the chest on the forward movement and touch the ears while moving up. Stretch the arms back in the backward movement and touch the sides of the trunk while coming down. Do it ten times clockwise and ten times counter-clockwise.

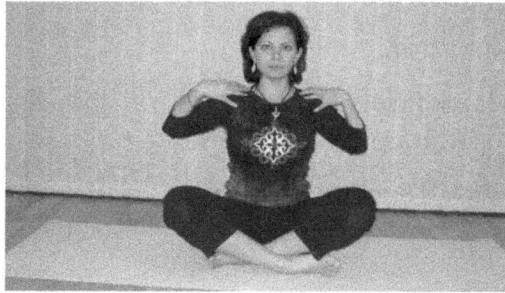

Focus—On the breath, mental counting and the stretching sensation around the shoulder joints.

Breathing Pattern—Inhale as you raise your arms and exhale as you lower your arms.

Physical Benefits—Maintains the flexibility of the shoulders and strengthens your pectoral (chest) muscles and brings stability in the upper body/torso.

Psychological Benefits—Teaches mindfulness and concentration.

Contraindications—If you are suffering from a frozen shoulder.

Value Addition—When you feel terribly restless, hug a tree or at least touch the bark. Check it out! There will be a certain amount of change in your mood.

Thought for the Day

A man without a goal in life is like a ship without a rudder.

Goolf Chakrasan
(Ankle Circles)

Aim—To release tension and stiffness from the ankles.

Time Span—Two minutes.

Technique—Sit with legs outstretched in front. Keep sufficient distance between the two legs. Keeping the heels on the floor, rotate the right foot clockwise and counter-clockwise ten times. Repeat the same with the left foot. Slowly rotate both feet together in the opposite direction. Do not allow the knees to move. Practice ten times. Repeat.

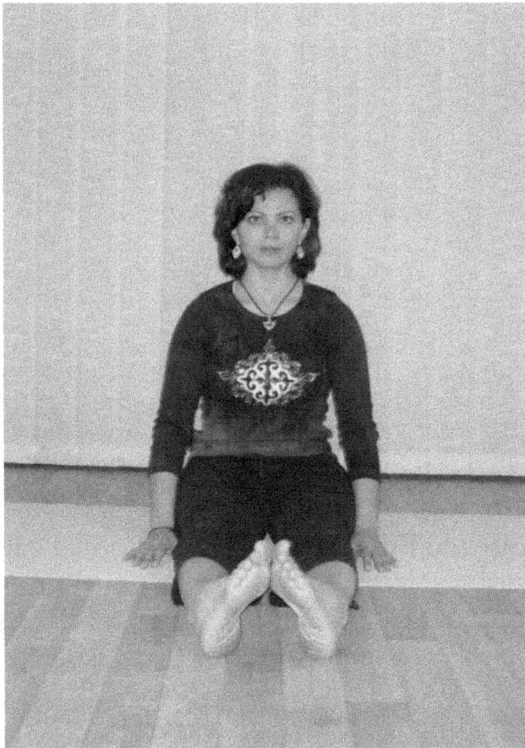

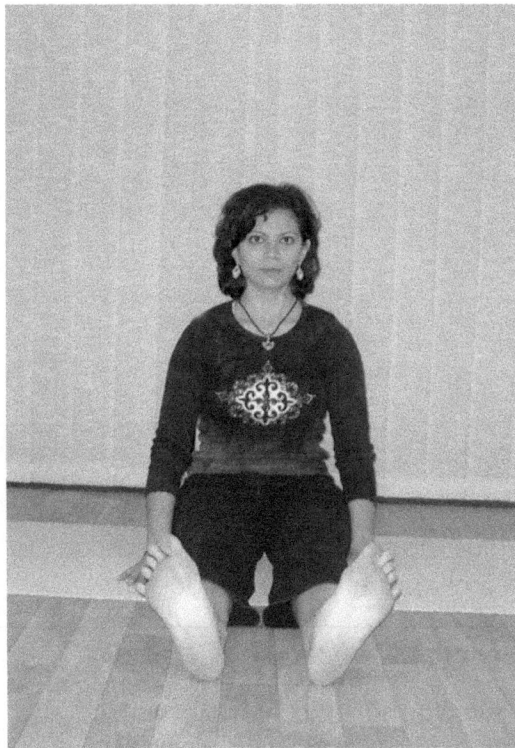

Focus—On the breath, mental counting and rotation. Rotate the ankles consciously and dramatically and your feet will respond to you favourably.

Breathing Pattern—Normal.

Physical Benefits—Releases tension and stiffness from the weight bearing joints. This helps in reviving the stagnant lymph and venous blood. Relieves tiredness, cramps and prevents venous thrombosis.

Psychological Benefits—Your feet become so flexible that they feel like hands, feather-light, lithe and lissom.

Contraindications—Avoid if the ankle is sprained.

Value Addition—Try foot massage on your own with any diluted essential oil like chamomile or lavender oil.

Thought for the Day

Always be kind to your ankles and feet. Previously women in the desert regions used to wear anklets and walk miles and miles in search of water. Walking in the sand is not easy. One must have strong feet and ankles, somewhat like the strong and flexible hooves of camels. The weight of the anklets would strengthen the leg muscles so that walking extensively was not too taxing.

<table>
<tr><td>16</td><td>**Janu Karshan**
(Knee Press)</td></tr>
</table>

Aim—To prevent any ailments of the knees and abdomen.

Time Span—Two minutes.

Technique—Sit in the squatting position with feet apart and the hands on the floor. Breathe normally, place your right hand on the right knee, press and bring it close to the floor. Take it back to the normal position. Now place your left hand on the left knee, press and bring it close to the floor. Take it back to the normal position. If you balance well, continue keeping your right hand on the right knee and the left hand on the left knee. Use your hands as a lever and gently push the knees one by one. Try to squeeze the lower abdomen with pressure from your inner thighs. Those who have difficulty in balancing yourself, support your back against the wall. Take care not to overstretch the knees.

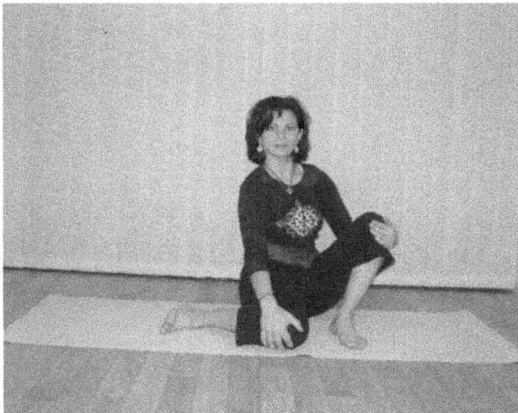

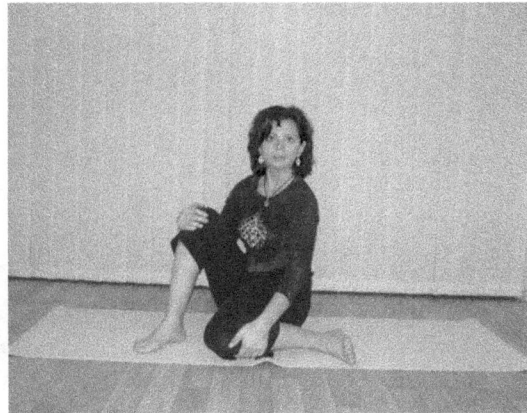

Focus—On the smooth movement of the knees.

Breathing Pattern—Normal.

Physical Benefits—Opens your hip/pelvic bone and allows in fresh prana/energy which helps in improving bone density in the hip area and blood circulation in the legs. The three energy centres below the navel; the Solar Plexus (Manipur Chakra), the Pelvis Plexus (Swadhishthan Chakra), and the Basic centre (Mooladhar Chakra) are revitalised and gradually the pain in the legs and knees disappears. This also relieves constipation or any abdominal ailment.

Psychological Benefits—Stored emotions like fear, guilt, hostility or hatred get dissolved and eventually disappear.

Contraindications—People suffering from any knee, ankle or hip disorder.

Value Addition—Cultivate the art of walking as it is Nature's ideal exercise. Especially for ladies: try a fresh fruit facial either at home on your own or at your favourite beauty saloon.

Thought for the Day

Do not be 'too particular' or peculiar and picky about everything in life as such an attitude creates stress and anxiety. This attitude is popularly known as an 'anal retentive' attitude. Learn to release all your stress and anxiety as it is not worth to be so 'propah'.

Udar-Karshanasan
(Rolls—Side to Side in Sitting Position)

Aim—To compress and stretch the organs and muscles of the lower body.

Time Span—Two to three minutes.

Technique—Sit with knees bent and feet on the floor and arms by your side. Drop both the knees on the right side, placing your hands on the floor behind you for support. Then drop both the knees on the left side. Knees move side to side keeping the torso right in the centre. You can do this alternate movement with your arms stretched out. Repeat it for about eight to ten times.

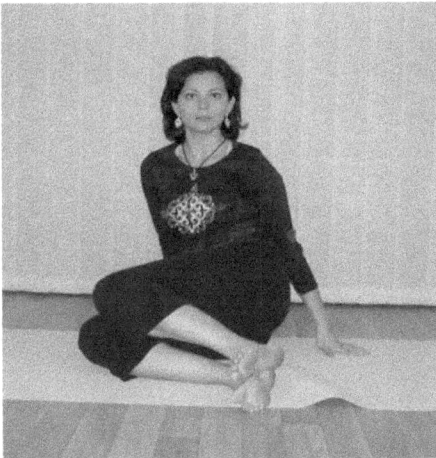

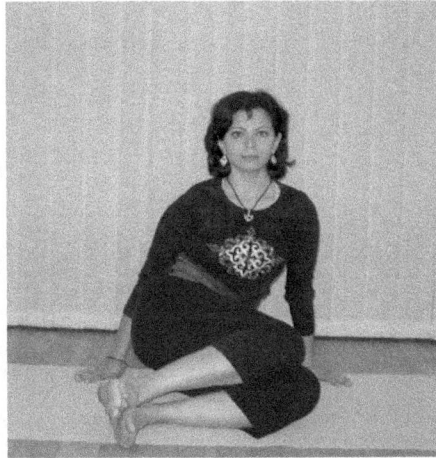

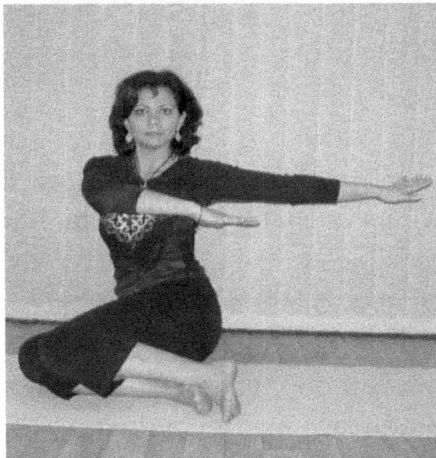

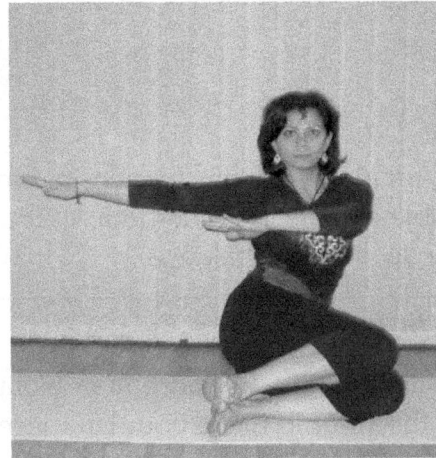

Focus—On the movement and the alternate stretch and compression of the lower abdomen.

Breathing Pattern—Normal.

Physical Benefits—Brings pressure on the spleen (left side) and the liver (right side). The spleen being the major entry point of prana/energy, energises the spleen chakra and tones the other abdominal organs. This also releases flatulence.

Psychological Benefits—This makes you feel physically and mentally light. The mind feels uncluttered without unwanted thoughts. This teaches you to make the necessary changes in your old pattern of thinking and make new adjustments in your planning.

Contraindications—People suffering from any knee, ankle or hip disorders.

Value Addition—Laugh whenever you can as laughter activates certain favourable chemicals in the body that place us in a very joyous state. Laughter restores our sense of balance.

> ### *Thought for the Day*
>
> If you are sleeping for more than eight hours a day, sleep one hour less and invest this hour to make your life more productive and rewarding.

18	**Janu Sanchalan/Chakra** **(Knee Crank)**

Aim—To strengthen the knee joint which has no strong muscles for support but bears the whole weight of the body and is most vulnerable to injuries, sprains and osteoarthritis.

Time Span—Two to three minutes.

Technique—Sit with your legs stretched in front. Bend the right leg with the knee pointing upward. Place the hands under the right thigh interlocking the fingers to support the right thigh. Inhale, raise and straighten the right leg. Exhale and bend it back to the normal position. Repeat the same with the left leg. You can also try some variations by rotating the leg. Keep the torso and the upper body upright and still.

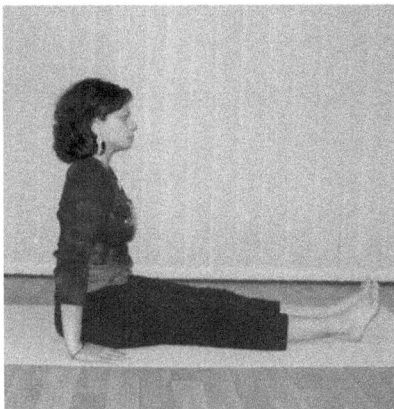

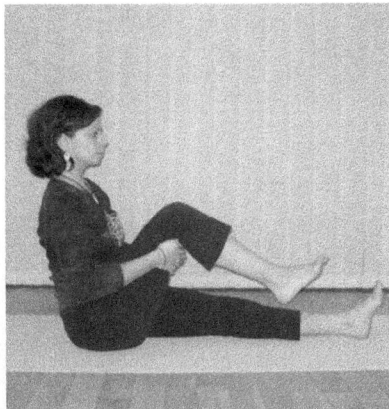

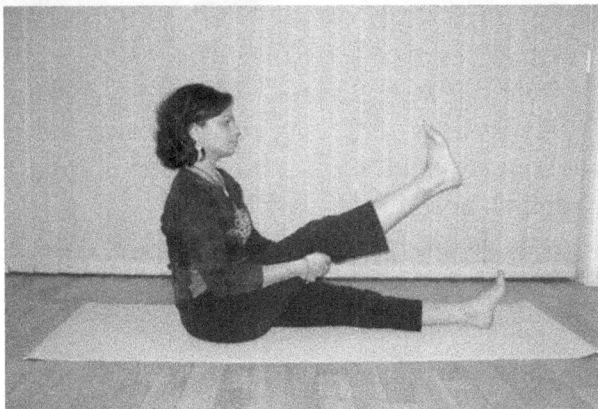

Focus—On the breath, mental counting, bending and stretching movement and perfection of circular rotation.

Breathing Pattern—Inhale on the upward movement; exhale on the downward movement in knee rotations.

Physical Benefits—Strengthens the quadriceps muscles and the ligaments around the knee joints.

Psychological Benefits—This asana rejuvenates and activates the healing energy in us.

Contraindications—People suffering from knee disorders.

Value Addition—Try fasting one day every two weeks and during these fasts, drink water and fruit/vegetable juices. Eat fresh fruits and vegetables only. You will feel more energetic, cleansed and alert.

Thought for the Day

Enhance your will power. Exercise it to enhance your self-esteem and then push it away before it gets stronger and enhances your ego.

19

Supta Prasarita Padasan
(Extended Stretch in Lying Down Position)

Aim—To improve the immune system.

Time Span—Two to three minutes.

Technique—Lie down on your back. Stretch the legs on the floor. Inhale, join and raise both legs upward at 90 degrees. Exhale and spread them outward/ sideways. Once again inhale and join the legs in the centre and exhale and lower them back to the normal position.

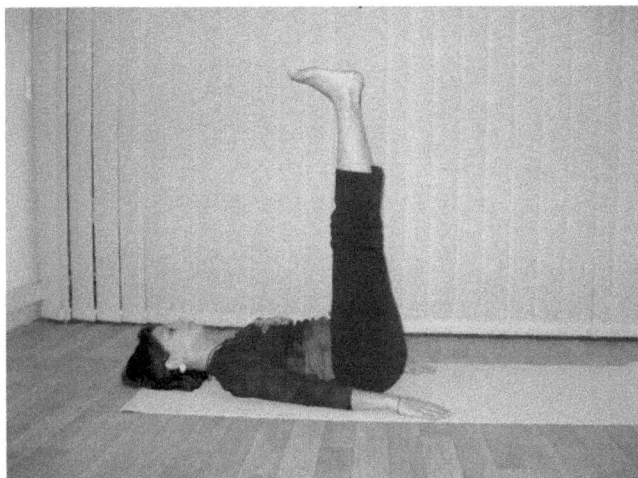

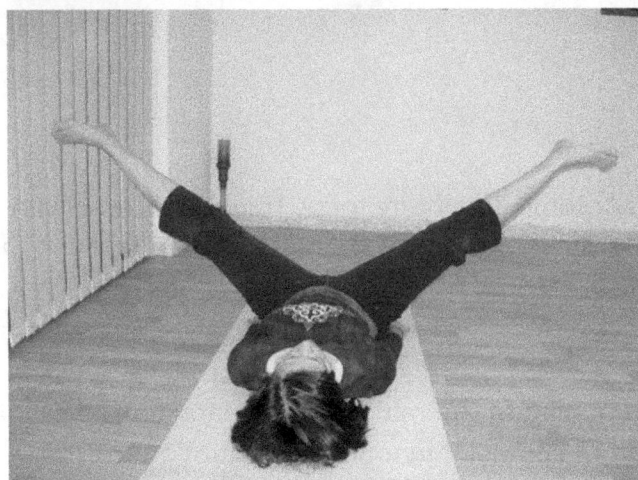

Focus—On breathing and steadying the nerves.

Breathing Pattern—Inhale and raise both legs upward. Exhale and spread them outward. Once again inhale and bring the legs in the centre and exhale and lower them back to the normal position.

Physical Benefits—This exercise eliminates accumulated toxins in the legs, boosts the immune system and improves circulation in the legs.

Psychological Benefits—It boosts confidence as your strong legs convey an assurance of physical and mental strength.

Contraindications—Any ailment or disorder of the legs, ankles and knees.

Value Addition—Try some adventure today but always do it with utmost caution and without foolhardiness. Try bike riding or power walking. Tune into your body, mind and soul.

Thought for the Day

Courage is not a quality of the mind, it is a characteristic of the soul. Check your own strength of character in unfamiliar situations.

20

Pad Sanchalan
(Leg Scissors)

Aim—To strengthen the leg muscles and the hip joint.

Time Span—Two to three minutes.

Technique—Lie down on your back. Inhale and raise your legs to 90 degrees. Exhale and point your toes. Inhale and stretch the legs wide apart. Exhale and cross your legs as if you are making scissors of your legs. Breathe normally and cross each leg alternately.

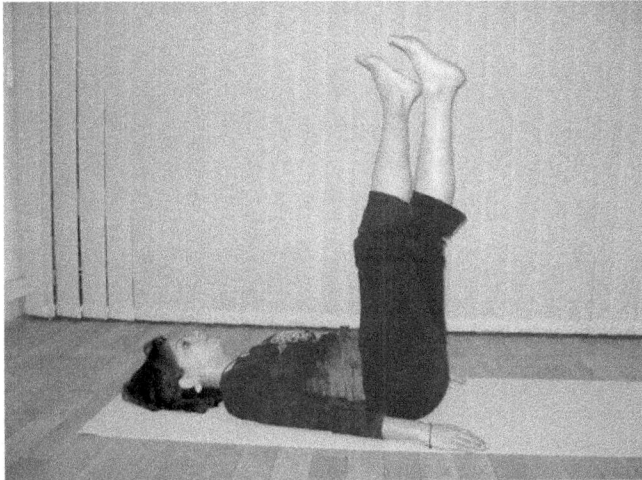

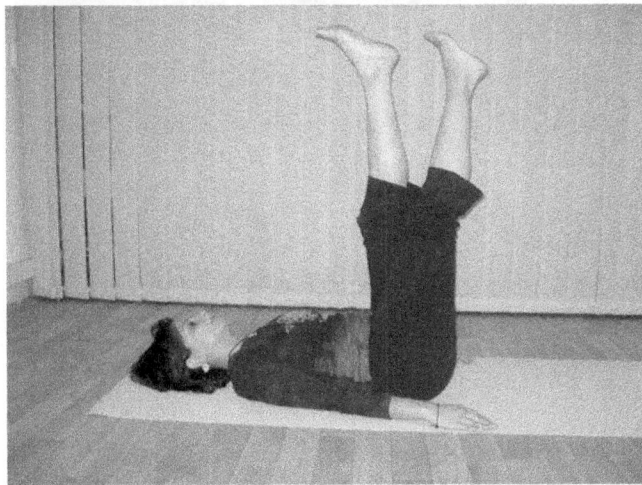

Focus—On synchronising the movement.

Breathing Pattern—Normal.

Physical Benefits—Improves blood circulation in the legs and in the lower part of the body. The pelvic organs and the muscles are massaged. It is also useful for relieving flatulence. Good for strengthening the hip joint, slims down heavy thighs. Tones the abdominal and spinal muscles.

Psychological Benefits—Teaches mindfulness and makes your reflexes swifter.

Contraindications—Those suffering from high blood pressure, serious heart conditions, back problems, sciatica, slipped disc or soon after any abdominal surgery.

Value Addition—Cup your hands joining the thumbs together and joining the little fingers. Create a buttercup flower with your fingers artistically. Make a wish keeping your palms upward. The Almighty grants your wish. It works.

Thought for the Day

Life is not a matter of milestones but of precious moments.

21

Supta Urdhva Hastasan
(The Breath Coordination)

Aim—To check whether you are relaxed or rigid/tense. If you are relaxed, you will feel the weight of your arms. If you are rigid or tense, all your energy is focused on your thoughts and you will not feel the weight of your arms.

Time Span—Two to three minutes.

Technique—Lie flat on the back. Inhale and stretch the arms overhead till they touch the floor. Exhale and bring the arms back to the normal position. Repeat it ten times.

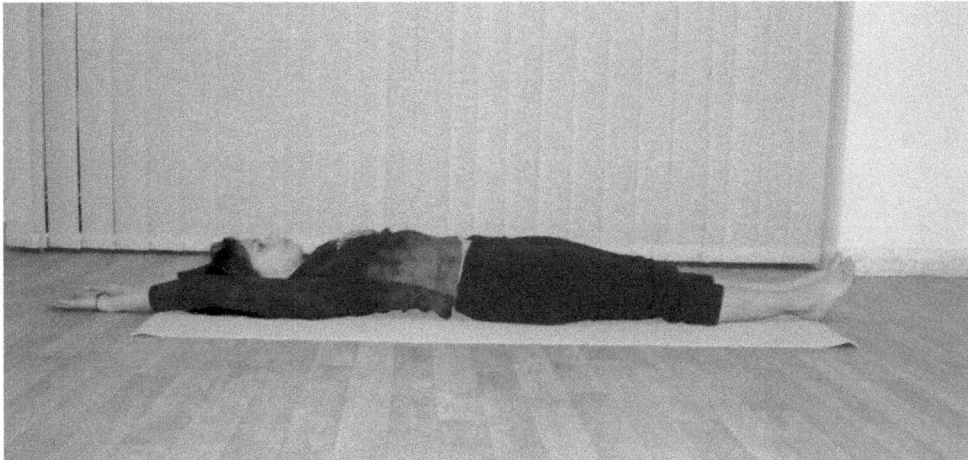

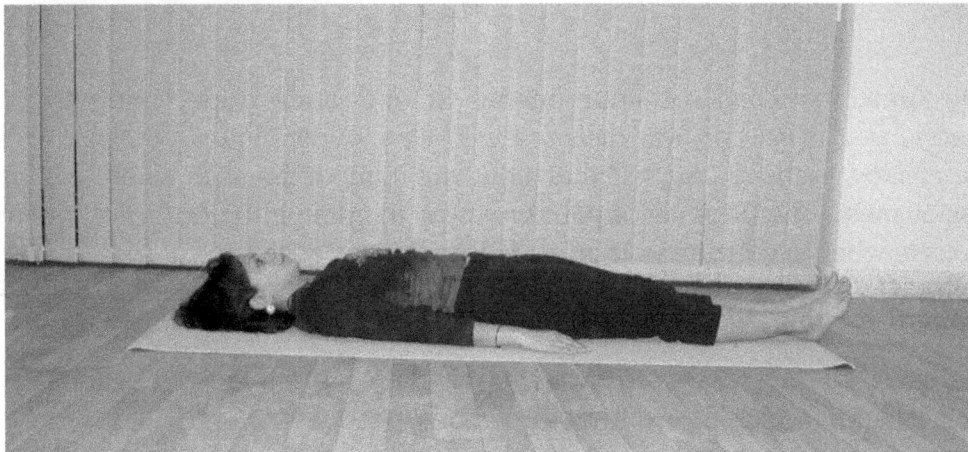

Focus—On breathing and synchronising the arm movements.

Breathing Pattern—Gentle and steady.

Physical Benefits—Eliminates nervous tension and brings about deep relaxation. It restores freshness which lasts throughout the day.

Psychological Benefits—Improves coordination and reflexes.

Contraindications—Nil.

Value Addition—Think of your enemy. If you have none, bring to mind someone you dislike or you disagree with or a public figure you hold in low esteem. Now remind yourself that you and him or her still share the same consciousness. The purpose of your enemy is to come into your life in the form of your teacher to educate you on something new.

Thought for the Day

The level of awareness in two people can be different but universal consciousness which dwells in both persons is the same.

22

Sharir Sanchalan
(Sixteen Point Upper Body Stretch)

Aim—To establish a state of concentration and calm.

Time Span—Two to three minutes.

Technique—Stand upright and inhale. Exhale and twist to the right side. Inhale and return back to the centre. Exhale and twist to the left side. Inhale and return to the centre. Exhale and stretch the arms in front at the shoulder level. Inhale and raise the arms over the head. Exhale and bend to the right side. Inhale and come back to the centre. Exhale and bend to the left side. Inhale and come back to the centre. Exhale and bend forward, touching the floor. Inhale and come back to the centre, raising the arms all the way up. Exhale and bring the arms to the normal position.

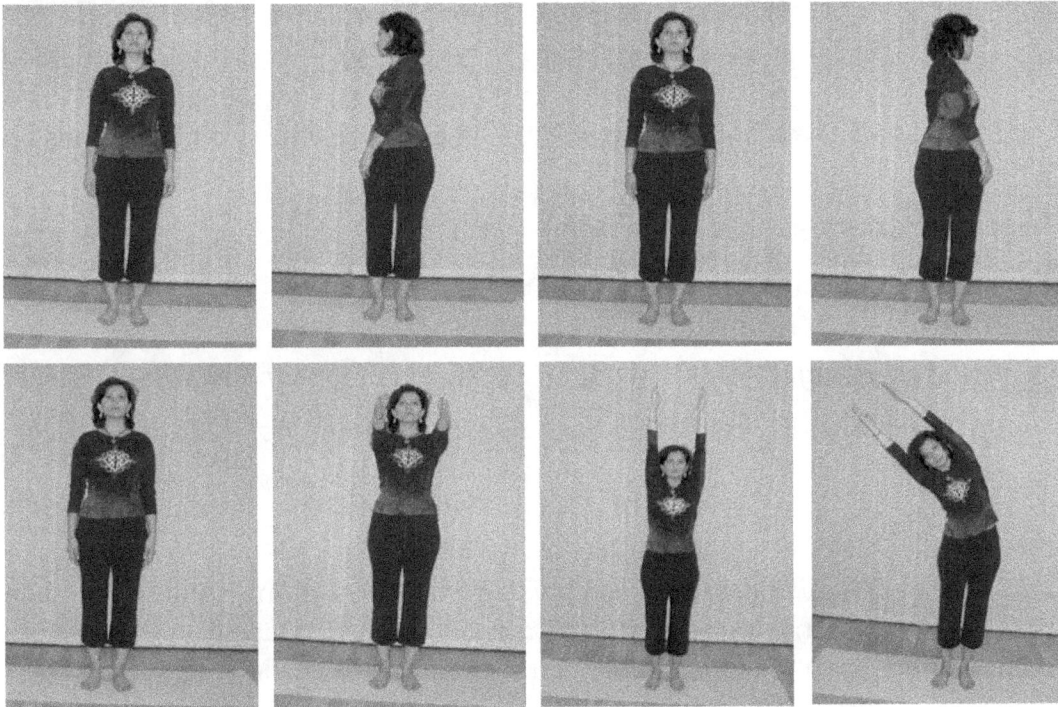

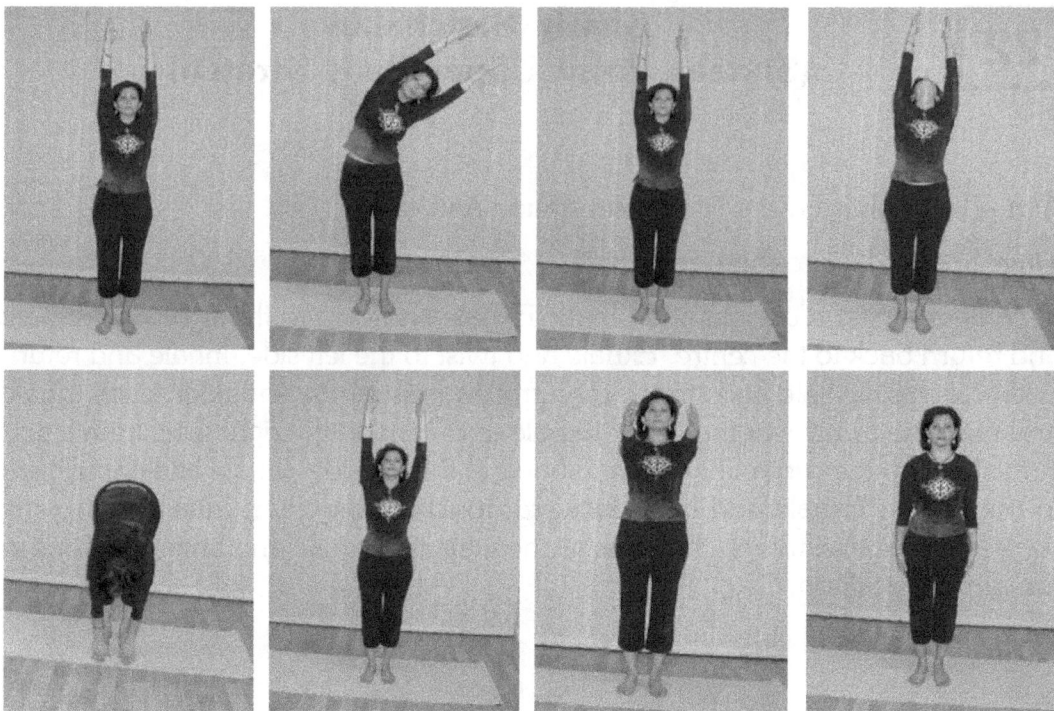

Focus—On each stretch, synchronise breathing and be aware of the expansion of the lungs.

Breathing Pattern—As described in the 'Technique'.

Physical Benefits—This is like cleansing all the chakras with a shower of fresh prana energy throughout the body.

Psychological Benefits—Body alignment and uprightness, confidence.

Contraindications—People with a back condition should not bend forward.

Value Addition—Everyday try to get away from the noise, the crowds, the rush, traffic and pollution. Spend a few moments alone in peaceful introspection, deep reading, deep breathing or any form of simple relaxation.

Thought for the Day

Everybody is beautiful so respect every creation of God.

23

Pad Sanchalan
(Sixteen Point Lower Body Stretch)

Aim—To improve circulation in the legs and the lower body.

Time Span—Two to three minutes.

Technique—Stand with both legs 12" apart for a good balance. Keep your hands on the hips. Inhale and raise the right leg forward. Exhale and bring it back to the normal position. Inhale and raise your right leg backward. Exhale and bring it back to the normal position. Inhale and raise the left leg forward. Exhale and bring it back to the normal position. Inhale and raise your left leg backward. Exhale and bring it back to the normal position. Inhale and raise the right leg sideways to the right side. Exhale and bring it back to the normal position. Inhale and raise the left leg sideways to the left side. Exhale and bring it back to the normal position. Inhale, take your right leg in a semicircular motion, crossing the left leg and touching the floor lightly with your right foot. Exhale and bring it back to the normal position. Inhale and take your left leg in a semicircular motion to the right side in the same manner as the right leg. Exhale and bring it back to the normal position.

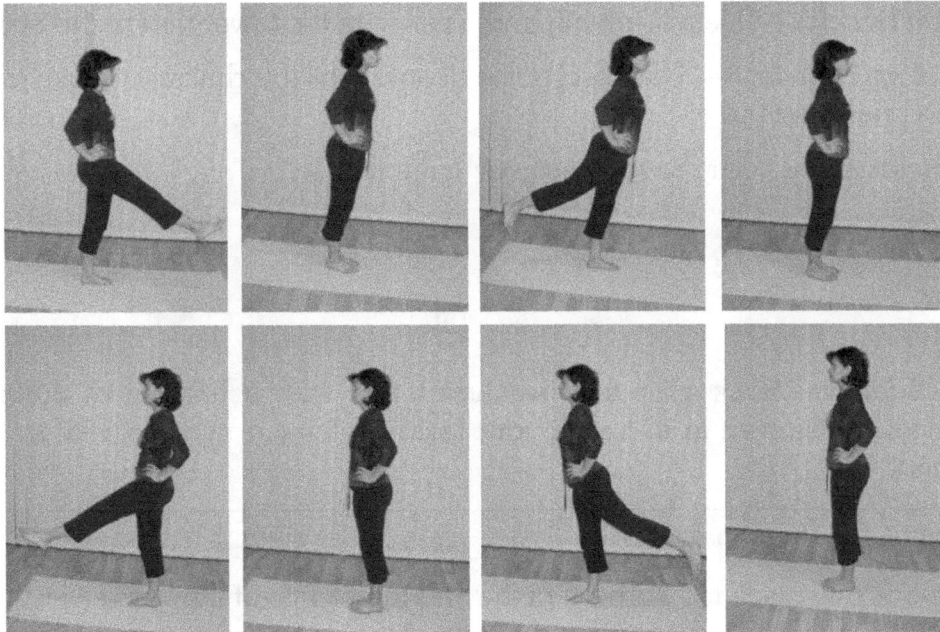

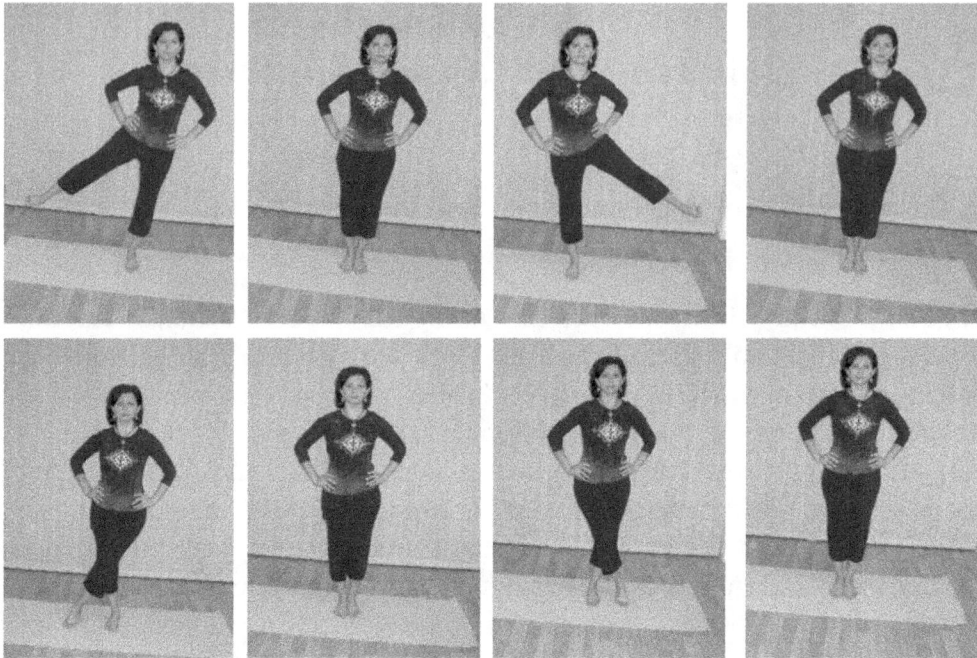

Focus—On the breath, mental counting and on smoothness of the movement and proper coordination.

Breathing Pattern—Check 'Technique'.

Physical Benefits—Overall strength and balance in the lower part of the body.

Psychological Benefits—The effect is like cleansing all the chakras with a shower of fresh prana energy.

Contraindications—Any severe leg/knee complaint.

Value Addition—Soak your feet in warm water with a handful of ordinary cooking salt dissolved in it. Leave your feet in it for ten minutes and see the difference.

Thought for the Day

Everyone must seek the purpose of life and the source of the being.

Janu Karshan
(Knee Press—Front (Standing))

Aim—To learn balance and strengthen the leg muscles.

Time Span—Two minutes.

Technique—Stand with feet together. Inhale, raise and bend the right knee. Exhale and hold the knee with both hands by interlocking the fingers. Balance on the left leg. Repeat the same with the left leg.

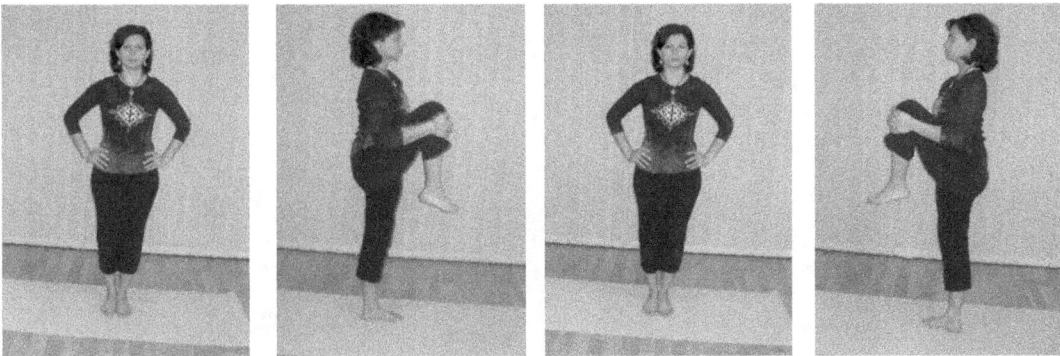

Focus—On breathing and balancing.

Breathing Pattern—Check the 'Technique'.

Physical Benefits—This teaches physical balance, composure, concentration and coordination and strengthens the leg muscles.

Psychological Benefits—Balances the cerebral hemispheres and you can be as realistic as you are artistic and vice versa.

Contraindications—People suffering from any acute knee injury.

Value Addition—Start a group discussion on 'Balance'.

Thought for the Day

Any balancing posture helps in balancing the brain hemispheres so that both the faculties are utilised equally, for instance, logic and magic or practicality and creativity.

---

25 Janu Karshan
(Knee Press—Back (Standing))

Aim—To learn balance and strengthen the leg muscles.

Time Span—Two minutes.

Technique—Stand with both feet together. Inhale and raise the right leg at the back, bending the knee. Exhale and hold the right ankle with the right hand or with both hands. Pull the leg backward and make sure both the knees are in line. Balance on the left leg. Repeat the same with the left leg.

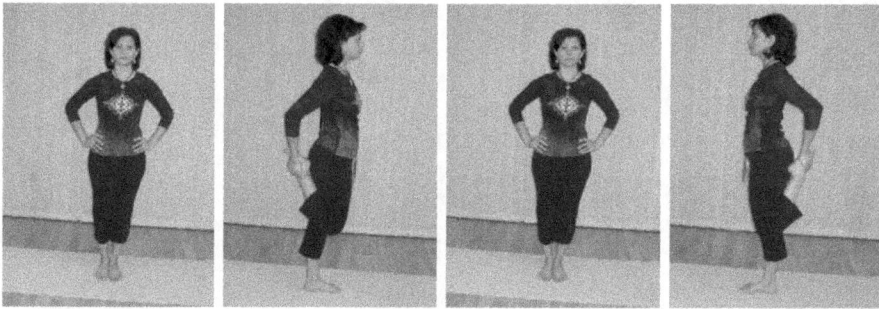

Focus—On breathing and balancing.

Breathing Pattern—Check the 'Technique'

Physical Benefits—This teaches physical balance, composure, concentration and coordination and strengthens the leg muscles.

Psychological Benefits—Balances the cerebral hemispheres and you can be as realistic as you are artistic and vice versa.

Contraindications—People suffering from any acute knee injury.

Value Addition—Think about living 'frugally'. Frugal living is a humble attempt to save our earth. Extravagant culture is a wasteful load on this earth.

Thought for the Day

Any balancing posture helps in balancing the brain hemispheres so that both the faculties are utilised equally. For instance, logic and magic or practicality and creativity.

Uthak-Baithak
(The Yogic Sit-ups)

Aim—To strengthen the knees and improve balance, coordination and concentration.

Time Span—Two minutes.

Technique—Stand with feet hip-width apart. It helps you to balance better rather than with feet together. Raise the heels, inhale and stretch your arms in front at the shoulder level, palms facing downward. Exhale and squat, keeping the heels raised. Inhale and stand up. Exhale and bring the arms and heels down to normal position. Repeat ten times.

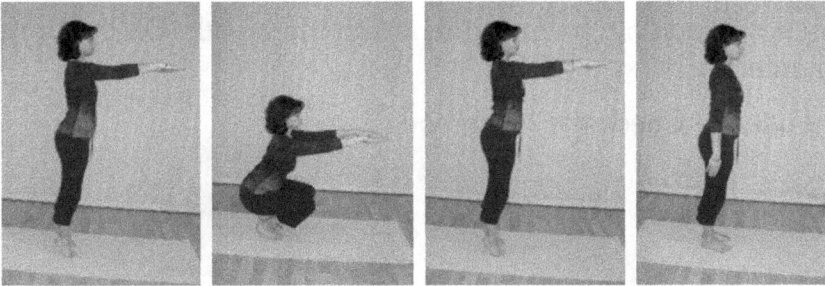

Focus—On breathing and synchronising the movements.

Breathing Pattern—Slow and steady.

Physical Benefits—Are good for physical balance and coordination; strengthens your ankles and prevents arthritis of the knees.

Psychological Benefits—Improves mental equilibrium, self-control and improves your reflexes. This conveys that the 'ups' and 'downs' in life are natural and teaches you to deal with them calmly and efficiently.

Contraindications—Acute knee problem/pain.

Value Addition—This weekend find out three people who you think have genuine humility.

Thought for the Day

Humility is a strange thing. The moment you think you've got it, you've lost it.

Pad Sanchalan
(Leg Kicking—Standing
(A) Front—Corresponding (B) Front—Cross)

Aim—To strengthen the leg muscles and improve balance.

Time Span—Two to three minutes.

Technique—(A) Stand with feet together and arms stretched in front at shoulder level with palms facing downward. Inhale and kick up with your right leg touching the right palm. Exhale and bring it down. Inhale and kick up with your left leg touching the left palm. Exhale and bring it down.

(B) The same exercise can be done with the opposite limbs—kicking the right leg up and touching the left palm and the left leg up touching the right palm.

Focus—On synchronising the movement with the breath. On the stretch in the legs and mental counting.

Breathing Pattern—Check the 'Technique'.

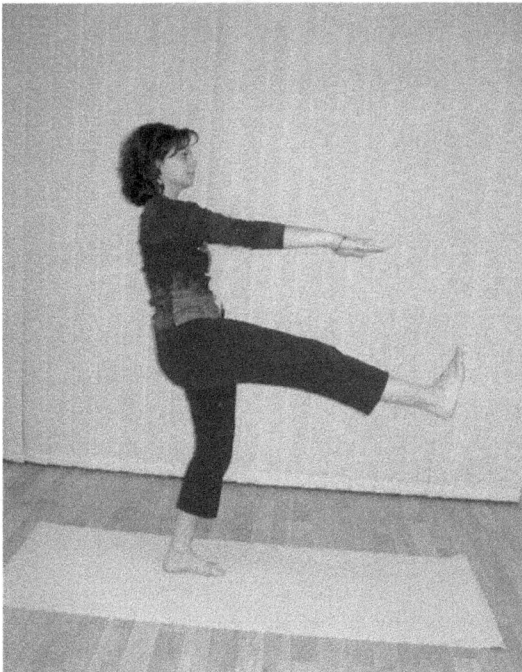

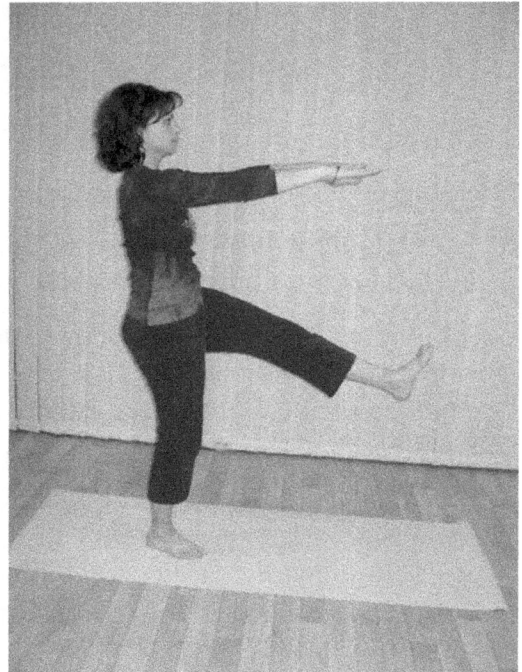

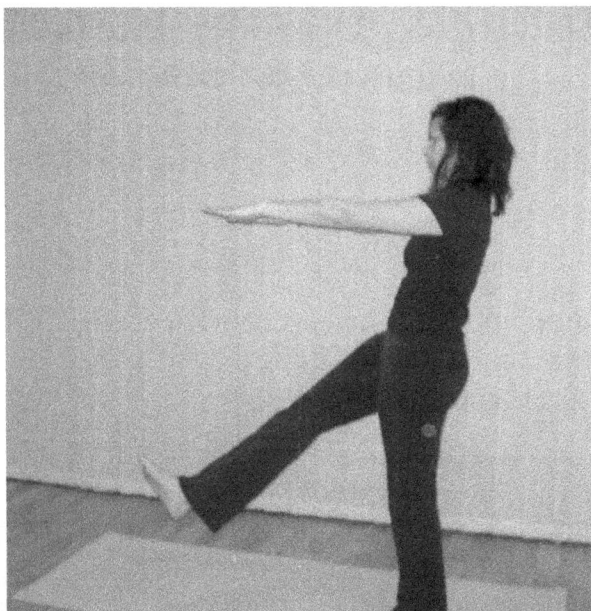

Physical Benefits—This is extremely good for obesity, tones the abdominal muscles and the lower region of the spine. The nerves and muscles connected to the legs and knees are strengthened.

Psychological Benefits—This improves your reflexes and coordination.

Contraindications—Nil.

Value Addition—From now on change your eating habits. Bring your palms together in a gesture of receiving (palms up, pinkies touching). At least once a week, take as much food as fits in your cupped hands. Ayurvedic tradition teaches that this is the perfect serving size for your body and can be digested in one sitting.

Thought for the Day

Super diets are super failures as they tempt you to indulge in compensation.

---

28 | Gatyatmak (Dynamic) Jhulana (Swinging) (Dynamic Stretch and Swing)

Aim—To rejuvenate all the muscles and to promote good circulation.

Time Span—Two minutes.

Technique—Stand upright. Inhale, mentally verbalising 'SO' and stretch arms overhead. Exhale, mentally verbalising 'HUM' and swing your arms down and back, bending your knees slightly.

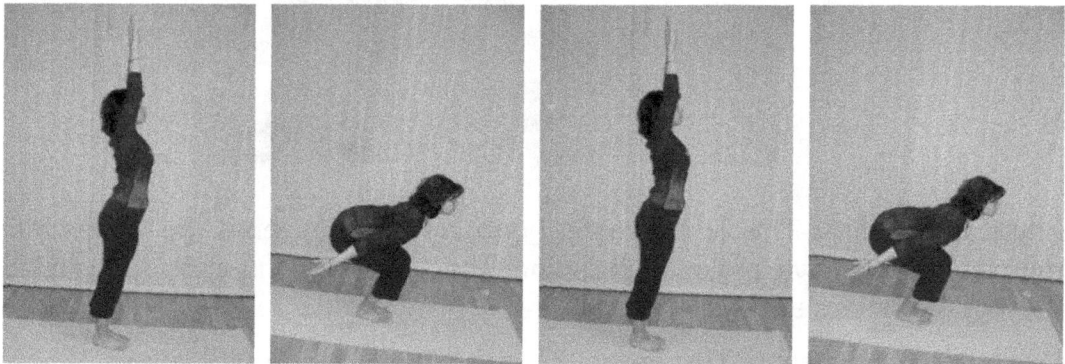

Focus—On breathing and synchronising the movements.

Breathing Pattern—Breathe in Ujjayi.

Physical Benefits—Energises the body.

Psychological Benefits—Energises the mind and makes it alert. Quickens your reflexes.

Contraindications—Heart condition, high blood pressure.

Value Addition—Today, try whether you can drink your food and eat your liquids.

Thought for the Day

Group discussion on the experience of how you feel more hungry on the days you do not workout or practice yoga.

Hasta Sanchalan
(Arm Scissors with Arms Right from the Centre, Upward and Downward)

Aim—To energise your body and mind.

Time Span—Two to three minutes.

Technique—Stand with feet hip-width apart. Stretch arms in front at shoulder level and shoulder-width apart. Breathe normally. Inhale and stretch the arms sideways expanding your torso. Exhale and cross your arms in front. Repeat this in quick succession, taking your arms upward and downward.

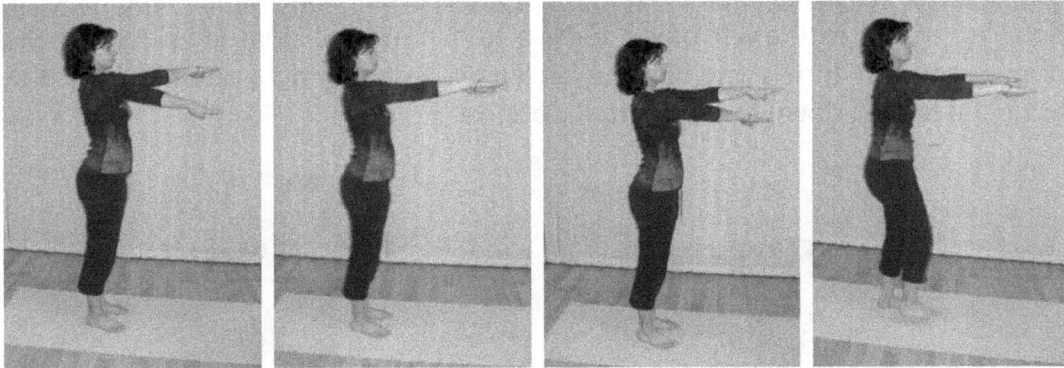

Focus—On the breathing and synchronisation of the scissor movement.

Breathing Pattern—Normal.

Physical Benefits—Energises the body.

Psychological Benefits—Energises the mind and makes it alert, quickens your reflexes.

Contraindications—Acute shoulder joint pain.

Value Addition—Try origami with paper and scissors using your creativity.

Thought for the Day

Greatness lies not in being strong but in the right use of strength at the right time.

Pad Sanchalan
(Leg Kicking—Sideways—
(A) Corresponding (B) Cross)

Aim—To strengthen the leg muscles and improve the balance.

Time Span—Two to three minutes.

Technique—Stand with feet together and arms stretched out sideways, palms facing downward. Hold the arms at shoulder level. Inhale and kick up the right leg sideways till it touches the right palm. Exhale and bring the right leg down to the normal position. Repeat the same with the left leg till it touches the left palm.

The exercise (B) is to kick the leg in the opposite direction—Inhale and kick the right leg across to the left palm. Exhale and bring the right leg down to the normal position. Inhale and kick the left leg across to the right palm. Exhale and bring the left leg down to the normal position.

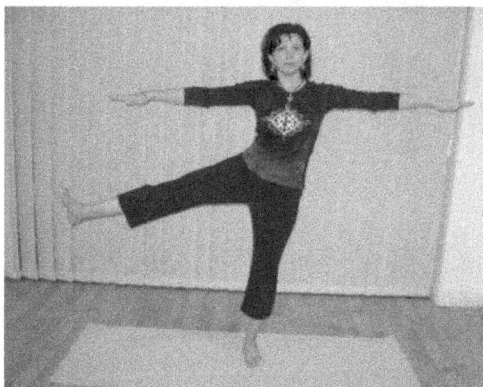

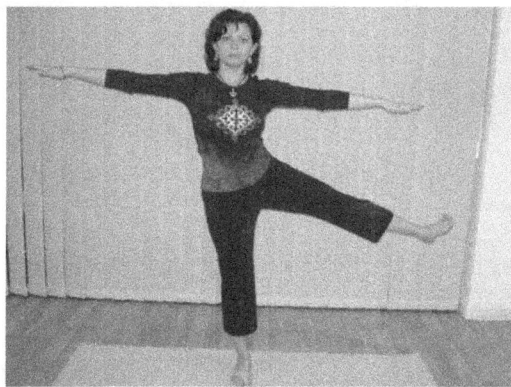

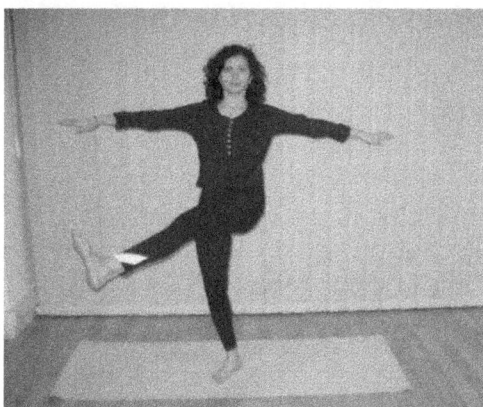

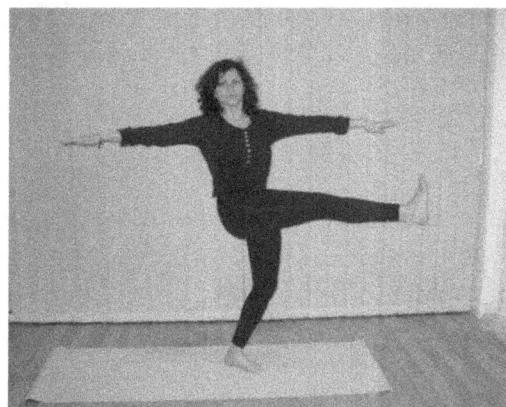

Focus—On synchronising the movement with the breath. On the stretch in the legs and mental counting.

Breathing Pattern—Check the 'Technique'.

Physical Benefits—This is extremely good for obesity, tones the abdominal muscles and the lower region of the spine and the nerves. Strengthens the muscles connected to the legs and knees.

Psychological Benefits—This improves your reflexes and coordination.

Contraindications—Nil.

Value Addition—Find out who you think is your best teacher.

> **Thought for the Day**
>
> Try to wipe your mind like a clean slate. The loaded mind cannot accept anything more. One who believes he cannot learn anything new, will stagnate quickly and not move to higher levels. Even the teachers have teachers.

SECTION–III

Standing Postures

1 | Parvatasan
(The Mountain Posture—Hands Over the Head)

Aim—To give a good stretch to the spine and to be aware of the symmetry of the body.

Time Span—Two minutes.

Technique—Stand with feet wide apart. Feel your feet firmly planted on the floor. Inhale and raise your arms over the head by joining the palms in Namaste position. Exhale, drop your head backward and look up at your thumbs. Breathe four times in the same pose.

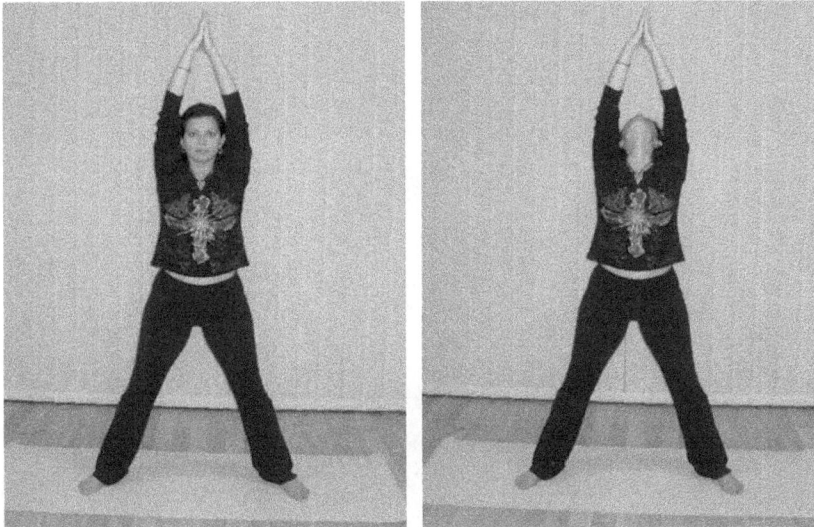

Coming Out of the Pose—Inhale, bring your head back to the normal position looking straight in front. Exhale and lower your arms back to the normal position. Once again breathe gently.

Focus—With total concentration on your thumbs and keeping the body straight in the centre without tilting on any one side.

Breathing Pattern—Refer to the 'Technique'.

Physical Benefits—This pose makes you steady, sturdy, strong and hardy like a mountain. The entire body is stimulated with positive energy. This stretch helps in adjusting the body alignment.

Psychological Benefits—It becomes effortless to achieve your aspiration as you build inner strength and mental clarity. It encourages you to reach the top of your goals and brings astounding results with each successive day. If you are going through any unpleasant situation, this pose teaches you to use that situation as a catalyst to bring out your hidden strength. If your life is smooth and happy, this pose leads you to further your spiritual growth.

Contraindications—People suffering from neck ailments should not attempt this pose.

Value Addition—Look at the mountain if you have one in the neighbourhood and check what thoughts come to your mind. Do you feel aware of your ambitions or feel encouraged to start some new venture today?

For Leisure Activity—How about mountain trekking?

Thought for the Day

Life is governed by a multitude of forces.

2

Prasarita Padottanasan–I
(The Wide Angle Forward Bend Posture–I)

Aim—To strengthen the quadricep muscles (the inner and outer thighs), including the hamstrings.

Time Span—Two to three minutes.

Technique—Inhale and stand with feet wide apart. Exhale, bend forward and keep your palms on the floor in the centre. Breathe four times. Inhale and hold the right ankle with both hands. Exhale. Breathe four times once again and on your last exhalation release your ankle. Inhale and hold the left ankle with both hands. Exhale. Breathe four times and on your last exhalation, release it. Inhale and keep the hands on the floor in the centre and exhale. Breathe four times.

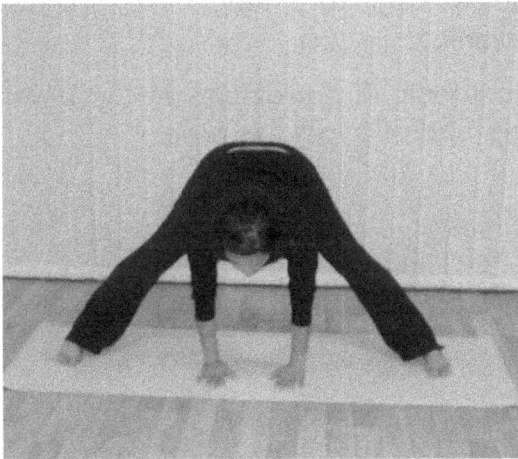

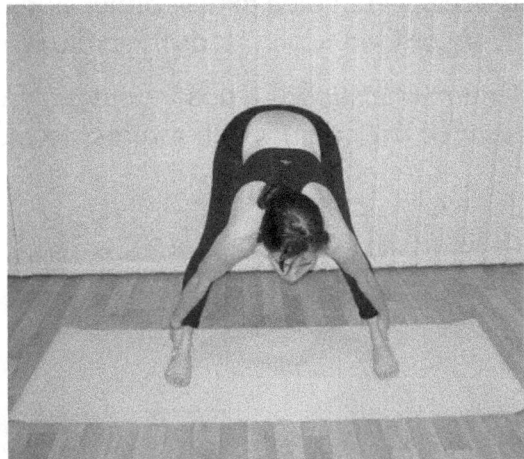

Coming Out of the Pose—Inhale and roll up raising both arms over the head. Exhale and bring the arms by your sides back to the normal position and bring your feet together.

Focus—On breathing and the step by step going into and coming out of each position.

Breathing Pattern—Check the 'Technique'.

Physical Benefits—The hamstring muscles, which are like the backbones of the legs, are stretched and strengthened. These muscles usually have a bad habit of storing tension and shrinking with age. With this posture they become strong through proper blood circulation and steady nerves. This also eases fatigue in the legs and the lower body. The other point is that in this pose, the position of the head is downward, sometimes almost touching the floor. Therefore the head, neck and the throat get a good amount of blood supply. The chakras like Sahasrara (the Crown), Ajna (the Third Eye) and Vishuddhi (the Throat) are activated.

Psychological Benefits—This pose calms the mind and instils the feeling of 'let-go'. It teaches resilience and mental flexibility. The range of your 'forward bend –stretch' symbolises the mental flexibility or the state of your mind. Rigidity in your stretch indicates rigid thinking so this pose teaches you to broaden your mindset by untangling certain inner mental knots. It sweeps away narrow-minded thinking. Practising this pose adequately, broadens your thought process, expanding to new dimensions and you begin to surrender to the Higher Truth or God which leads to spiritual awakening.

Contraindications—Those suffering from chronic disc problems in the lower back or back pain which radiates to the legs should avoid this pose.

Value Addition—If you have lower back pain, check whether you are sitting properly at your work place. Long hours of sitting in one place at work without any foot support brings pressure on the lower back. Always keep a foot-rest under your feet to prevent back problems.

> ### Thought for the Day
>
> Man cannot elevate himself by searching outside as the real scope for growth lies within.

3

Tadasan
(The Palm Tree Posture)

Aim—To stretch the spine and boost the energy centres.

Time Span—Two to three minutes.

Technique—Stand with feet 10–12 inches apart. Feel the body weight equally on both the feet. Inhale, raise the heels and simultaneously raise the right arm upward, stretching it up as much as possible. Hold the breath for a couple of seconds. Your gaze should be on the floor 8 feet away. This helps you in standing erect without being shaky.

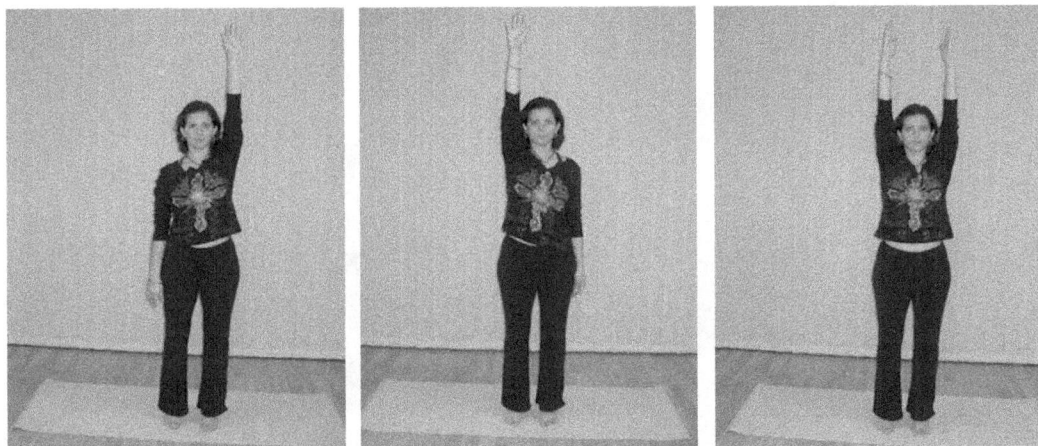

Coming Out of the Pose—Exhale and lower your heels and bring the right arm back to the normal position.

Repeat the same pose with the left arm.

Finally repeat the same with both arms simultaneously. Breathe gently.

Repeat the entire sequence once again.

Focus—On breathing and stretching up.

Breathing Pattern —Check the 'Technique'.

Physical Benefits—This stretches your spine and strengthens and massages the nerves, muscles and the mammary glands. It boosts the nervous system which brings neuro-muscular control. It is very good for children to gain height.

95

Psychological Benefits—This pose teaches you to strive till you reach the top through sheer determination. It rejuvenates all the energy centres or chakras; also makes you adequately ambitious (not over-ambitious) and brings clarity to your ambition. This inspires you to venture out wisely in your endeavour. You cannot succeed if you are shaky, tense or anxious about your goals. You need to be steady and sturdy, only then will your confidence come alive. This pose has the power to awaken your innate skills. Your struggle to reach the top brings astounding results. Soon it becomes effortless to achieve your aspiration (desire) or goal.

Contraindications—People with weak knees or too weak to balance the body.

Value Addition—Write down your goals and prioritise them.

Thought for the Day

Your physical state is the reflection of your mental state.

---

4 | Hasta Karshanasan
(The Forward Bending Palm Press Posture)

Aim—To activate your acupressure points in the fingertips.

Time Span—Two to three minutes.

Technique—Inhale and stand with feet apart and hands on your hips. Exhale and bend forward placing your palms on the floor. Press the fingertips on the floor breathe normally for four breaths. In case you cannot reach the floor, increase the distance between your feet and see the difference.

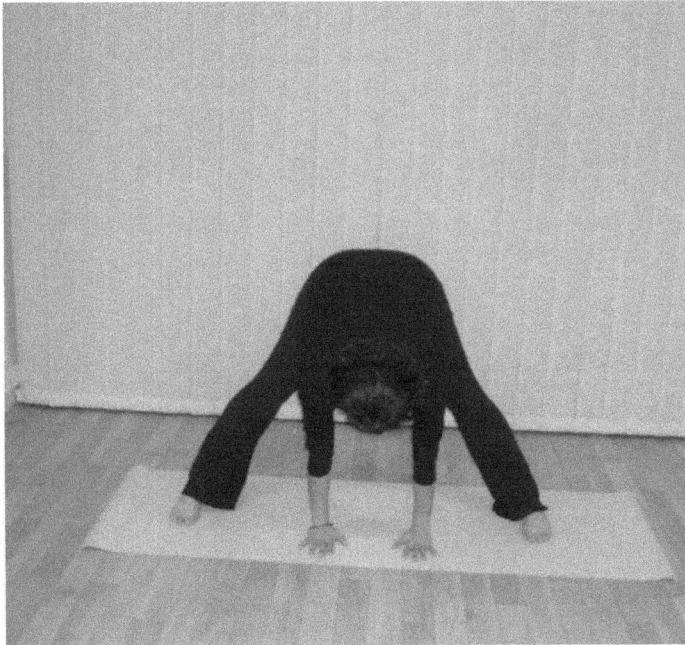

Coming Out of the Pose—Inhale and release the pressure from your fingertips; exhale and let go of your hands from the floor. Inhale and roll up and stand in the initial position. Exhale and bring the feet together. Breathe gently.

Focus—On the fingertips and pressing them on the floor gently.

Breathing Pattern—Check the 'Technique'.

Physical Benefits—Strengthens the legs, hamstring muscles, inner thighs, the back muscles and arms.

Psychological Benefits—This pose is very important and is one of my favourite postures. It opens the tiny receptors on your fingertips and awakens your psychic powers, creativity, sense of humour, intuition, ESP or the sixth sense. This activates your premonition and you gain new insights.

Contraindications—Those suffering from disc problems or lower back pain which radiates to the legs and makes it difficult to bend forward.

Value Addition—To intensify your concentration, press your little fingers, ring fingers, middle fingers and the index fingers with the thumb individually and utter/chant '*sa, ta, na, ma*'.

Thought for the Day

Every day is a gift from God and therefore it is called a 'present'. Make good use of this present.

---

5 Triyaka Tadasan or Ardha Chakrasan (The Swaying Palm Tree Posture—Sideways Stretch (Holding the Opposite Wrist—Optional))

Aim—To detect the stiffness of the oblique muscles and to unblock the energy flow around the shoulder area.

Time Span—Two to three minutes.

Technique—Stand erect with feet slightly apart. Inhale and raise your arms over the head. Exhale and stretch to the right side. You can also hold the opposite wrist and stretch. Inhale and stretch both hands upward as much as you can. Make sure your hip does not stick out from any side while stretching. Breathe four times in the same position.

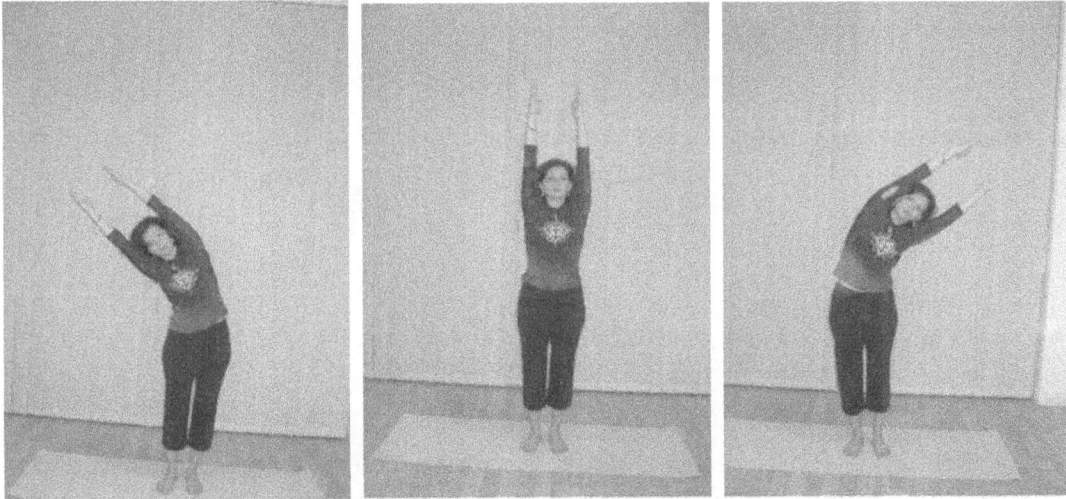

Coming Out of the Pose—Inhale and bring the arms overhead again. Exhale and bring the arms back to the normal position. Breathe gently.

Repeat the same stretching to the left side. You can also hold the opposite wrist and stretch.

Focus—On breathing, stretching and on keeping the balance.

Breathing Pattern—Inhale while stretching and exhale while bending.

Physical Benefits—This improves physical balance and coordination. This pose stretches the spine sideways, tones the back muscles and redistributes excess weight from the waistline. This energises the upper body 'obliques'. Each side is recharged with fresh prana-energy especially the spleen located on the left side which is the major entry point of prana-energy and the liver on the right side. This pose prevents constipation, gas, acidity, indigestion, urinary infection, obesity and helps considerably in diabetes as the pancreas begin to respond positively.

Psychological Benefits—The stiffness in the upper body determines whether your emotions are bundled up in a tight knot and whether you need to loosen up and be willing to reach out more to people. With regular practice, certain suppressed and unwanted emotions get released from the system. You begin to feel cheerful after the practice.

Contraindications—People suffering from acute shoulder pain or backache, severe heart conditions, nephritis.

Value Addition—Think about your favourite colour today and wear it. Throughout the day, check your surroundings to see where else you spot the same colour.

Do you know something about colours? The colour that you like today may not necessarily be your favourite after a few years as your moods and perceptions change from time to time and your choice of colour depends largely on your mood and perception.

Thought for the Day

There is no quick and easy way to lose weight. Retain your dietary and exercise habits to maintain your weight.

6

Dolasan
(The Pendulum Posture)

Aim—To strengthen the spine and the knees and to improve balance.

Time Span—Two to three minutes.

Technique—Stand with feet about 30–36 inches apart. Inhale, interlock your fingers and keep your hands on the nape of the neck. Exhale and bend forward towards the right foot. Breathe steadily for four times and settle down in this pose by keeping your feet firmly planted on the ground and the body weight distributed equally on both the feet. Check whether you can bend slightly more by bringing the forehead as close to the right knee as possible. Breathe four times.

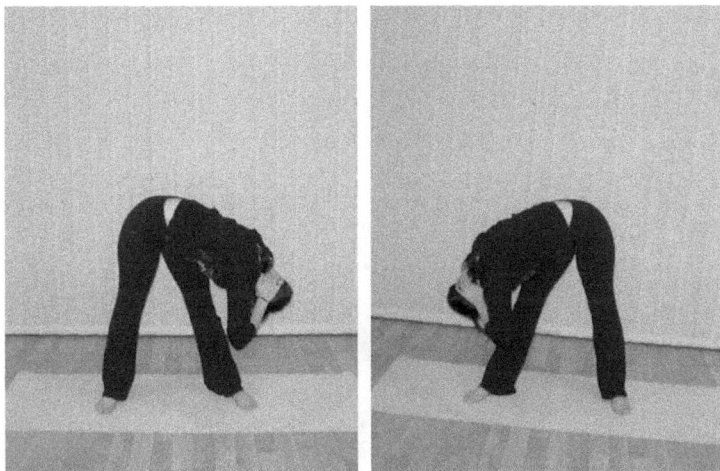

Coming Out of the Pose—Inhale and roll up raising the arms and torso. Exhale and bring your hands and the feet together back to the normal pose. Breathe gently.

Repeat the same, bending forward towards the left foot.

For the pendulum effect, you can swing the head and torso from the right knee to the left knee and from the left knee to the right knee. Repeat four times breathing steadily. Inhale and return to the centre and the upright position.

Focus—On stretching the spine and the hamstring muscles.

Breathing Pattern—Steady and normal.

Physical Benefits—This pose improves the back muscles, the connective tissues of the spine and the hamstring muscles in the legs. Tones the spinal nerves and improves blood circulation in the entire body.

Psychological Benefits—It improves your sense of balance which has a profound effect in improving your emotional balance as well.

Contraindications—People suffering from backache, vertigo, pregnancy.

Value Addition—Check how many times you practice patience in difficult situations. Your regular yoga practice makes it easy to observe patience.

Thought for the Day

To practice patience, it is important to recognise impatience first.

7

Utkatasan
(The Chair Posture)

Aim—To strengthen the leg muscles, learn balance and concentration.

Time Span—Two minutes.

Technique—Stand with feet hip-width apart. Inhale and stretch the arms in front at shoulder level and shoulder-width apart with palms facing downwards. Exhale and bend the knees as if you are sitting on a chair. Breathe four times.

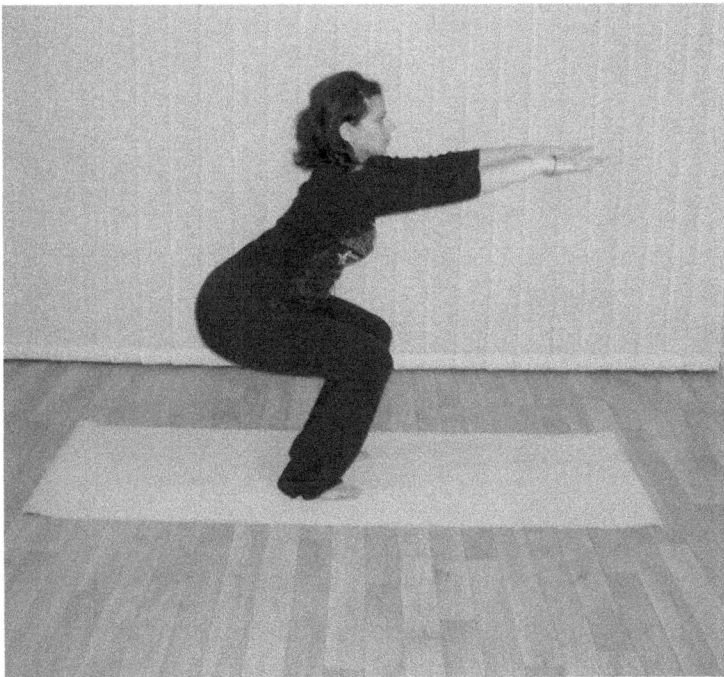

Coming Out of the Pose—Inhale and straighten the legs and stand in the normal position. Exhale and bring the arms down, back to the normal position.

Focus—On breathing and bringing steadiness to the legs.

Breathing Pattern—Check the 'Technique'.

Physical Benefits—Strengthens the muscles of the middle of the back, the pelvis and the uterus and also the thighs, knees and ankles; strengthens the feet, ankles and the quadricep muscles that support the knee.

Psychological Benefits—This teaches you emotional stability. The proper alignment teaches you to have the correct perspective. You quickly learn to balance your emotions well by balancing or mastering this pose. If you bend too much forward in this pose, it indicates that you are unduly anxious about your future. By improving your pose, you stop worrying about your future and build up confidence in yourself and in others. This boosts the circulation of prana energy in the body.

Contraindications—Prolapsed uterus, pregnancy.

Value Addition—Find out in which situations you use your head, heart and hands. The head related situations are mental or intellectual, the heart related situations are emotional and the hands related situations are either social or personal.

Thought for the Day

A gift always brings happiness to most therefore I offer you the precious gift of yoga because all you yogis and yoginis know that everything you need for true happiness is already inside your heart and the gift of yoga can help you achieve it through your head, heart and hands.

---

8 Hasta-Padangushthasan
(The Forward Spine Stretch with Hooked Thumbs)

Aim—To stretch the important muscles in the lower back, legs and arms.

Time Span—Two to three minutes.

Technique—Inhale and stand with feet hip width apart. Exhale, bend forward and hook the big toes with your thumbs, index and middle fingers. Breathe normally and bend forward as much as possible. Breathe four times.

Coming Out of the Pose—Inhale and release the thumbs and stand up. Exhale.

Focus—Bending forward and on breathing.

Breathing Pattern—Check the 'Technique'.

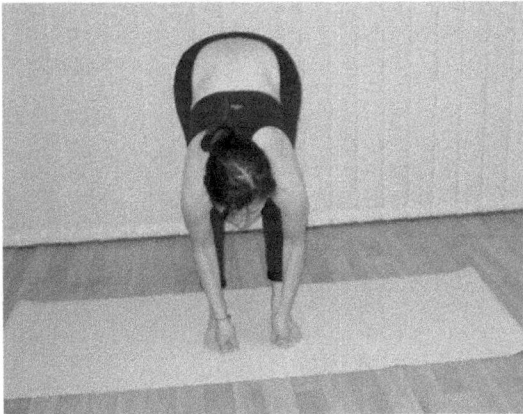

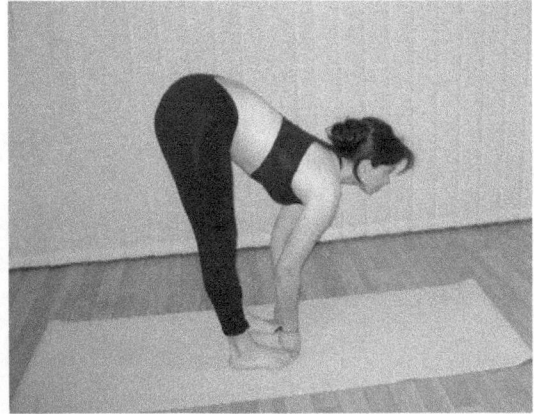

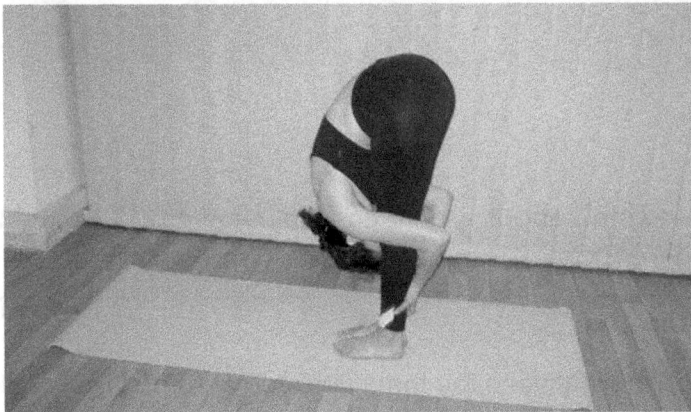

Physical Benefits—This gives a good stretch to your hamstrings, lumbar region and the triceps in your arms. It strengthens the back muscles and the spine. It also releases tension from the hamstrings and tones the quadriceps.

Psychological Benefits—This intense stretch teaches you to let go of accusations and criticism. This surrender teaches softening of attitude, humility, acceptance and resilience. It is believed that this is an antidote for mental rigidity.

Contraindications—People suffering from acute back pain or stiff/tight hamstrings.

Value Addition—Think about a new concept—have you thought of financing any needy child's educational expense at least for a year?

Thought for the Day

There is a difference between the family burden and the family responsibilities.

Devi Asan
(The Goddess Posture)

Aim—To learn balance and elegance.

Time Span—Two to three minutes.

Technique—Stand with feet 24 inches apart. Inhale, raise your arms and bend your arms at the elbows keeping them at shoulder level with the palms facing outward and close to the shoulders. Exhale and bend the knees, turning the feet outward at either 10 o'clock and 2 o'clock or at 9 o' clock and 3 o' clock positions. Breathe four times in the same position.

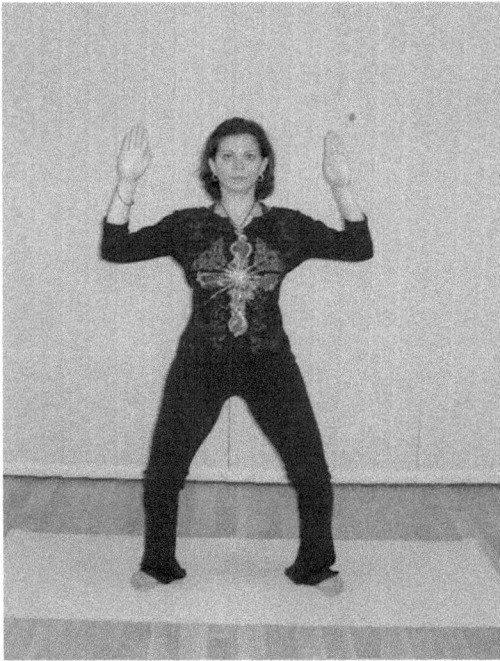

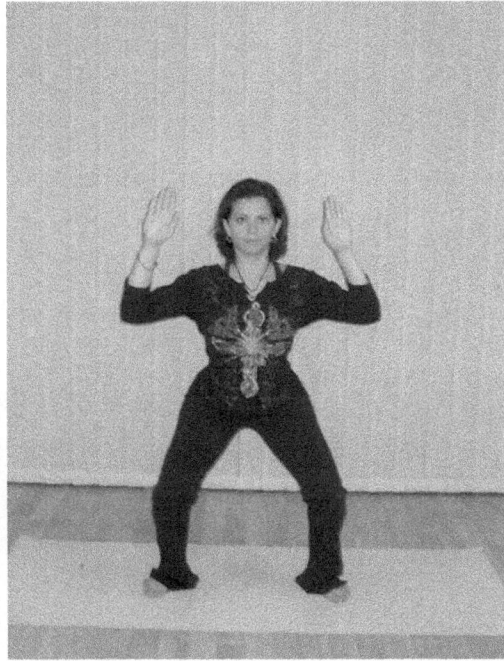

Coming Out of the Pose—Inhale and straighten the knees and bring your feet inward. Exhale and bring the arms and feet back to the normal position.

Focus—To improve our focus in life.

Breathing Pattern—Check the 'Technique'.

Physical Benefits—This is good for your knees and the spine.

Psychological Benefits—To create balance and elegance in our lives, it requires that we study physical imbalance which is manifested in certain weak spots and reflects mentally or emotionally. This pose teaches you that only strength is not enough in life and that you need flexibility as well. Only force is not adequate but sustained duration is also important. This fosters resilience, perseverance, focus and balance.

Contraindications—Acute or painful conditions of the hip joint.

Value Addition—Make sure that when you are not well, you see a doctor who believes that the medicine should be 'patient specific' as the cure takes place depending on the efficacy of the vital force or spiritual energy in the body.

Thought for the Day

Death is a fact of life but disease should not be the cause of death.

---

10   Sulabha Konasan
(The Simplified Angle Posture)

Aim—To activate the muscles of the sides of the trunk and to tap the unused parts of the lungs for better breathing.

Time Span—Two to three minutes.

Technique—Inhale and stand with legs wide apart. Exhale and put your right foot outward and the left foot slightly inward. Inhale and stretch your arms sideways at the shoulder level with palms facing downward. Exhale and bend the right knee. Inhale and stretch your left hand upward with your arm touching your ear. Exhale and bend sideways to the right, placing your right elbow on the right knee with the forearm stretched out at a right angle to the knee. Breathe four times looking straight ahead.

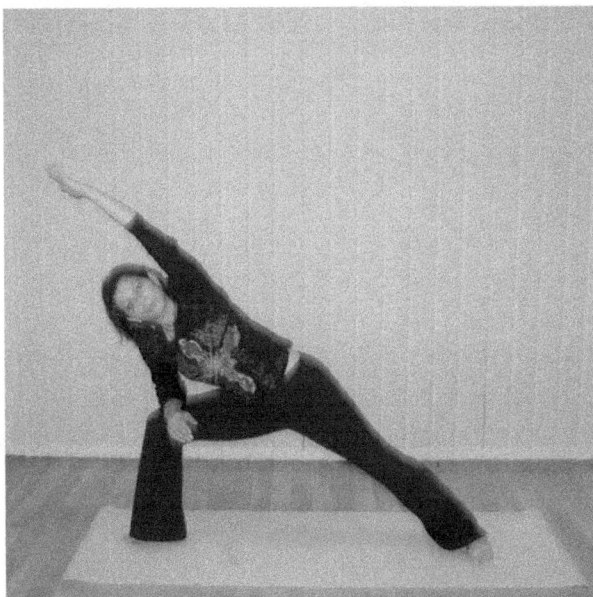

Coming Out of the Pose—Inhale, lift the right elbow from the right knee and straighten your torso. Exhale and lower your left arm. Inhale and straighten your right knee. Exhale and bring your right and left feet to the normal position. Inhale, exhale and bring the feet together. Repeat on the left side.

Focus—In maintaining the sideways stretch.

Breathing Pattern—Deep and rhythmic or Ujjayi.

Physical Benefits—This pose is excellent for the muscles on the sides of the trunk, the waist and the back of the legs which are not used often. It stimulates the nervous system and alleviates nervous depression. It improves digestion, activates intestinal peristalsis and alleviates constipation. Strengthens pelvic area and tones the reproductive organs. Also reduces flab from the waistline.

Psychological Benefits—This teaches balance and focus. It makes you realise the importance of Trinity and interdependence. This pose improves your public relations or inter-personal relationships.

Contraindications—People suffering from acute back conditions.

Value Addition—Make a family tree using your creativity.

Thought for the Day

Simplicity cannot be affected or destroyed if it is either innate or ingrained in one's nature.

---

11 | Parivritta Parvatasan (The Twisting Mountain Posture)

Aim—To twist the spine and the waist to bring in fresh prana energy.

Time Span—Two to three minutes.

Technique—Stand with feet hip width apart. Inhale and raise your arms over the head. Interlock the fingers. Exhale and twist the torso to the right side, looking in that direction. Breathe four times.

Coming Out of the Pose—Inhale once again and bring the torso to the centre. Exhale and bring the arms down. Repeat the same twisting the torso to the left side.

Focus—On steady breathing and maintaining the twist to feel the stretch in the spinal muscles.

Breathing Pattern—Slow and steady.

Physical Benefits—This pose tones the spine, waist, back and the hips. It helps a great deal in reducing a stiff back.

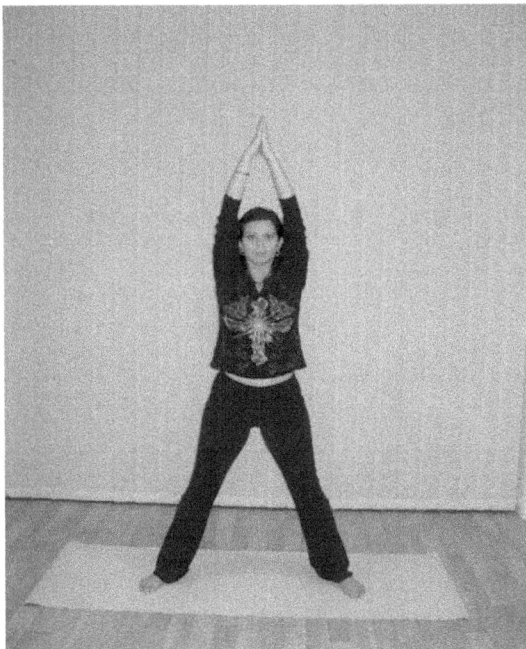

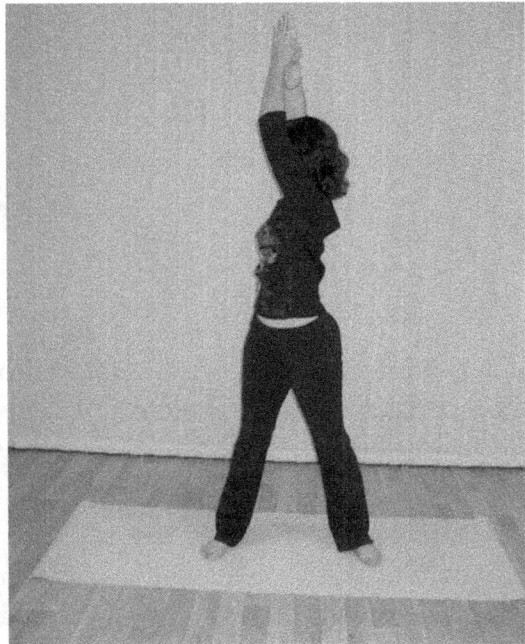

Psychological Benefits—The stiffness in the back also indicates the rigidity in thinking therefore by loosening up the spinal muscles, the thought process can be free from rigidity.

Contraindications—People suffering from any spinal injury should avoid this pose.

Value Addition—If possible, read Mahatma Gandhi's biography. It can change your perception for the better.

Thought for the Day

Today the world seems to run on pragmatic fuel which postulates that everything has only a relative value and nothing is permanently good or bad. It is not as much as 'survival of the fittest' but 'survival at any cost'.

---

12 | **Virbhadrasan–II (The Warrior Posture–II)**

Aim—To prepare you for the advanced pose of Virabhadrasan III with ease.

Time Span—Two to three minutes.

Technique—Inhale and stand with feet wide apart. Exhale, turn your right foot out and the left foot slightly in. Inhale and stretch your arms out sideways, palms facing down. Exhale and bend the right knee. Inhale, keep the torso in the centre and do not move it to either side. Exhale and turn the head toward the right hand. Breathe four times.

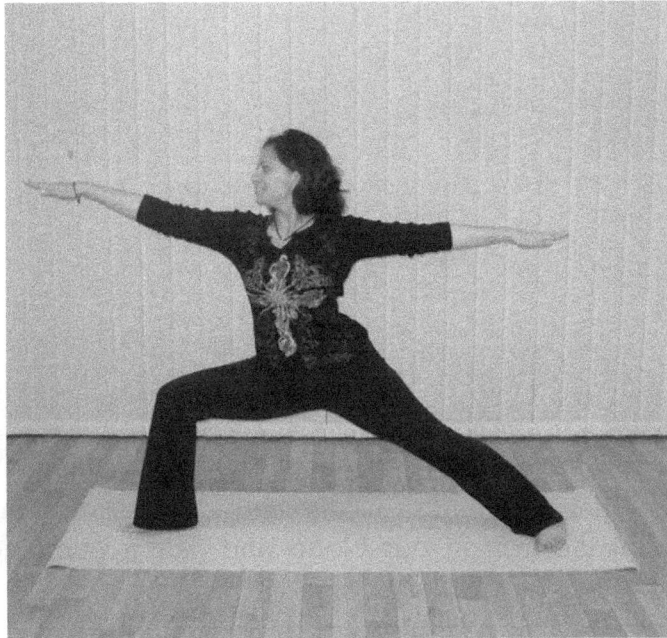

Coming Out of the Pose—Inhale and look straight in front. Exhale and straighten your right knee. Inhale and bring the feet back to the normal position. Exhale, bring the arms down and feet together.

Repeat the same using the left leg.

Focus—On breathing and synchronising the movements.

Breathing Pattern—Normal and steady.

Physical Benefits—This pose strengthens the leg muscles and relieves cramps in the calves and thigh muscles, brings elasticity to the legs and lower back muscles. This also has a toning effect on the abdominal organs. Expanding the rib cage helps to feel the balance between the right and left ribs.

Psychological Benefits—This pose awakens your innate powers and courage. It builds up your confidence and will power.

Contraindications—In acute or painful conditions of the hip joint.

Value Addition—Have you tried 'Magnet Therapy' anytime? Magnets can reduce menstrual pains, arthritis, ulcers and depression. Magnets have a whirlpool effect on the iron in our blood and gets it pumping much more efficiently than usual.

Thought for the Day

What has the most attractive properties in this world? The answer is a 'Magnet'. It is believed that in the next 5–10 years, magnets will be seen in first aid boxes for their healing properties. There will be magnetic hair brushes to stimulate hair growth, magnetic facial masks to reduce wrinkles, magnetic insoles to boost 'chi' energy in the feet and magnetic jewellery to ward off negativity.

13

Ek Pad Bakasan or Marulasan
(The Flamingo Posture)

Aim—To assess your sense of balance and prepare yourself for the more advanced balancing poses like the Tree Pose, the Balance Pose, etc.

Time Span—Two to three minutes.

Technique—Stand with feet together and hands on the hips. Inhale, raise your right leg, bending your right knee. Exhale and keep your right foot on the left knee like a flamingo bird. Balance on the left leg and breathe four times normally.

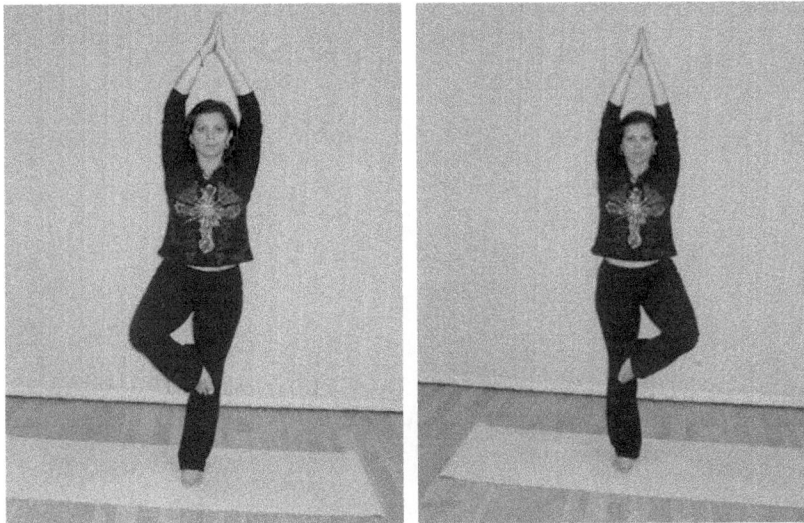

Coming Out of the Pose—Inhale and release the right foot from the left leg. Exhale and bring the right leg down on the floor. Repeat the same with the left leg.

Focus—On steady breathing and balancing. To make your balance easy, keep a steady gaze on the floor about 8 feet away from where you are standing.

Breathing Pattern—Slow and steady.

Physical Benefits—This pose improves blood circulation in the lower body strengthening your hamstrings, the legs and the ankle joints. It also stimulates digestion which eases constipation.

Psychological Benefits—All balancing poses improve your attention span, concentration, coordination and balance. When your physical balance improves your mental or emotional balance gets better.

Contraindications—People with any ailment like sciatica, slipped disc, hernia, weak legs, high blood pressure, pregnancy.

Value Addition—Try moon bathing at night on a full moon day which has a cooling and calming effect. This also dissolves your suppressed anger/hostility to a certain extent.

Thought for the Day

If at all you must get angry, initially direct your anger at those who have deserved it, (towards your target) and not towards those you fear will offend you in the future. The best thing would be not to get angry. Get even... still better..... get over it.

14

Utkatasan-Prasarita Padottanasan
(The Spiderman Posture/the Shoulder/
Inner Thigh Stretch)

Aim—To strengthen your inner thighs, knees and ankle joints.

Time Span—Two to three minutes.

Technique—Inhale and stand with your feet wide apart. Exhale and squat walking your hands back in between your legs. Inhale and tuck your hands around your ankles and hold on to your feet, looking straight ahead. Let your inner knees rest on your elbows. Exhale and stretch your thighs further with this extra support. Bounce gently with your hips. Breathe four times.

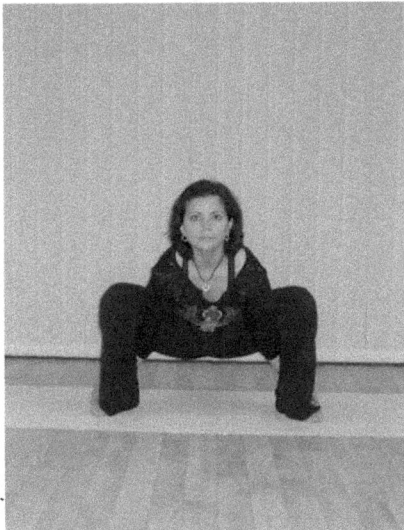

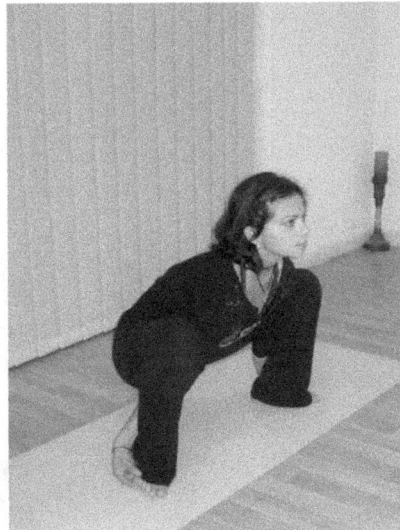

Coming Out of the Pose—Inhale and release your hands from the ankles. Exhale and keep the hands on the floor. Inhale and roll up. Exhale and bring your feet together.

Focus—On bouncing your buttocks.

Breathing Pattern—Normal.

Physical Benefits—Strengthens your hamstrings which are like the backbones of your legs. This loosens the shoulders as well. Resting your knees on the elbows and bringing each elbow and knee together eases energy blocks in the shoulders and knees.

Psychological Benefits—You create a harmonious circuit of energy around yourself.

Contraindications—People suffering from knee or ankle pain, during pregnancy.

Value Addition—Find out which prayer calms you down and brings contentment.

Thought for the Day
May all beings be happy. May all beings be healthy. May all beings receive the strength from God to treat happiness and unhappiness alike.

15

Vrikshasan
(The Tree Posture)

Aim—To stimulate digestion, to remove constipation, improve blood circulation, strengthen the leg muscles and to improve balance.

Time Span—Two to three minutes.

Technique—Stand with feet hip-width apart. Inhale and raise the right knee. Exhale and place the right foot on the inner side of the left thigh. If you feel comfortable, you can also fold the leg and place the foot on top of the left thigh. Inhale and join the palms in Namaste position. Exhale and look at the floor 8 feet away. This helps in steadying your nerves and balancing. Inhale and raise your arms over the head with palms joined in Namaste position. Breathe in this position for four times.

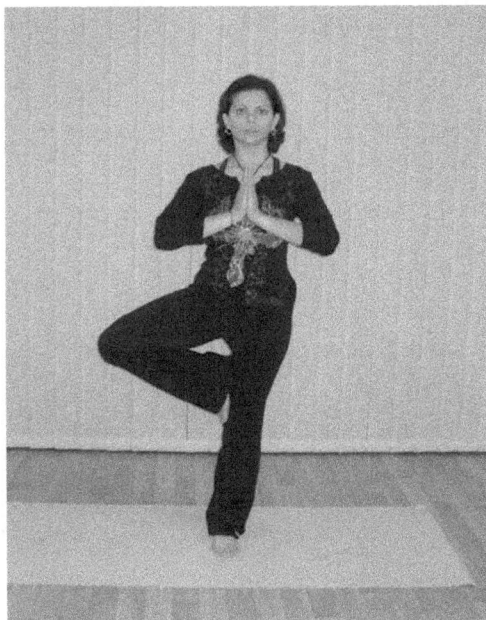

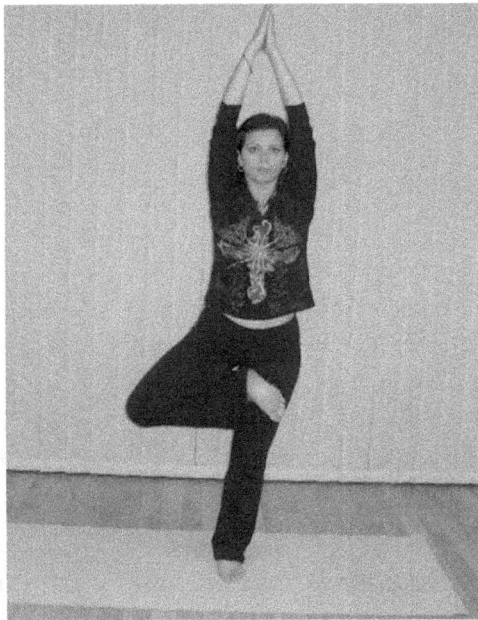

Coming Out of the Pose—Inhale and get ready to come out of the position. Exhale and bring the arms down to the Crown Chakra. Inhale and wait. Exhale and bring the hands to the Heart Chakra. Inhale and take your arms back to the normal position. Exhale and place the foot/leg back to the normal position. Repeat with the left leg.

Focus—On maintaining balance and also on steady breathing.

Breathing Pattern—Check the 'Technique'.

Physical Benefits—To stimulate digestion, to remove constipation, improve blood circulation, strengthen the leg muscles and to improve balance.

Psychological Benefits—Improves your ability to take independent or the right decisions quickly. When mastered, this pose will decide whether you can be self-reliant and survive without support.

Contraindications—People with sciatica, slipped disc, hernia, very weak legs or high blood pressure.

Value Addition—Find out what your reaction is when you receive unconditional love from someone?

Thought for the Day

There is only one action which has no motive and that is unconditional love, every other action has some motive or the other.

| 16 | **Tolasan**
(The Balance Posture) |

Aim—To acquire physical and mental balance.

Time Span—Two to three minutes.

Technique—Stand with feet together. Inhale and bend the right leg at the back, bringing the right foot close to the right hip and keep the knees together. Exhale and hold the right ankle with the right hand. Inhale and raise the left arm upward, keeping the inner arm close to the left ear. Exhale.

Breathe four times.

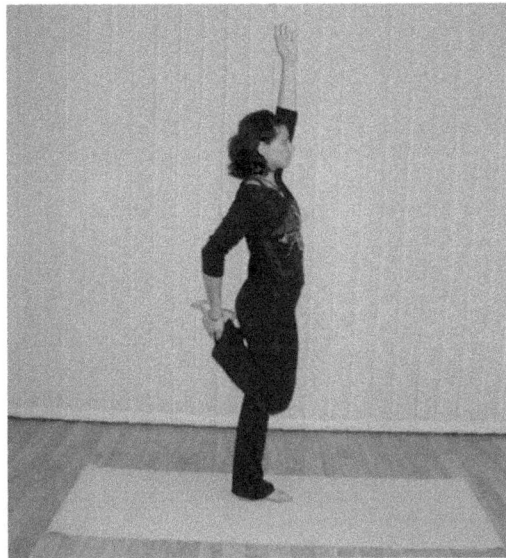

Coming Out of the Pose—Inhale and release the right ankle and keep the right foot down on the floor. Exhale and bring the left arm down to the normal position. Repeat the same using the other side.

Focus—On breathing and maintaining the balance.

Breathing Pattern—Slow and steady.

Physical Benefits—It improves physical balance. It strengthens the leg muscles and stretches the torso. It also develops overall strength and flexibility and promotes the cardio vascular and respiratory systems.

Psychological Benefits—Physical balance teaches mental and emotional discipline. You cannot succeed if you are shaky, tense and anxious about your goals. You need to be steady and sturdy physically. Your physical state is the reflection of your mental state. This pose particularly encourages you to remain unaffected by any negative and baseless criticism about yourself.

Contraindications—People with sciatica, slipped disc, hernia, very weak legs or high blood pressure.

Value Addition—Find out situations in your life where you have to use the three ingredients given below to succeed.

Thought for the Day

Success in life is very important and there are three factors to make success successful—Integrity, Maturity and Mentality.

---

17 | Prasarita Padottanasan or Parshvottanasan–I, II (Extended Legs or Flank Posture–I, II)

Aim—To relieve stiffness in the legs, hip muscles and the spine.

Time Span—Two to three minutes for each—I and II.

Technique–I. Stand with your feet together and hands on the hips. Inhale and put your right foot forward about 24–30 inches. Exhale and put your body weight on your left leg. Inhale and stretch your arms upward. Exhale and bend forward, dropping your hands on either side of your right foot (if possible, place your palms on the floor). Settle down in the position. See if you can bring your forehead closer to the knee. Breathe four times.

Coming Out of the Pose—Inhale, release your hands from the floor and roll up. Exhale and bring your right foot back in the normal position keeping feet together.

Repeat the same with the left leg.

Technique–II. Stand with feet together and hands on the hips. Inhale and put the right foot forward. Exhale and bend your right knee. Inhale and join your hands at the back in Namaste position. Draw the shoulders and elbows back. Exhale, bend forward as much as you can, stretching the spine gradually. Your ultimate goal is to rest your forehead on the right knee. Breathe four times in the same position.

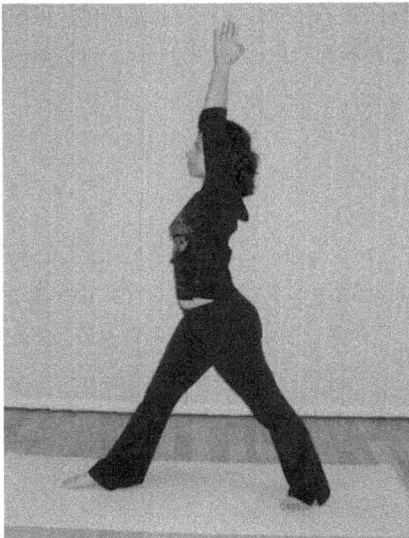

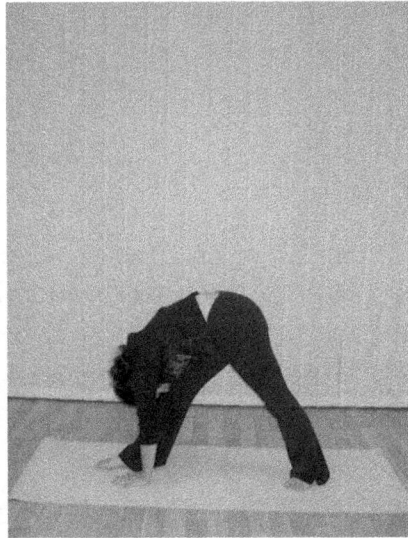

123

Coming Out of the Pose—Inhale and stand up. Exhale and straighten your knee. Inhale and release your hands from the Namaste. Exhale and bring the right leg back to the normal position.

Repeat the same with the left side.

Focus—On balancing the upper body and the lower body.

Breathing Pattern—Steady and deep (Ujjayi).

Physical Benefits—The shoulders are stretched down in (I) or drawn back in (II) which corrects any defect in the shoulders and removes stiffness.

Psychological Benefits—This instils poise and alertness or caution. You learn to overcome obstacles in the journey of life.

Contraindications—People suffering from vertigo, high blood pressure, hernia or acute shoulder problem.

Value Addition—A group discussion on the meaning of 'being lucky' (at the right place, at the right time, surrounded by the right people and the right kind of energy and blessings). Find out what lucky people contribute to the less privileged people?

Thought for the Day

Not getting what you want is sometimes a wonderful stroke of luck.

Veer Garudasan
(The Eagle Warrior Posture)

Aim—To prepare for the advanced poses.

Time Span—Two to three minutes.

Technique—Stand with feet apart like the Warrior Posture–II. Inhale and stretch the arms sideways. Exhale and turn the right foot outward and left foot slightly inward. Inhale and bend the right knee. Exhale and bring the right arm upright to the centre of your torso and entwine the left arm around the right arm bringing the palms together. Look straight ahead and breathe four times.

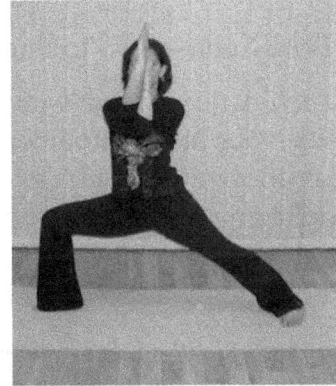

Coming Out of the Pose—Inhale, release your arms and stretch the arms sideways. Exhale and straighten the knee. Inhale, and bring the right and left foot to their normal positions. Exhale and bring the arms back to the normal position.

Focus—On breathing and synchronising the movements.

Breathing Pattern—Normal and steady.

Physical Benefits—This pose strengthens the torso and releases any tension around the shoulders. It strengthens the leg muscles and relieves cramps in the calves and thigh muscles, brings elasticity to the legs and to the lower back muscles. It also has a toning effect on the abdominal organs.

Psychological Benefits—This pose awakens your innate powers of courage and focus.

Contraindications—In acute or painful conditions of the shoulders or hip joint.

Value Addition—Choose your words carefully when you say anything so that it will be far from a lie or even a white lie and they do the least harm and the most good to the listeners/others.

Thought for the Day

The yogic practice of 'Satya'—truthfulness, focuses on speaking the truth.

Utthitha Trikonasan
(The Triangle Posture)

Aim—To tone the entire body.

Time Span—Two to three minutes.

Technique—Stand with feet comfortably apart. Inhale and stretch the arms sideways at the shoulder level. Exhale and turn the right foot outward and the left foot inward. Inhale and stretch the right arm outward leaning towards the right side as much as possible. Exhale and bend to the right side, placing the right hand on the right foot or holding the right ankle. Breathe four times, looking upward at the left thumb.

Coming Out of the Pose—Inhale and look straight in front. Exhale and release your right hand from the right foot/ankle. Inhale and return to the upright position, keeping both the arms stretched sideways. Exhale and bring the arms back to the normal position. Inhale and bring the right foot and left foot back to the normal position. Exhale and bring your feet together.

Repeat the same pose using the other side. This completes one round. You can practice variations in this pose.

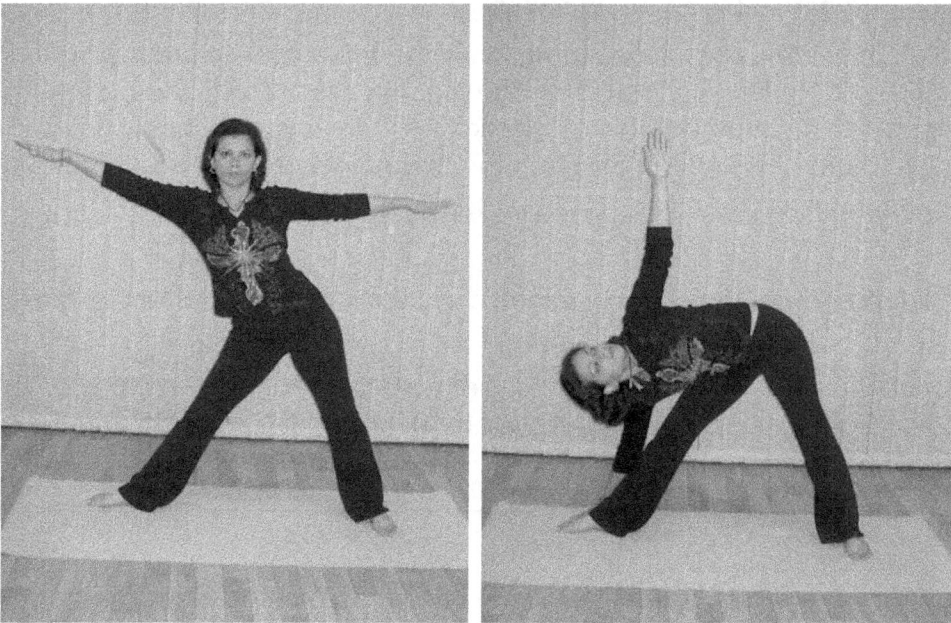

Focus—On coordination of movement, balance and the stretch on the side of the trunk in the final position.

Breathing Pattern—Normal and steady.

Physical Benefits—This pose is excellent for the muscles on the sides of the trunk, the waist and the back of the legs which are not used often. It stimulates the nervous system and alleviates nervous depression. It improves digestion, activates intestinal peristalsis and alleviates constipation. Strengthens the pelvic area and tones the reproductive organs. Also reduces flab from the waistline.

Psychological Benefits—This teaches balance and focus. It makes you realise the importance of Trinity and interdependence. This pose improves your public relations and inter-personal relationships. It also makes you aware of the correct focus when you look upward at the thumb.

Contraindications—People suffering from acute back conditions.

Value Addition—Find out the difference between independence and freedom. How do you use your freedom? It should not be at the expense of someone's basic rights.

Thought for the Day
Independence is a great virtue which leads to your personal victory but interdependence is a greater virtue which leads to your public victory.

20

Parshvottanasan
(The Backward Spine Stretch)

Aim—To stretch the spine backward to strengthen it and bring a flush of oxygenated blood supply to the connective tissues of the spine.

Time Span—One to two minutes.

Technique—Stand with your feet 30–36 inches apart. Place your hands on the hips. Inhale and stretch the spine upward. Exhale and bend backward as much as you can, staying well within the limits of your flexibility. Breathe four times in this position.

Coming Out of the Pose—Inhale and bring the torso back to the normal. position. Exhale and bring the hands down and feet together.

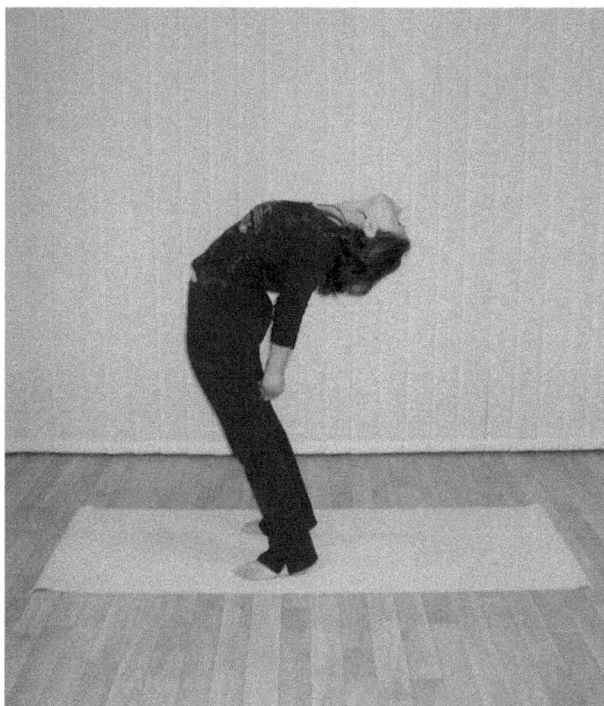

Focus—On breathing and bending backward gently without loosing your balance.

Breathing Pattern—Normal and steady or Ujjayi breathing.

Physical Benefits—This pose serves as a heart opener which stretches and strengthens the throat, shoulders and torso and boosts energy to the whole upper region. This also creates a strong foundation by strengthening the lower body as the strength required for the bend comes from the lower body. Therefore you strengthen the lower body as well. This helps to improve the respiratory system and reduce conditions such as asthma. It also improves the mobility of the spine and improves posture.

Psychological Benefits—This relieves you from anxiety and other unnecessary tension. It develops concentration in the face of challenges.

Contraindications—Neck (especially disc injury) or lower back injury, migraine or tension headaches, high or low blood pressure, pregnancy.

Value Addition—Write your own experience where yours or somebody else's absentmindedness cost you a fortune.

Thought for the Day

The root of carelessness is in absentmindedness and the antidote to this is mindfulness.

---

21 — Parshvakonasan (The Angle Posture)

Aim—To rejuvenate the hamstring and quadricep muscles.

Time Span—Two to three minutes.

Technique—*Parshva* means side or flank and *kona* means angle so this is the extended lateral pose. Stand with feet wide apart. Inhale and stretch the arms sideways at the shoulder level. Exhale. Inhale and turn the right foot outward and the left foot slightly inward. Exhale and bend the right knee. Inhale. Exhale and bend to the right side bringing the right hand close to the right foot or holding the right foot with the right hand. Inhale and stretch the left arm upward. Exhale and bring the left hand downward parallel to the floor. Breathe four times steadily.

Coming Out of the Pose—Inhale and bring the left arm upward. Exhale and release your right arm from the right foot/ankle. Inhale and raise your torso bringing your arms sideways. Exhale and straighten the knee. Inhale and position the feet back to the normal position and exhale and bring the arms down.

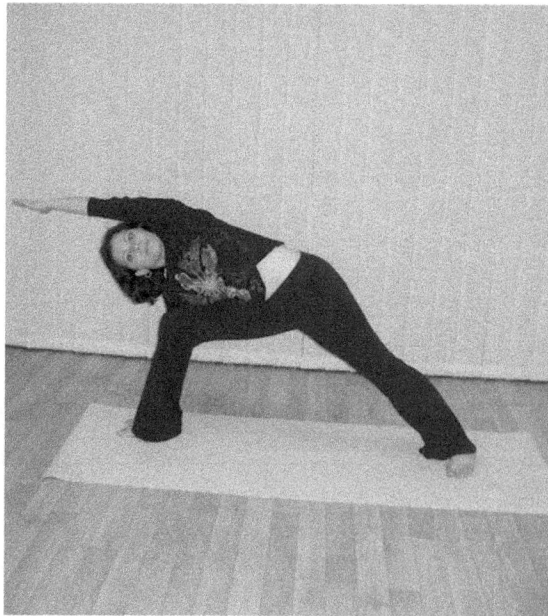

Repeat the same sequence using the other side.

Focus—On breathing and stretching the leg.

Breathing Pattern—Steady and normal or ujjayi breathing.

Physical Benefits—This pose strengthens the ankles, knees and thighs. It corrects defects in the calves or legs. It is excellent for reducing fat around the hips and relieves arthritis, sciatica, varicose veins. This also helps in constipation by increasing the peristaltic activity.

Psychological Benefits—This teaches you survival techniques to succeed in life.

Contraindications—Acute back condition or painful condition of the shoulder joint.

Value Addition—Introspect when you lose. Spend some time alone everyday.

Thought for the Day
When you lose, do not lose the lesson.

22 Dwikonasan–I or Setu Bandhanasan
(The Bridge Posture)

Aim—To stretch the shoulders and the chest.

Time Span—Two to three minutes.

Technique—Stand with feet hip-width apart. Inhale and stretch the arms sideways at the shoulder level. Exhale and extend the arms behind at the back and interlock the fingers. Inhale and look forward keeping the spine erect. Breathe four times while in the position. Please remain in the natural limits of your flexibility. The arms act as a lever to accentuate the stretch.

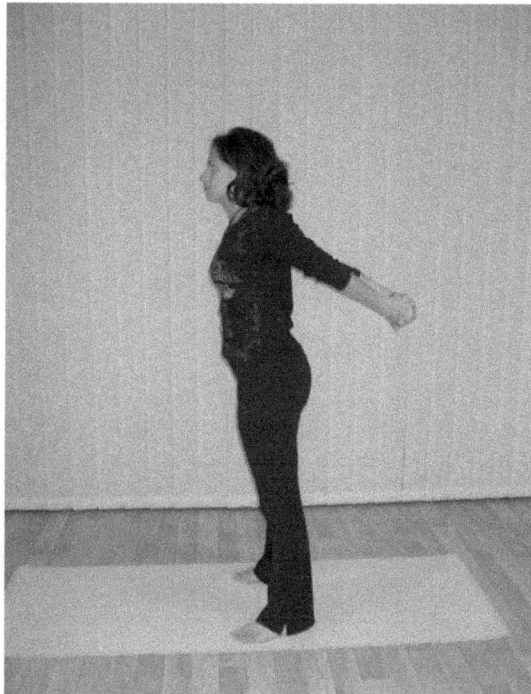

Coming Out of the Pose—Inhale and raise your torso to stand upright. Exhale and release the interlocked fingers. Inhale and bring the arms back to the normal position. Exhale and bring your feet together.

Focus—On the stretch of the arms, shoulders and upper back.

Breathing Pattern—Check the 'Technique'.

Physical Benefits—Stretches and strengthens the upper body—the spine, torso and arms.

Psychological Benefits—This pose opens the heart chakra, the centre of higher and refined emotions and makes you discerning in giving your love and affection to others. It strengthens the Thymus gland which helps fight infections. This also strengthens your lungs.

Contraindications—In acute or painful conditions of the shoulder joints.

Value Addition—Find out whether you have at least five or six good friends. If not, what kind of friends do you have at the moment?

Try to establish contact with at least five or six friends from various walks of life. A school friend is for sharing simple joys and confiding your emotions. A college friend is for exchanging experiences of similar situations in life who may perhaps share similar interests and careers; a neighbour who may challenge or stimulate you to broaden your mental boundaries. A work colleague who may shoulder similar responsibilities like yours and help you get charged with positive energy or resourcefulness; a mother or father figure who would serve as a source of inspiration and guidance for you; a partner who would be reliable and dependable. Finally you should have a mentor for your emotional support and practical advice.

Once you have them by your side, how would you reciprocate with these people?

Thought for the Day

Five friends that everyone must have to improve the quality life for instance, a school friend, a college friend, a work colleague, a mother/father figure and a mentor.

133

Dwikonasan–II
(The Anxiety/Fear-Free Posture)

Aim—To strengthen the pectoral muscles and the shoulder joint.

Time Span—Two to three minutes.

Technique—Stand with feet hip-width apart. Inhale and stretch the arms sideways at shoulder level. Exhale and extend the arms behind at the back and interlock the fingers. Inhale and look forward keeping the spine erect. Exhale and bend forward from the hips while simultaneously raising the arms behind the back as high as possible without strain. Breathe four times while in the position. Please remain within the natural limits of your flexibility. The arms act as a lever to accentuate the stretch.

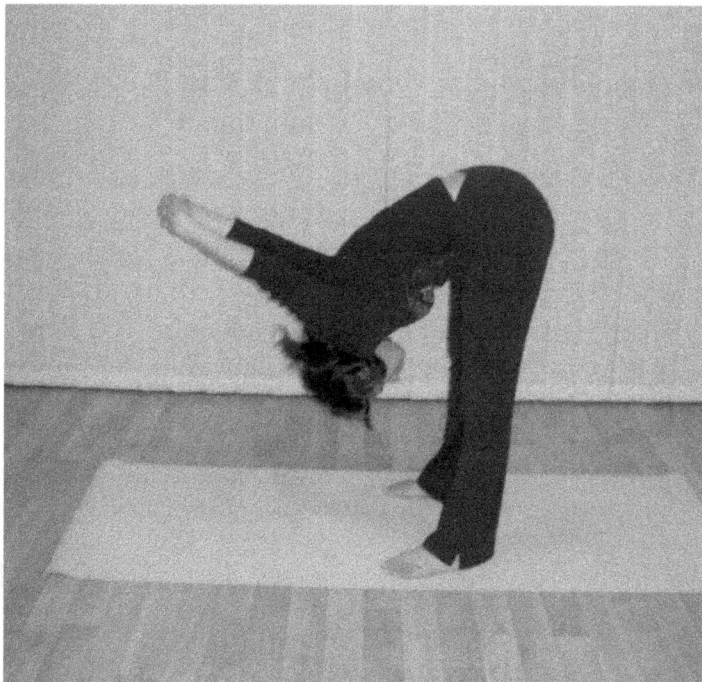

Coming Out of the Pose—Inhale and raise your torso to stand upright. Exhale and release the interlocked fingers. Inhale and bring the arms back to the normal position. Exhale and bring your feet together.

Focus—On the stretch of the arms, shoulders and upper back.

Breathing Pattern—Steady and normal.

Physical Benefits—This pose strengthens the connective tissues of the spine, shoulder-blades and upper back.

Psychological Benefits—It encourages you to remain down-to-earth in any situation. This frees you from real or imaginary fears. You also recover from certain traumas and phobias. This also activates your psychic awareness and you gain new insights which help solve your problems. Frees you from anxiety, insecurity and negative thoughts. When the chest expands, it empties out fear and anxiety.

Contraindications—In acute conditions of the spine or shoulder joints.

Value Addition—Follow the 3 R's : Respect for self, Respect for others, Responsibility for all your actions.

Thought for the Day

The practice of yoga discourages emotional indulgence and encourages spiritual enhancement.

| 24 | **Chakorasan**
(The Flying Balance Posture) |

Aim—To achieve good balance, coordination and concentration.

Time Span—Three to four minutes.

Technique—Stand with feet 30–36 inches apart. Inhale and stretch the arms sideways at the shoulder level. Exhale. Inhale and twist to the right side. Exhale and twist to the left side. Repeat the same once more to get a good momentum. Inhale and twist to the right side once more, turning your right foot out. Exhale and bend forward standing on the right leg and arms outstretched sideways like a flying bird. Inhale and raise the left leg parallel to the floor. Exhale and steady your gaze in front. Breathe four times in the same position.

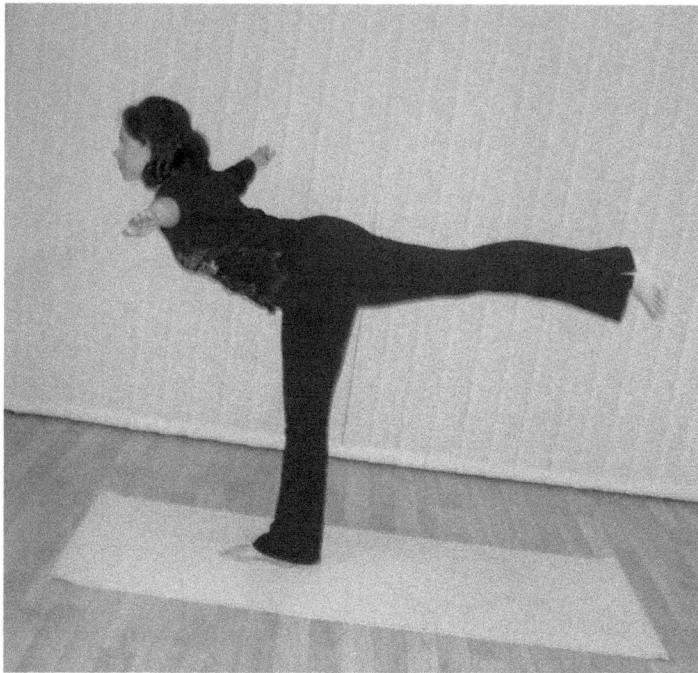

Coming Out of the Pose—Inhale and look straight ahead. Exhale and bring your left leg down. Inhale and bring your torso upright with the right foot back to the normal position. Exhale and bring the arms back to the normal position.

Repeat the same with the left leg.

Focus—On breathing and maintaining balance.

Breathing Pattern—Steady and normal.

Physical Benefits—This pose balances the nervous system and equalises the brain hemispheres. It also develops control of the body.

Psychological Benefits—This teaches you about your willingness to be resilient and perseverant. This also teaches you to balance your emotions. It trains you in the single or one-pointedness of an eagle and mental concentration and soon you learn to zero in on your target. This teaches aim in life and the willingness to spring into action.

Contraindications—People suffering from vertigo or high blood pressure.

Value Addition—Think of 'Human Values' and let them reflect in your personality.

Thought for the Day

(The Source—Internet) *(Take it in a lighter vein)*

A worldwide survey was conducted by the UN. The only question asked was:

"Would you please provide your honest opinion about solutions to the food shortage in the rest of the world?"

The survey was a huge failure, because:

    In Africa they didn't know what "food" meant
    In India they didn't know what "honest" meant
    In Europe they didn't know what "shortage" meant
    In China they didn't know what "opinion" meant
    In the Middle East they didn't know what "solution" meant
    In South America they didn't know what "please" meant
    And in the USA they didn't know what "the rest of the world" meant.

25

Tolasan
(The Trefoil Clover Posture)

Aim—To help in concentration, balance and coordination.

Time Span—Two to three minutes.

Technique—Stand with feet together. Inhale and stretch your right arm upward touching your right ear. Exhale and stretch your left arm sideways to the left side at the shoulder level. Inhale and lift your right leg backward. Exhale and focus the gaze on a fixed point at eye level. Breathe four times balancing on the left leg.

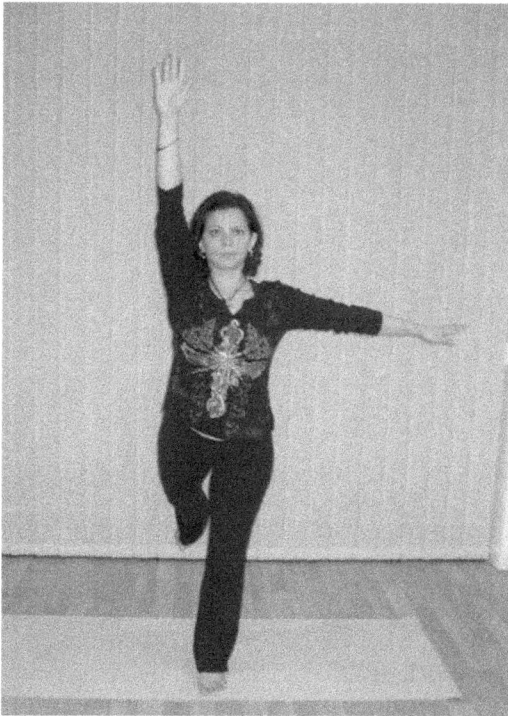

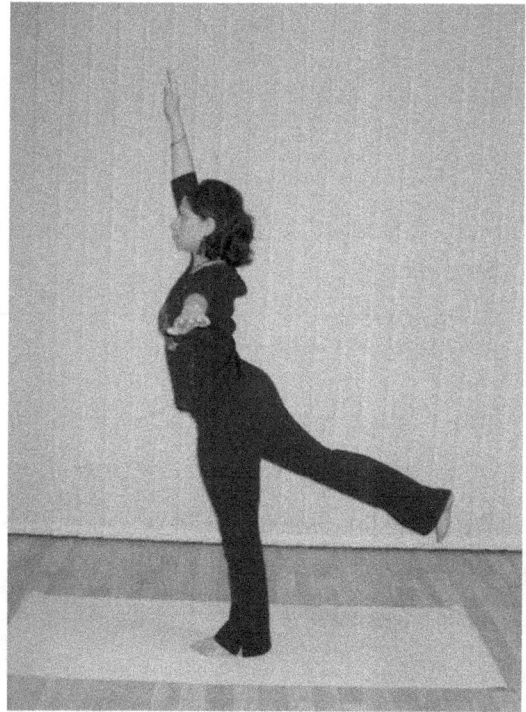

Coming Out of the Pose—Inhale and get ready to come out of the pose. Exhale and bring the right leg back to the normal position. Inhale and bring the left arm down. Exhale and bring the right arm down to the normal position. Repeat the same with the left side.

Focus—On maintaining the balance and on steady breathing.

Breathing Pattern—Steady and normal.

Physical Benefits—This clears the respiratory passage and prevents mucous formation, improves circulation, strength and balance. It stimulates blood circulation in the legs and strengthens the leg muscles.

Psychological Benefits—This improves your 'ABC'—Attention span, Balance and Coordination.

Contraindications—People suffering from sciatica, slipped disc, weak legs or high blood pressure.

Value Addition—Be alert and find out what gives you happiness or who brings you joy today.

Thought for the Day

Enjoying life comes with doing one thing at a time with total mindfulness. Simple things bring maximum joy.

Virbhadrasan–I
(The Warrior Posture–I)

Aim—To remove stiffness from the shoulders, neck, back, knees and the ankles.

Time Span—Two to three minutes.

Technique—Stand with feet together and hands on the hips. Inhale and put your right foot about 24–30 inches forward. Exhale. Inhale and stretch your arms over the head and join the palms together in Namaste position. Exhale and bend the right knee, putting your weight on the left leg. Breathe four times steadily.

Coming Out of the Pose—Inhale and straighten the right knee. Exhale, bring your right foot back and lower the arms to the normal position.

Repeat the same thing with your left foot forward.

Focus—On the smooth controlled movement and balance.

Breathing Pattern—Steady.

Physical Benefits—This pose gives a good stretch to the quadricep muscles and to the entire body.

Psychological Benefits—This pose improves concentration and a sense of balance. This also boosts confidence and creates a powerful and protective shield around your aura or the energy field.

Contraindications—This pose is tough and should not be performed by those who are weak and with a heart condition.

Value Addition—To boost your immune system just kick off your shoes and take a stroll on the earth or on the grass so that the acupressure points on your feet get stimulated and induce the secretion of hormones evenly from the corresponding organs.

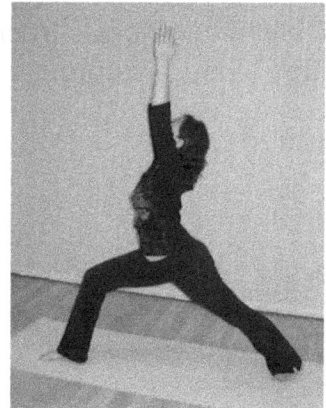

Thought for the Day

Yoga's IDEA is
'Self-**I**mprovement', 'Self-**D**iscipline', 'Self-**E**xperience, 'Self-**A**wareness'

Virbhadrasan–III
(The Warrior Posture–III)

Aim—To learn balance, concentration and coordination.

Time Span—Two to three minutes.

Technique—Stand with your feet together and hands on the hips. Inhale and put your right foot 24–30 inches forward. Exhale and keep your left foot firmly planted on the floor. Inhale and raise your arms overhead and interlock your fingers. Exhale and bend the right knee. Inhale and stretch the arms upward slightly to stretch your spine. Exhale and bend forward, straightening the right leg and stand on it, raising the left leg parallel to the floor. Inhale. If you feel wobbly, bring the left leg down on the floor and adjust the distance between the feet to start off a good balance while standing on the right leg again. Exhale and settle down in this pose. Breathe four times in this position. Repeat with the other side.

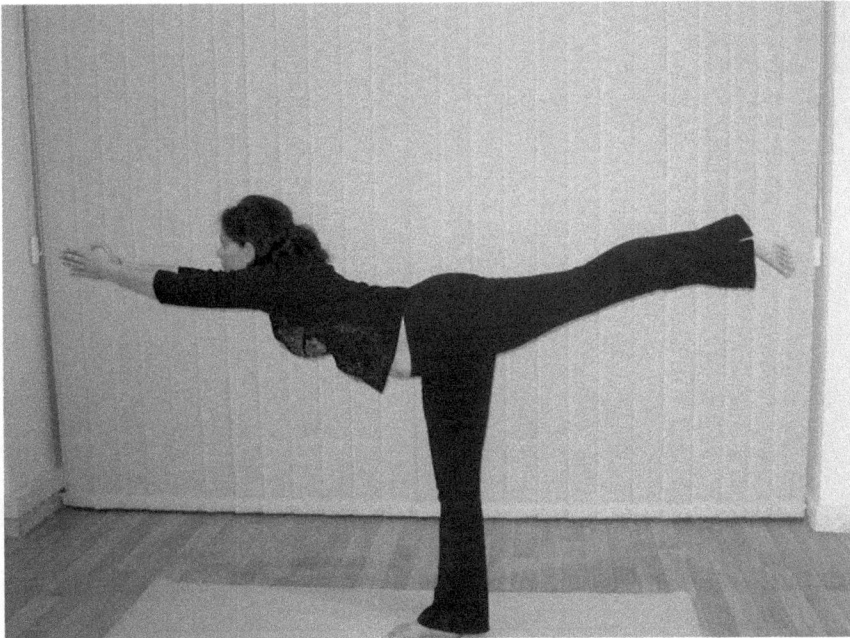

Focus—On balancing the pose.

Breathing Pattern—Ujjayi.

Physical Benefits—Relieves stiffness in the shoulders and back. This strengthens the legs, ankles and arms and tones the abdominal muscles and internal organs.

Psychological Benefits—This improves concentration and coordination, attention span and agility, making your reflexes swifter and improving poise.

Contraindications—People suffering from vertigo, high blood pressure, leg injury and during pregnancy.

Value Addition—Find out whether you take responsibility for your commitments.

Thought for the Day
Life is not an option but an obligation. It is a contract between you and God.

28 | Triyaka Tadasan
(The Swaying Palm Tree Posture—Lateral Stretch)

Aim—To loosen up the sides of the waist because we normally do not bend sideways.

Time Span—Two minutes.

Technique—Stand with feet about 24–30 inches apart. Keep the torso in the centre all throughout the posture. Inhale, stretch the arms overhead and interlock your fingers. Exhale and bend to the right side from the waist. Do not bend in front or at the back. Do not twist the torso. Hold the position for four breaths.

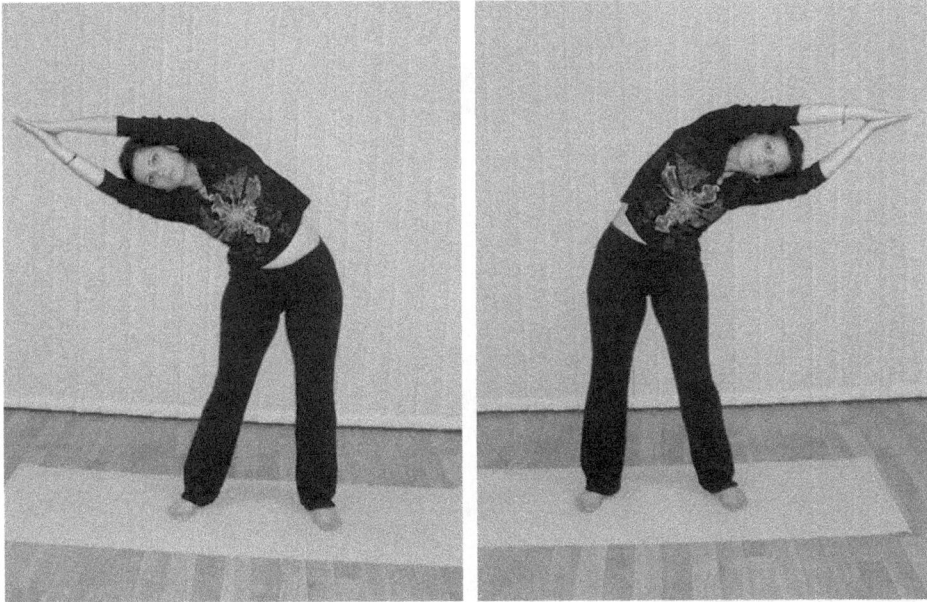

Coming Out of the Pose—Inhale and come back to the centre. Exhale and bring the arms down, back to the normal position.

Repeat the same with the left side.

Focus—On breath synchronisation, on the stretch along the side and maintaining the balance.

Breathing Pattern—Steady.

Physical Benefits—This is one pose which stretches the sides of the lungs, waist and the postural muscles which are not stretched otherwise. This stretch loosens up, massages and balances the right and left sides of the body and brings fresh oxygenated blood to these sides.

Psychological Benefits—Bending sideways detects stiffness in the sides of the chest/waist area. This particular stiffness denotes that your emotions are tied up in a tight knot and that you need to loosen up in order to avoid being stifled.

Contraindications—People suffering from vertigo or high blood pressure.

Value Addition—Check out through your own breathing pattern whether you are tired or relaxed. If you are tense, your breathing will be either short or shallow. If you are relaxed you will inhale with great effort and if you are tired you will exhale with great effort.

Thought for the Day

Being a yogi is about having the wisdom to remove anything that stifles your consciousness.

Sulabha Malasan
(The Garland Posture—Simplified)

Aim—To stretch the spine and the connective tissues.

Time Span—One or two minutes.

Technique—From the Forward Bending Posture, inhale and put your hands around and behind your ankles and interlock your fingers. Exhale, open your knees sideways and squat, sliding your torso in between your knees. Inhale. Exhale and lower your head and rest your forehead on the feet or the floor. Breathe four times.

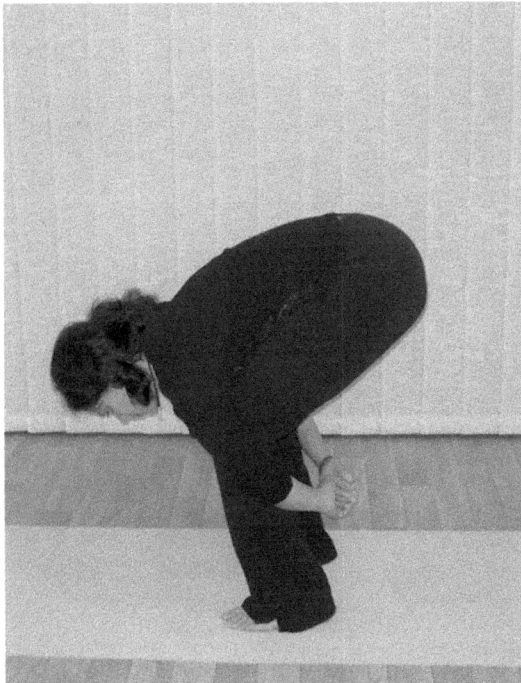

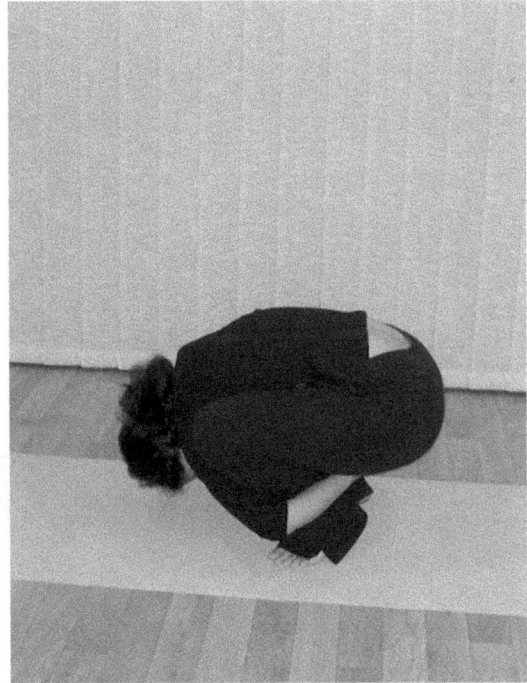

Coming Out of the Pose—Inhale and look up straight. Exhale, release your hands and place them on the floor in front of your feet. Inhale and start rolling up. Exhale and stand in the normal position.

Focus—On steady breathing and holding the pose.

Breathing Pattern—Normal and steady. Try ujjayi breathing.

Physical Benefits—This is especially good for ladies for menstrual or menopausal problems, also for colon problems, arthritis, sciatica, varicose veins and improved peristalsis for digestion and elimination.

Psychological Benefits—This pose brings you close to the earth and prepares you to have a 'down-to-earth' attitude.

Contraindications—People suffering from any back problem.

Value Addition—Have you made any flower garland? In Hindu culture, young girls and ladies make colourful garlands to offer to their deity.

> **Thought for the Day**
>
> When the body and mind are in sync, truth rises to the top.

30 Adhomukha Shvanasan (Simplified) (The Tendon Stretch/The Heels Up and Down)

Aim—To activate your tendons and strengthen the calf muscles and hamstrings.

Time Span—Two to three minutes.

Technique—Inhale and stand with feet together. Exhale and go on all fours on the floor, placing your hands in front of you at a comfortable distance. Inhale and walk your hands way out in front of you. Exhale, straighten both legs backward, raising your hips. Breathe normally. Keeping your feet on the floor, raise your right heel, dropping the right knee close to the floor. Bend your right leg, swing your right knee inward bending your leg and curling your toes and swing it outward straightening the right leg. Repeat four times and switch to the left leg and repeat the same. Breathe normally all throughout.

You can do this by alternating the right and left leg as well.

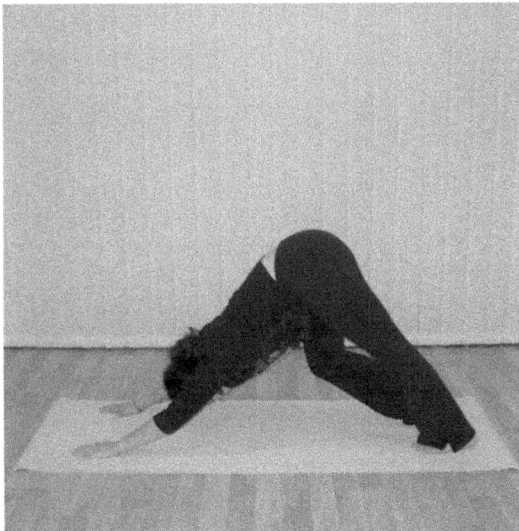

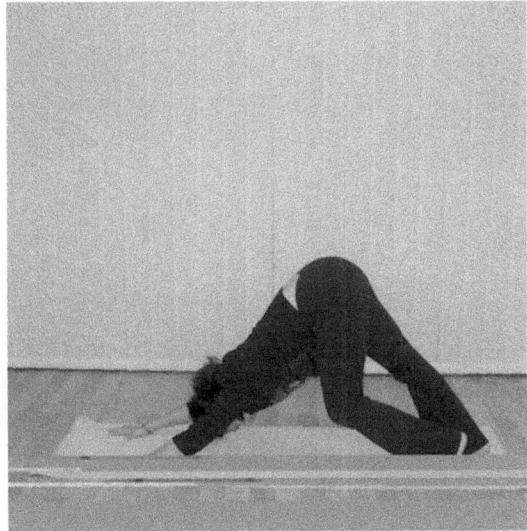

Coming Out of the Pose—Inhale. Go on all fours. Exhale and walk your hands back closer to your feet. Inhale, roll up and stand. Exhale.

Focus—Synchronising the movements.

Breathing Pattern—Normal.

147

Physical Benefits—When you do various stretches and moves in yoga poses, Lactic acid sometimes accumulates in the muscles giving rise to muscle cramps or contractions. With this stretch, you get rid of the lactic acid or any impurity in the calves and ankles.

Psychological Benefits—This invigorates all your chakra systems, energising you and making you light footed.

Contraindications—Sprained ankle or foot.

Value Addition—Make a nice family collage with your latest family pictures.

Thought for the Day

Don't blame! Your life is your responsibility so take ownership of it and make it work by overcoming obstacles.

---

31 Adhomukha Shvanasan
(The Downward Facing Dog Posture)

Aim—To strengthen your arms and legs.

Time Span—Two to three minutes.

Technique—Stand with feet hip-width apart. Inhale and stretch both arms upward. Exhale and bend forward bringing the hands on the floor. Inhale and step back with the right foot. Exhale and bring the left foot back beside the right foot. Simultaneously, raise the buttocks and lower the head between the arms. Breathe gently for four breaths. Straighten your arms and legs. Try to touch the floor with your heels and in the traditional Downward Facing Dog Posture, you try to bring your head towards the floor.

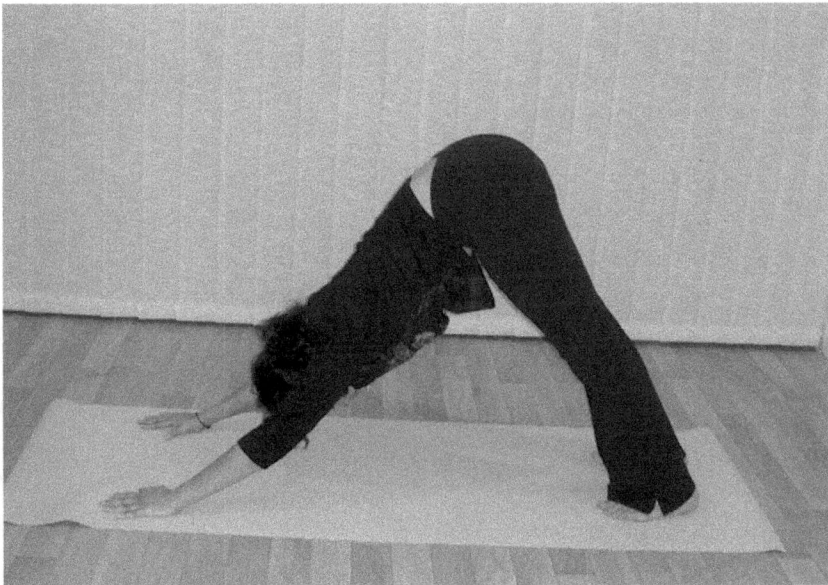

Coming Out of the Pose—Inhale and bring the right foot forward, near your right palm. Exhale and bring the left foot forward, near your left palm and come into the Forward Bending Posture. Inhale and roll up, bringing your torso and head upward. Breathe gently.

Focus—On breathing and raising the buttocks and lowering the head.

Breathing Pattern—Slow and steady.

Physical Benefits—This pose strengthens the nerves and muscles in the arms and legs, improves the circulation and tones the spinal nerves. This makes your shoulders also more flexible along with the upper body. It tones the muscles of the back, massages and strengthens the abdominal organs; this also builds endurance in your upper body and removes stiffness in the neck or shoulder area.

Psychological Benefits—This brings energy to the Vishuddhi chakra or the throat chakra and promotes agility, perseverance, grace, poise, purity. It changes your perspective for the better and corrects your perception.

Contraindications—High blood pressure or any complaint in the legs. Those having a tendency towards dislocation of shoulders or chronic shoulder injuries, pregnancy, unmanaged high/low blood pressure, herniated lumbar discs, positional vertigo.

Value Addition—Can you name one influential person in your life who has been responsible in teaching you moral values.

Thought for the Day

Moral values do not depend on power, position, person, pelf (money) or period (time) but they depend on integrity.

Ek Pad Adhomukha Shvanasan
(The Downward Facing Dog Posture with One Leg Up)

Aim—To strengthen your legs and arms.

Time Span—Two to three minutes.

Technique—Stand with feet hip-width apart. Inhale and stretch both arms upward. Exhale and bend forward bringing the hands on the floor. Inhale and step back with the right foot. Exhale and bring the left foot back beside the right foot. Simultaneously, raise the buttocks and lower the head between the arms. Breathe gently for four breaths. Straighten your arms and legs. Try to touch the floor with your heels and in the traditional Downward Facing Dog Posture, you try to bring your head towards the floor.

With One Leg Upward: Exhale and settle down distributing your body weight equally on your hands and feet. Inhale and raise your right leg up as much as possible. Ideally the leg should be in line with your upper body. Breathe four times looking at the inner side of your right arm. In this pose, you balance your body on three limbs that is your two arms and one leg.

Inhale and look down on the floor for balance and exhale and bring the right leg down on the floor.

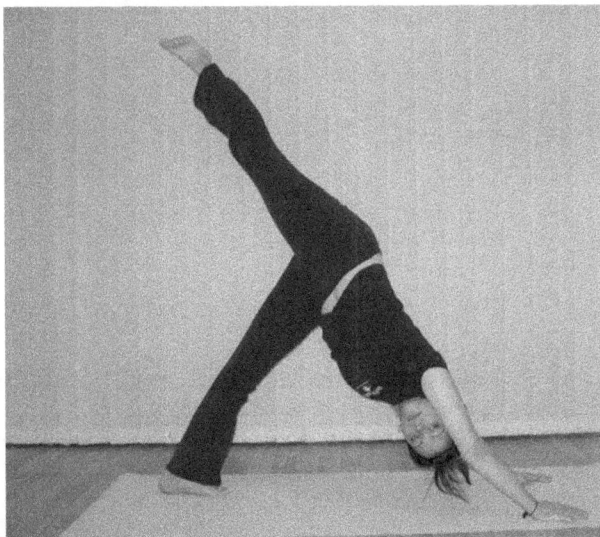

Repeat the same with the left leg.

Coming Out of the Pose—Inhale and bring the right foot forward, near your right palm. Exhale and bring the left foot forward, near your left palm and come into the Forward Bending Posture. Inhale and roll up, bringing your torso and head upward. Breathe gently.

Focus—On breathing and balancing.

Breathing Pattern—Slow and steady.

Physical Benefits—Raising one leg gives a good stretch to that particular side as compared to the traditional Downward Facing Dog. It also teaches you balance and simultaneoulsy strengthens the other three limbs which take the whole body weight. It makes you stronger in your upper as well as in the lower body. It makes you more flexible. It tones the spine, massages and strengthens abdominal organs, makes your shoulders more flexible, strengthens arms and legs and builds endurance and removes stiffness in the neck or shoulder area.

Psychological Benefits—The 'one leg extended upward pose' teaches correct balance, agility, perseverance, grace, poise and purity. It changes your perspective and corrects your perception.

Contraindications—High blood pressure or any complaint in the legs. Those having a tendency to dislocate their shoulders or chronic shoulder injuries, pregnancy, unmanaged high/low blood pressure, herniated lumbar discs, positional vertigo.

Value Addition—Find beauty in everyone and everything including yourself.

> **Thought for the Day**
>
> Life is lived forward and understood backward.

33	**Surya Namaskar**
	(Sun Salutation)

The Sun represents life force energy and has been worshipped since ancient times. Having 12 names, the complete sequence of the sun salutation includes 12 steps in the form of different postures which also represent 12 months or the 12 zodiac signs. The solar energy which flows within the right nostril is called 'Surya Nadi' or 'Pingala'. It has warm, energising and vitalising qualities. Generally men are drawn towards the solar energy as it represents masculine force.

Ideally, the Sun salutations are performed in the morning facing the Sun in the East which generates dynamic life-force energy and has a transforming effect on life but can also be practised at sunset. However, given the constraints faced these days, it may be practised whenever possible. The only point to be noted is that it should be practised on an empty stomach and the bowels should be clear. This practice serves like a meditation as it includes different postures, deep breathing and chanting of the Sun's 12 names.

The Sun Salutation is a series of 12 postures performed in a graceful fluid movement which is coordinated precisely with either inhalation or exhalation.

Hope you enjoy practising the Sun Salutation which is also known as Solar Revitalisation that brings vigour and vitality within.

Aim—To balance and energise all the chakras.

Time Span—One minute for one sequence of 12 poses.

Technique—There are 12 poses in this salutation, the first and the last ones being in the form of a Namaste position to begin and to complete the salutation. In this form of salutation, the body is considered to be two joined halves. Therefore, one Sun Salutation consists of two complete sequences of 12 poses each, one for the right side of the body and the other for the left which are performed along with the chanting of the 12 names of the Sun.

This serves like a gentle meditation when the focus is on all the three factors i.e. Postures, Breathing and Mantra Chanting:

Pose 1:   Om Mitraya Namaha—stand with feet together in Namaste position—Prarthanasan.

Pose 2:   Om Ravaye Namaha—inhale and stretch your arms upward—Hastha Utthanasan.

Pose 3: Om Suryaya Namaha—exhale, bend forward and place your palms on the floor—Paad-hastasan.

Pose 4: Om Bhanave Namaha—inhale, stretch your right foot backward and squat on your left leg—Ashwa Sanchalanasan.

Pose 5: Om Khagaya Namaha—exhale and stretch your left leg backward to join the other foot and bend forward touching the floor—Adho-mukha Shvanasan.

Pose 6: Om Pooshne Namaha—inhale, lean forward to get ready to prostrate, exhale and go into the Saashtang Namaskarasan.

Pose 7: Om Himyagarbhaya Namaha—inhale and raise your torso into Urdhwa-mukha Shvanasan.

Pose 8: Om Maricchaya Namaha—exhale and raise your lower body and drop you head down just like in pose 5—Adhomukha Shvanasan.

Pose 9: Om Aadiyaaya Namaha—inhale and bring your right leg forward between your hands just like in pose 4—Ashwa Sanchalanasan.

Pose 10: Om Savitreya Namaha—exhale and bring your left leg/foot forward, close to the right foot, just like in pose 3 in the 'forward bend pose'—Paad-hastasan.

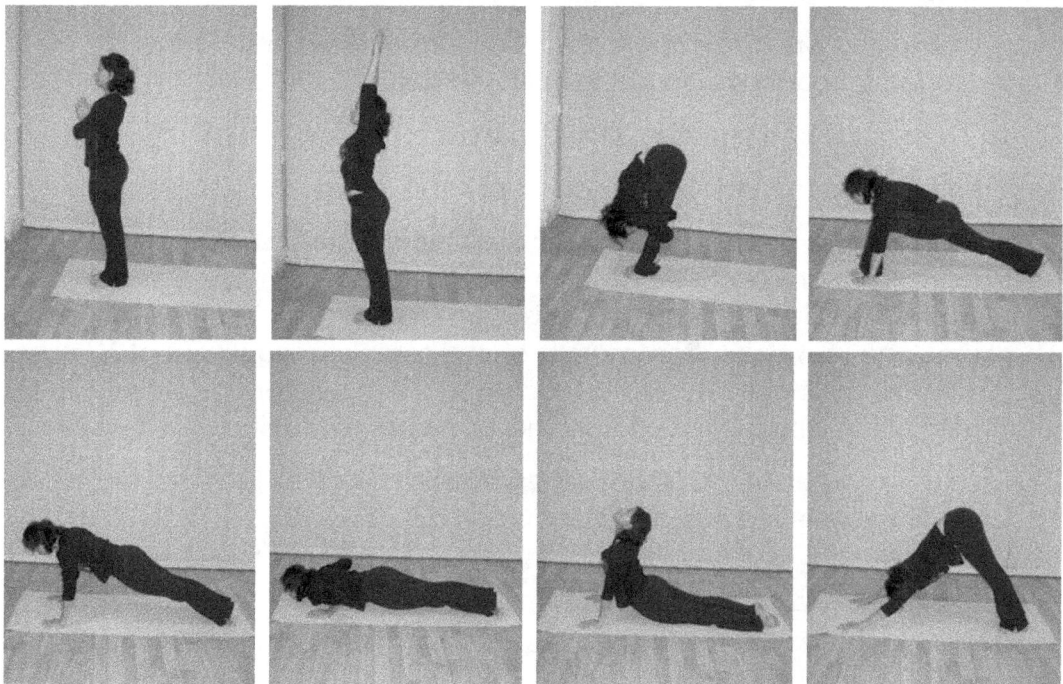

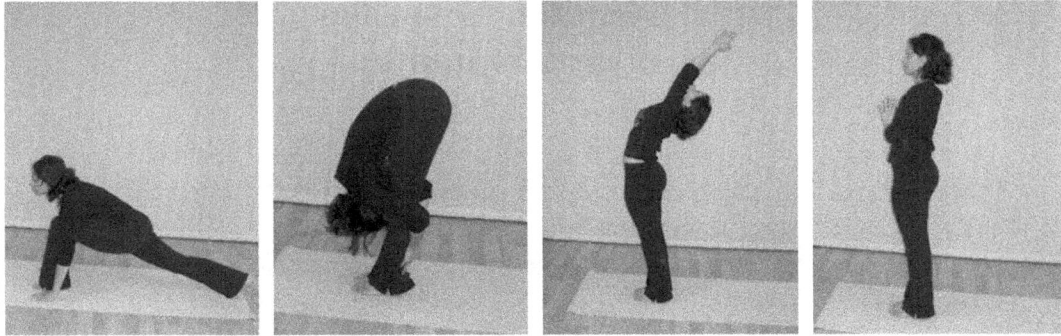

Pose 11: Om Arkaaya Namaha—inhale and stretch your arms upward just like in pose 2—Hasta Utthanasan.

Pose 12: Om Bhaskaraya Namaha—exhale and bring your arms downward into Namaste position just like in pose 1—Prarthanasan.

Repeat the same sequence using your left leg first.

Although the text describing the postures may seem tedious, they are not difficult to practice, especially when you begin to feel totally rejuvenated throughout the day.

Focus—On breathing.

Breathing Pattern—Slow and steady or ujjayi breathing.

Physical Benefits—Apart from balancing and stimulating all the chakras, it improves the endocrine, circulatory, respiratory and digestive systems. Its influence on the pineal gland and hypothalamus helps to prevent calcification and pineal degeneration. This removes carbon dioxide and impure/stale air from the lungs and replaces them with fresh oxygen. By supplying fresh oxygenated blood to the brain, it increases vitality and mental clarity.

Psychological Benefits—Its daily practice increases awareness through solar revitalisation. It brings the necessary heat/warmth to energise all the chakras.

Contraindications—People suffering from acute back problems, high blood pressure, coronary artery diseases, stroke, hernia or tuberculosis.

Value Addition—A group discussion on solar energy and the solar calendar.

Thought for the Day

Ideally one should perform 12 sun salutations at a time because the Sun God has 12 names and the number 12 is significant as it symbolises 12 zodiac signs whereas you will notice in the moon salutations that there are 14 steps as they symbolise 14 phases of the moon.

155

Chandra Namaskar
(Moon Salutation)

The moon has no light of its own but reflects the light of the sun, so the practice of the Moon Salutation too reflects that of the Sun Salutation. The sequence is the same as that of the Sun Salutation except that the Sun Salutation has 12 steps which represent 12 months or the zodiac signs whereas the Moon Salutation has 14 steps which represent 14 phases of the moon. If you notice the lunar calendar, you will know that there are 14 phases of the moon before the full moon (bright fortnight) and after the full moon (dark fortnight). The lunar energy flows within the left nostril and is called '*Chandra Nadi*' or '*Ida*'. It has cool, relaxing and creative qualities. Generally women are attracted to the full moon as the lunar energy represents feminine force.

Before performing the Moon Salutation, it is advisable to practice the Sun Salutation. The Moon Salutation can be performed in the late evening when the moon is visible. However, you may perform them in the morning or evening as a learning practice. Practising Moon Salutations on a full moon day or in the moonlight is spiritually charging and ensures a magical effect on the psyche. It develops a sense of soothing balance and brings a lot of gentleness and contentment.

One salutation consists of two complete sequences of 14 poses each—one for the right side of the body and the other for the left. The actual difference between the Sun Salutation sequence and the Moon Salutation sequence is that after the 'Lunge Pose', there is an additional pose known as the Half Moon Pose.

Hope you enjoy practising the Moon Salutation and bring calmness within.

Aim—To balance and energise all the chakras.

Time Span—Two salutes for two minutes.

Technique—There are 14 poses in this salutation. The poses in the Moon Salutation are similar to those of the Sun Salutation. The only difference is an additional pose which is the Half Moon Pose.

---

* To add a little extra flavour to the Half Moon Pose you can accentuate it by stretching sideways to the right side when the right leg is forward and then stretching sideways to the left side when the left leg is forward. This is to characterise the crescent of the moon through your body movement. Refer to the picture that follows the Moon Salutation.

The Moon Salutation is a series of 14 postures performed in a single, graceful flow. Each movement is coordinated with the breath. The sequence is almost the same except that the Sun Salutation has 12 poses denoting 12 months or the zodiac signs whereas the Moon Salutation has 14 poses symbolising the moon's 14 phases and the lunar signs known as 'Chandra Raashis'. The lunar calendar shows 14 phases before and 14 phases after the full moon known as (Shukla Paksha-bright fortnight) and (Krishna Paksha-dark fortnight) respectively.

The Moon Salutation is a complete spiritual practice in itself for it includes several postures, deep breathing, (mantra) chanting and meditation. When one's attention is focused on the sound of the mantra, it serves as a gentle form of meditation.

Pose 1: Om Kameshvarayey Namaha—stand with feet together in Namaste Pose. Inhale and exhale—Pranamaasan.

Pose 2: Om Bhagamalinayey Namha—inhale and stretch your arms upward— Hastha Utthanasan.

Pose 3: Om Nityaklinnayey Namaha—exhale, bend forward and place your palms on the floor—Paad-hastasan.

Pose 4: Om Bherundayey Namaha—inhale and exhale: Inhale, stretch your right foot/leg backward and squat on your left leg—Ashwa Sanchlanasan.

Pose 5: Om Vahnivasinyey Namaha—inhale, stretch your right hand upward and backward so that the body movement characterises the shape of the crescent moon—Ardha Chandrasana.

Pose 6: Om Vajreshvarayey Namaha—exhale, stretch your left foot/leg to join the right foot and bend forward to touch the floor—Parvatasan.

Pose 7: Om Dutyayey Namaha—inhale and exhale: Inhale, lean forward to get ready to prostrate, exhale and go into the Saashtang Namaskarasan pose. Exhale—Ashtang Namaskar.

Pose 8: Om Tvaritayey Namaha—inhale, raise your torso into the Cobra pose—Bhujangasan.

Pose 9: Om Kulasundaryey Namaha—exhale, raise your body and bend forward to touch the floor as in pose 6—Parvatasan.

Pose 10: Om Nityayey Namaha—inhale, stretch your right hand upward and backward to make your body take the shape of the crescent moon just like in Pose 5—Ardha Chandrasana.

Pose 11: Om Nilapatakinyey Namaha—inhale and stretch your right foot backward and squat on your left leg just like it pose 4—Ashwa Sanchalanasan.

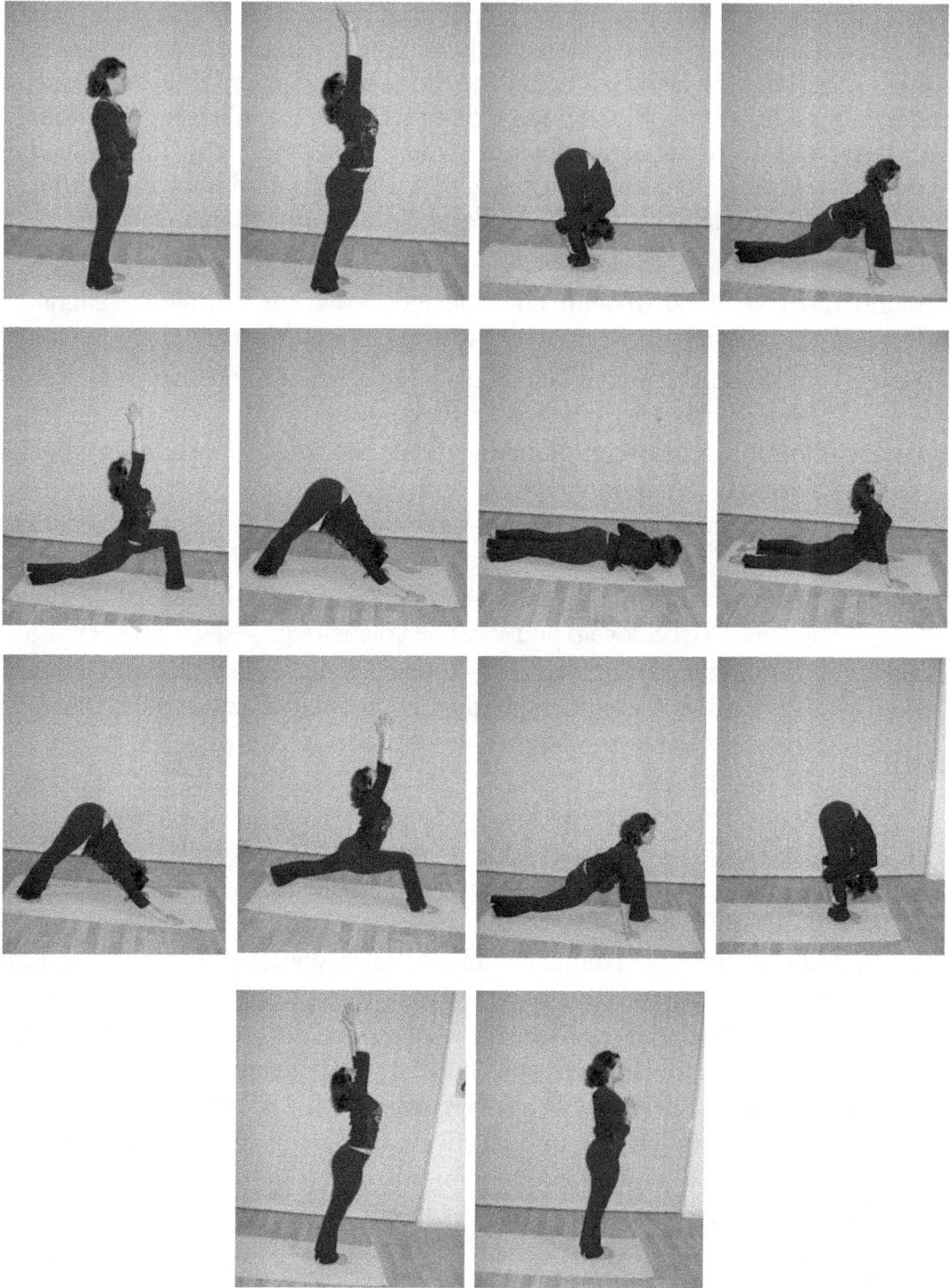

Pose 12: Om Vijayey Namaha—exhale, joining both feet, bend forward and place your palms on the floor just like it pose 3—Paad-hastasan.

Pose 13: Om Sarvamangalaye Namaha—inhale and stretch your arms upward just like in pose 2—Hastha Utthanasan.

Pose 14: Om Jvalamalinayey Namaha—exhale, bring your arms downward into the Namaste position just like in pose 1—Pranamaasan.

Focus—On breathing.

Breathing Pattern—Slow and steady.

Physical Benefits—Apart from balancing and stimulating all the chakras, it also improves the endocrine, circulatory, respiratory and digestive systems. Its influence on the pineal gland and hypothalamus helps to prevent pineal degeneration and calcification. This removes carbon dioxide and impure/stale air from the lungs replacing them with fresh oxygen. It increases mental clarity by supplying fresh oxygenated blood to the brain.

Psychological Benefits—The daily practice increases awareness through lunar revitalisation. It brings the necessary coolness and calmness in the body and mind. It also relaxes all the chakras.

Contraindications—People suffering from acute back problems high blood pressure, coronary artery diseases, stroke, hernia or tuberculosis.

Value Addition—A group discussion on lunar energy and the lunar calendar.

Thought for the Day

Ideally one should perform 14 moon salutations at a time because the number 14 symbolises 14 phases of the moon.

Additional Pose—
Half Moon Pose with Sideways Stretch

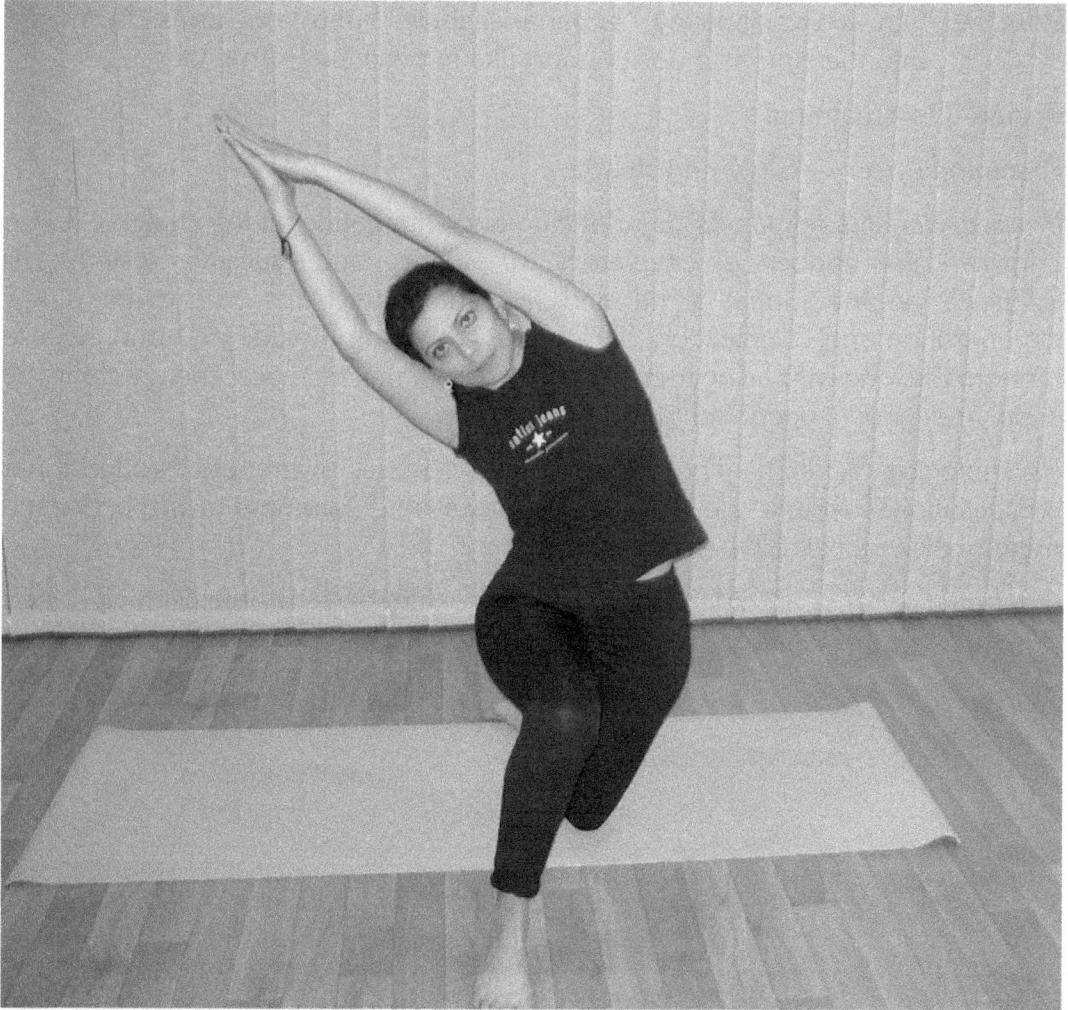

SECTION–IV

Sitting Postures

1. The Staff Posture
2. The Butterfly Posture
3. The Forehead to the Knee Posture
4. The Heron Posture
5. The Diamond Posture
6. The Warrior Posture
7. The Mountain Posture
8. The Simple Spinal Twist Posture
9. The Traditional Spine Twist Partial Posture–I
10. The Thread and the Needle Posture
11. The Seed Posture
12. The Forward Spine Stretch
13. The Divine Posture
14. The Namaste Posture
15. One Arm/Leg Stand
16. The Partial Camel Posture
17. The Spine Twist Posture–II
18. The Air Douche Posture
19. The Head to Knee Posture
20. The Cow Head Posture— Simplified
21. The Cow Head Posture–II
22. The Seated Archer Posture
23. The Dragon Posture–I, II, III, IV
24. The Wind Mill Posture
25. The Seated Triangle Posture
26. The Cross-Beam Posture
27. The Balancing Archer
28. The Backward Diamond Posture–I, II
29. The Royal Dove Posture
30. The Anchored Boat Posture—I, II and III
31. The Revolved Head to Knee Posture
32. Cradle the Baby Posture
33. The Prayer Posture— A Therapy
34. The Blossoming Lotus Posture
35. The Foetus/Child Posture as a Therapy
36. The Lotus Posture
37. The Easy Posture

1

Dandasan
(The Staff Posture)

Aim—To awaken and balance the Root (Mooladhar) Chakra.

Time Span—Two minutes.

Technique—Inhale, sit on the floor with the legs stretched straight in front and arms to the sides with palms on the floor. Exhale and make sure you straighten your arms by locking your elbows and pressing the palms on the floor which helps you to keep the back (spine) upright. Looking straight in the front, breathe four times.

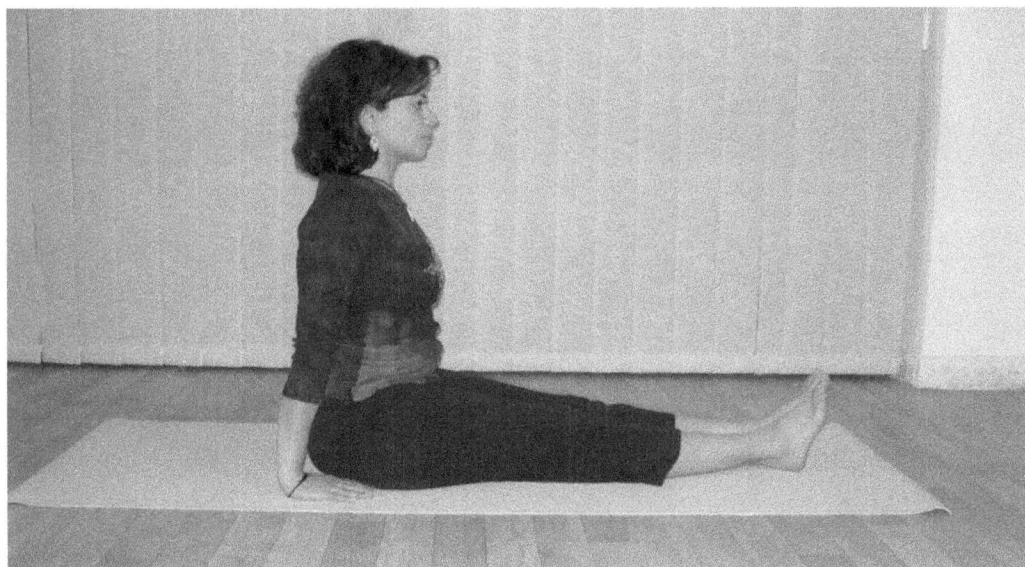

Coming Out of the Pose—Inhale and release the pressure from your arms. Exhale.

Focus—From the muscles at the perineum up to the seventh chakra—Sahasrara Chakra i.e. throughout the spine.

Breathing Pattern—Normal and steady.

Physical Benefits—Brings fresh prana energy to the spine. This relieves overall bloating sensation due to flatulence. It reduces flab around the waistline and tones the kidneys.

Psychological Benefits—Teaches you uprightness, steadiness and to have unshakable faith in yourself. It helps in breaking free from unhealthy patterns of old habits and encourages you to move toward a healthier lifestyle with a joyous future.

Contraindications—Nil.

Value Addition—Gently try foot stamping in the standing position. This is believed to open the mini, minor chakras in the feet.

Thought for the Day

When Mooladhar Chakra is healthy and balanced, we feel nurtured and experience a wholesome equation with the surroundings.

2

Bhadrasan/Baddha Konasan
(The Butterfly/Cobbler's Posture)

Aim—To awaken and work through imbalances in the second chakra called 'Swadhishthan'.

Time Span—Two to three minutes.

Technique—Sit with legs outstretched in front of you. Inhale and fold the legs bringing your feet together in such a way that both your soles and heels touch each other. Exhale, interlock your fingers and grasp your toes. Breathe normally for four times. You can move your knees up and down in a gentle movement like the flapping of butterfly wings which helps in loosening up the inner thighs.

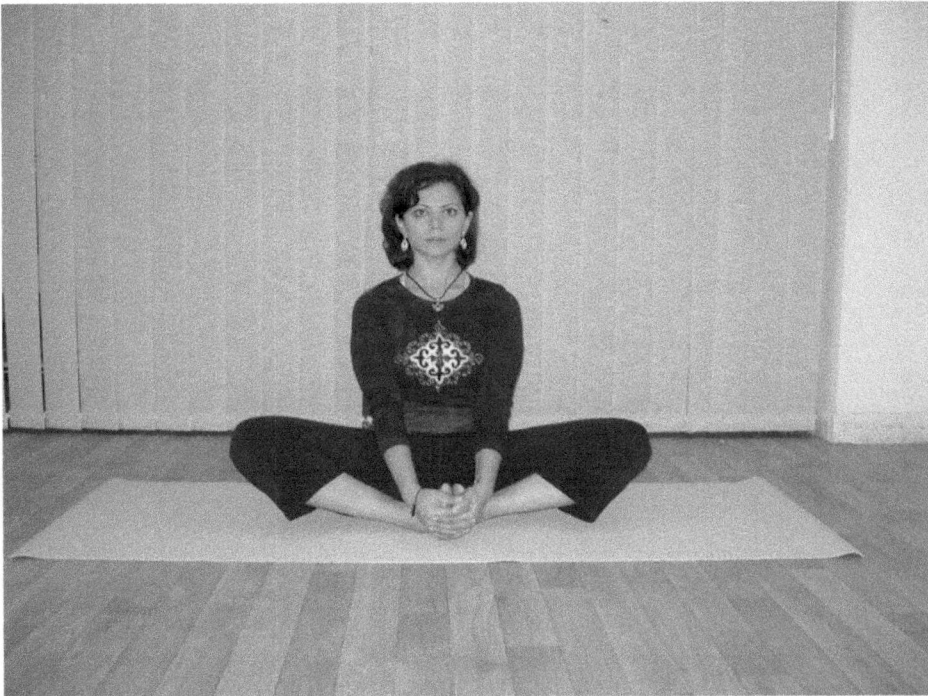

Coming Out of the Pose—Inhale and release your toes. Exhale and release the legs back to normal position.

Focus—On the second chakra: 'Swadhishthan' or The Pelvis Plexus.

Breathing Pattern—Normal.

Physical Benefits—This is an excellent pose for ladies which opens their pelvis and the hip joint. It is good for conception, improves the functioning of the kidneys, bladder and other urinary organs. This pose can be done during pregnancy for easy and natural delivery. This brings pressure on the pelvis chakra and promotes vaginal elasticity and firmness. This pose is also known as the Cobbler's Pose as in olden days, cobblers used to sit in this position to mend shoes for nearly 18 hours at a stretch without any backache.

Psychological Benefits—This teaches Patience, Tolerance and Perseverance— these virtues are required to stay in control and gain mastery over the emotions and also for working long hours without getting stressed out. This pose also promotes free, independent and original thinking.

Contraindications—Nil.

Value Addition—Set on a Nature Trail and fill your journey with passion towards a more balanced union with Nature.

Thought for the Day

Honour Divine Nature.

3

Janushirasan
(The Forehead to the Knee Posture)

Aim—To awaken and balance the third chakra—The Solar Plexus (Manipoor Chakra).

Time Span—Two to three minutes.

Technique—Sit with both legs outstretched in front of you. Focus on your right leg. Bend the left leg/knee to bring the left foot closer to the right inner thigh. Inhale and raise arms over the head. Exhale, bend forward and hold the right foot with both hands. Inhale, look forward and reach out, pausing to stretch your spine. Exhale and rest your forehead on the right knee.

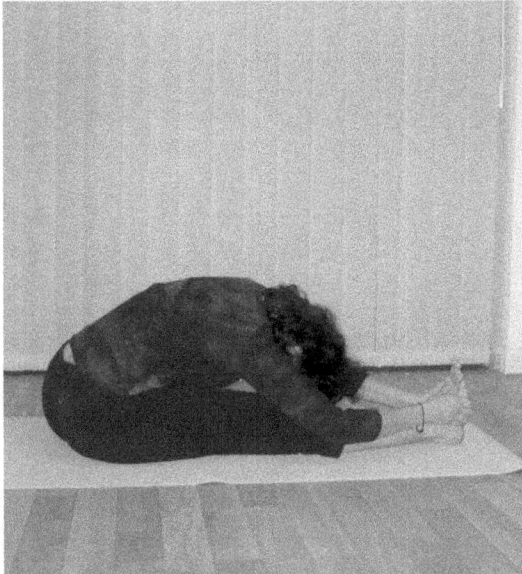

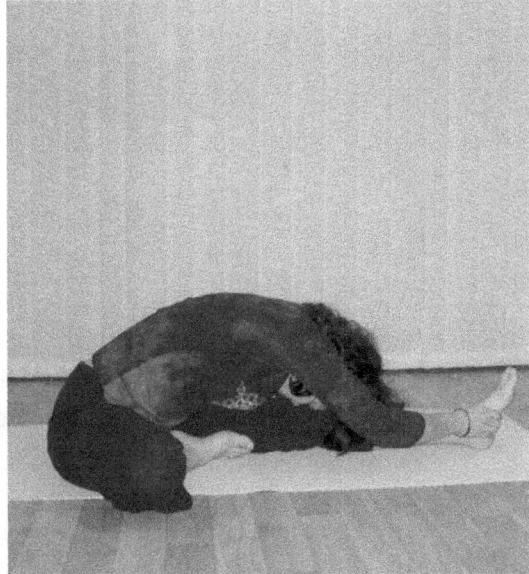

Coming Out of the Pose—Inhale, raise your forehead and look straight in the front. Exhale. Inhale and raise your arms over the head. Exhale, bring your arms back to the normal position.

Repeat the same with the left leg.

Focus—On bending forward with ease and remaining within the natural limits of your flexibility. On steady breathing and on the navel.

Breathing Pattern—Check the 'Technique'.

Physical Benefits—Energises your front and back solar plexus which is the second brain of the body. It reduces cholesterol, diabetes, arthritis, high blood pressure and alleviates many other ailments. It strengthens the kidneys, adrenal glands and the body's heating and cooling systems.

Psychological Benefits—This teaches you to trust in the future and march forward without turning back. This instils confidence and self-assurance.

Contraindications—People suffering from any spine injury, especially lower back injury, disc problems, sciatica pain, hamstring injury, sacroiliac pain or joint pain and pregnancy.

Value Addition—Check whether you have chronic fatigue or digestive problems. Move beyond what feels safe. Gently push yourself into something new. Weigh the risk in relation to your capacity and what seems appropriate. In a party get up and walk across the room to get a glass of water. If that is easy, plan to buy a house.

Thought for the Day

The power of the solar plexus is involved in self-esteem, courage and the power of transformation. When the chakra is balanced, we are able to make lasting changes, to take risks and feel a sense of inner power and self-confidence.

When the chakra is lacking in energy and balance, we have little energy, bad digestion, low self-esteem and often feel intimidated.

If this chakra is over-energetic, we become 'control freaks', competitive, stubborn and put too much emphasis on power and social status.

	Krounchasan (Modified)
4	**(The Heron Posture—**
	The Knee to the Forehead Pose)

Aim—To develop long and strong hamstrings, to give full extension to the leg muscles/joints. To rejuvenate the abdominal organs.

Time Span—Two to three minutes.

Technique—This pose is complementary to the 'Forehead to Knee pose'. Sit with legs outstretched in front of you. Inhale, bend your right leg, knee pointing upward, keeping your right foot on the floor and drawing it closer to your torso. Exhale and interlocking your fingers, grasp your right foot. Inhale and raise the right leg up with both hands, sitting upright. Exhale and bring the forehead towards the knee. Breathe four times in the same position.

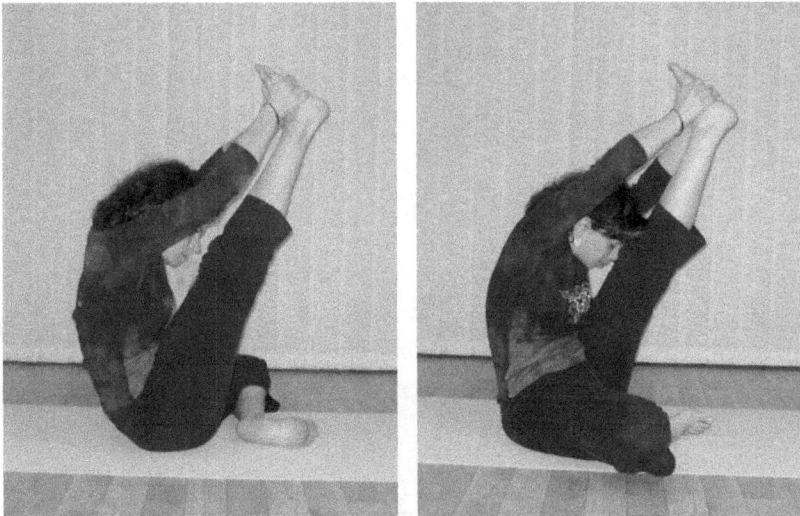

Coming Out of the Pose—Inhale and bring the forehead back to the centre in the normal position. Exhale, bend the right leg and lower it back to the normal position. Inhale, release your foot and keep your arms by your sides. Exhale and straighten your right leg back to the normal position.

Repeat the same with the left leg.

Focus—On stretching the leg upward. Most importantly, staying within the limits of natural flexibility and not over-stretching the leg.

Breathing Pattern—Inhaling on stretching and pausing when needed.

Physical Benefits—This pose relieves muscle tension, improves posture, increases the freedom of movement, reduces wear and tear on the lower back, builds hamstring strength in the lengthened position.

Energises your front and back solar plexus which is the second brain of the body. It reduces cholesterol, diabetes, arthritis, high blood pressure and many other ailments. Strengthens the kidneys, adrenal glands and the body's heating and cooling systems.

Psychological Benefits—This pose teaches you to be assertive, to trust in the future and not to fret about the past. This pose is challenging and needs concentration and in real life too this teaches you take up new challenges and improves your concentration.

Contraindications—People suffering from any spine injury, especially lower back injury, disc problems, sciatica pain, hamstring injury, sacroiliac pain or joint pain and pregnancy.

Value Addition—Review the day backward from sunset to sunrise.

Thought for the Day

Today, we have structured our lives in such a way that we don't need to be connected to Nature or to our surroundings, to each other or to our inner self anymore but life gets so much richer by being profoundly connected to this world. We can reinvent the 'Urban Almanac' to reconnect with Nature, our surroundings, each other and ourselves.

| 5 | **Vajrasan**
(The Diamond Posture) |

Aim—To stretch the ankles and quadriceps and to ease stiffness in the hips and groins.

Time Span—Two to three minutes.

Technique—Sit upright with both legs stretched in front. Inhale, bend the right leg and tucking your right foot beneath the right buttock, sit on the right heel. Exhale and similarly bend the left leg, sitting on the left heel. Keep both hands on the knees.

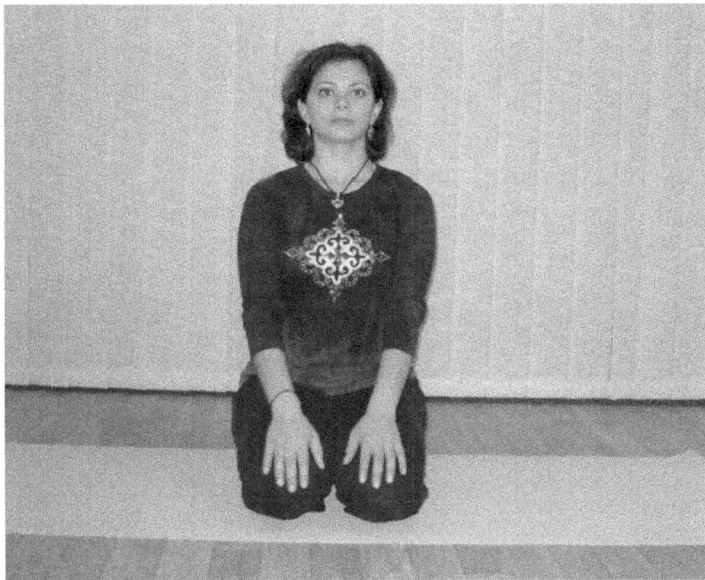

Focus—On the spine right from the Mooladhar to the Sahasrara Chakra.

Breathing Pattern—Gentle and steady.

Physical Benefits—Excellent to promote circulation in the feet and the lower body. Encourages digestion. This pose energises the basic chakra which serves as an anti-depressant to the state of mind. This pose reduces back pain by stretching and strengthening the spine. It stimulates the flow of prana/energy through the connective tissues of the spine. It also works on prostate gland disorders and activates pancreas and regulates the secretion of insulin.

171

Psychological Benefits—This teaches self-discipline. You will learn to deal with people and situations courageously and free of regrets.

This is excellent for concentration, prepares you for meditation and helps in relaxation.

Contraindications—Knee injury, sacroiliac pain, cardiac conditions.

Value Addition—Tonight before going to bed have a cup of hot chocolate or a small piece of dark chocolate.

Thought for the Day

One of the health journals claims that cocoa has anti-oxidants as it contains flavonoids which prevent the artery walls from narrowing and it also helps in Alzheimer's disease. Cocoa is good to cut down the risk of cancer and has the capacity to combat a stroke.

Veerasan
(The Warrior Posture for Auto Suggestion)

This exercise helps in relaying a direct order or a command from the conscious mind to the subconscious mind. Your mind is very receptive and super sensitive in this posture therefore the resolve gets firmly implanted in the mind and brings astounding results. While in this position, you should repeat a message that you would like to hear to fulfil your desires, dreams, ambitions or resolutions.

Aim—To become focused in life and fulfil your ambition.

Time Span—Two to three minutes.

Technique—Sit in the Staff posture (Dandasan); inhale, bend your right leg forward with your foot on the floor. Exhale, bend the left knee and sit on the raised left heel. The left knee should not touch the floor. Inhale and make fists and then keep them on each knee. Exhale and look straight ahead. Breathe four times gently and make a wish or a resolve.

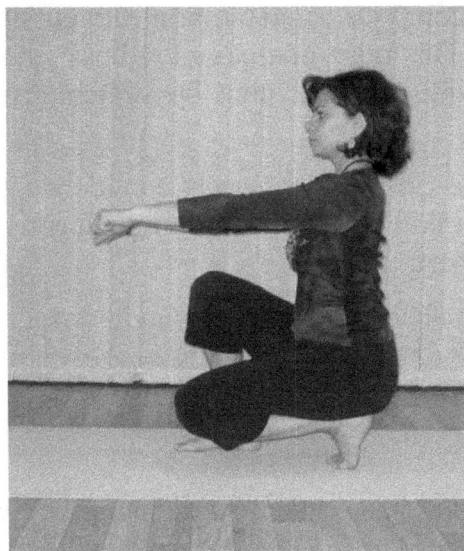

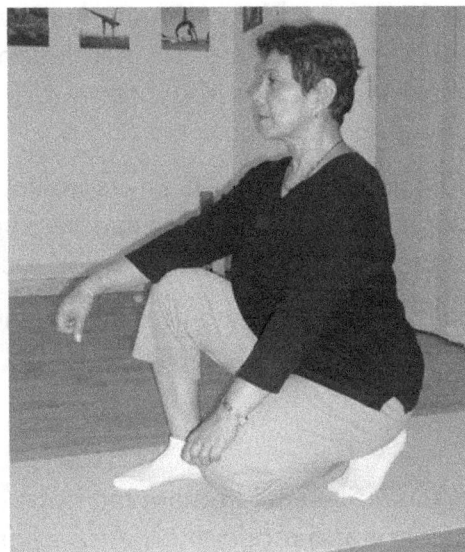

Coming Out of the Pose—Inhale and release the arms back to the normal position. Exhale and release both legs into normal position. In the Mahabharata, Lord Krishna counsels Arjuna who sits in this position and absorbs all that he hears.

Make a wish and say it clearly to yourself. Listen to your inner voice when you utter it and your wish becomes utterly clear. Verbalising mentally brings a lot of clarity to your wish serving like a subliminal message to your subconscious mind and your subconscious mind is then programmed to work towards fulfilling your wish.

Here are some very simple examples but you may alter them to suit your resolutions.

1. I will remember to breathe correctly today.
2. I will remember to eat sensibly today.
3. I will attain perfect health.
4. I will attain mental peace.
5. I will be true to myself and my conscience.
6. I will think positive and be dynamic.
7. I will be cheerful and spread happiness around me.

Focus—On the posture and on the mental resolution.

Breathing Pattern—Slow and steady.

Physical Benefits—Excellent for circulation in the feet and the lower body. It teaches balance and coordination and encourages concentration with ease and relaxation; prepares you for meditation. This pose energises the basic chakra which serves as an anti-depressant. It reduces back pain by stretching and strengthening the spine.

Psychological Benefits—It is a meditative pose which instils confidence and equanimity in you. This pose can help you find your own inner hero. It can also be used to practice Auto-Suggestion techniques.

Contraindications—Knee/foot injury, sacroilliac pain, cardiac-conditions.

Value Addition—Children are the hope of the future so communicate with them with balance and moderation, respect and sensitivity, firmness and clarity.

> **Thought for the Day**
>
> Group discussion on 'Hyperactivity stems out of an unsteady mind or boredom'.

7   Parvatasan
(The Mountain Posture—Seated)

Aim—To become sturdy and hardy like a mountain.

Time Span—Two minutes.

Technique—Sit in any cross-legged position. Ideally, it should be Padmasan or the Lotus Pose but you can sit in the Sukhasan—'the Easy Pose' or the Siddhasan—'the Adept Pose'. Inhale and raise both arms sideways over the head. Avoid bending the arms at the elbows and wrists. Exhale and join the palms. Inhale and drop the head backwards. Exhale and look at the thumbs. Breathe four times in the same position.

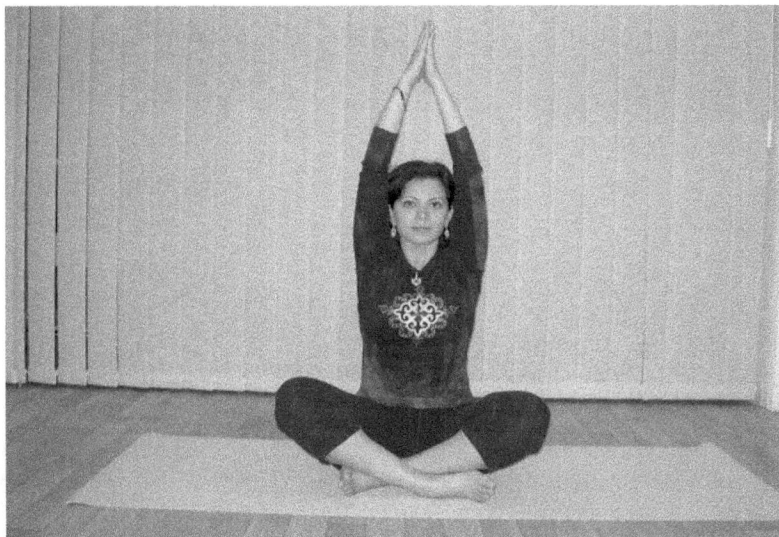

Coming Out of the Pose—Inhale and look straight ahead. Exhale and bring the arms down, back to the normal position.

Focus—On stretching the spine and arms upward.

Breathing Pattern—Slow and steady.

Physical Benefits—It stretches the spine and corrects minor defects in the body alignment. Since the chest expands fully, the breathing capacity increases making the lungs stronger. The spine and its connective tissues become supple and strong. The nervous system gets toned and digestion is improved.

Psychological Benefits—Teaches you to be hardy and sturdy like a mountain; although this pose may seem very passive, it brings about a lot of insight into thinking and helps in taking firm decisions.

Contraindications—Any neck injury.

Value Addition—Keep your elbows close to the torso/ribcage and open your palms facing your heart. Without touching your heart, fan your heart with your hands moving in quick motion. This creates vibrant energy for a more effective level of mental clarity and contentment.

Thought for the Day

There are many indiscretions you are unable to forget; there is aggression or resentment towards you or humiliation and injustice at every step. This situation may have drained your confidence but you will realise that somewhere deep inside your resolve to retaliate or attack may have strengthened. This is a basic survival instinct.

Meru Vakarasan
(The Simple Spinal Twist—
without crossing the leg over)

Aim—To equalise and balance the energy between each side of the ribcage.

Time Span—Four minutes.

Technique—Inhale and stretch the legs in front of you. Exhale, fold the right leg/knee and place the right foot close to the left knee. Simultaneously, place your right palm on the floor at the back. Inhale and stretch the left arm upward. Exhale and grab the right ankle with the left hand. Inhale and steady your gaze in the front. Exhale and twist the torso to the right side, looking over the right shoulder. Breathe four times in the same position.

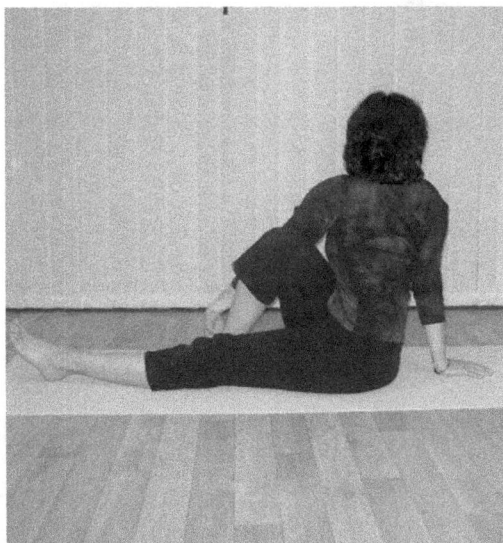

Coming Out of the Pose—Inhale and look straight in the front. Exhale and release your left hand bringing it to the normal position. Inhale and bring your right hand back to the normal position. Exhale and stretch your right leg back to the normal position.

Repeat the same using the other side.

Focus—On steady breathing and twisting the spine.

Breathing Pattern—Same as the 'Technique'.

Physical Benefits—Stretches the spine, loosens the vertebrae and tones the nerves. It alleviates backache, neck pain, lumbago, sciatica. It is believed that we have two sides of the ribcage and at times excess energy may build up in any one side. With this posture, the energy gets evenly distributed.

Psychological Benefits—This teaches re-adjustment in thinking. This makes you more sensitive, more conscious, more aware of your body and mind, your feelings, emotions and your very nature. As sensitivity increases, you can savour each individual moment and taste the unique flavour of each experience or situation. You are prepared to handle life's endless dilemmas elegantly, without feeling overwhelmed or fearful. This allows you to forget certain painful memories and look into the past fearlessly.

Contraindications—People with a severe back condition, stomach ulcers, hernia.

Value Addition—Check whether there are any friendships you may have neglected. Do not wait till they cross their expiry dates.

Thought for the Day
Some friendships are like a flower. You need to tend to it to make it flourish.

9 | Ardha Matsyendrasan–I (The Traditional Spine Twist Partial Posture–I)

Aim—To make your spine flexible.

Time Span—Four minutes.

Technique—Stretch your legs in front. Inhale and cross your right leg over the left leg, placing your right foot close to the left knee. Exhale and place the right palm at the back, close to your right hip. Inhale and raise your left arm over the head. Exhale and bring it down across the right knee and hold the outer side of the right foot/ankle. Inhale and look straight ahead. Exhale and turn the head looking over your right shoulder. Breathe four times in the same position.

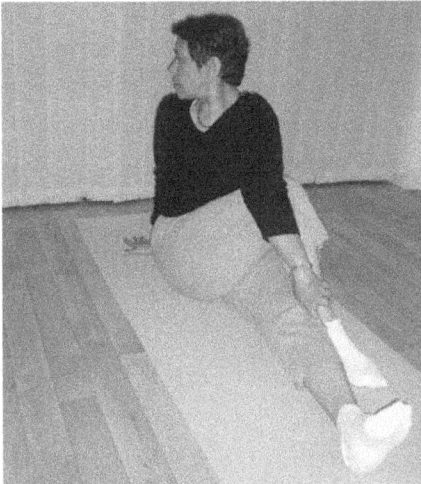

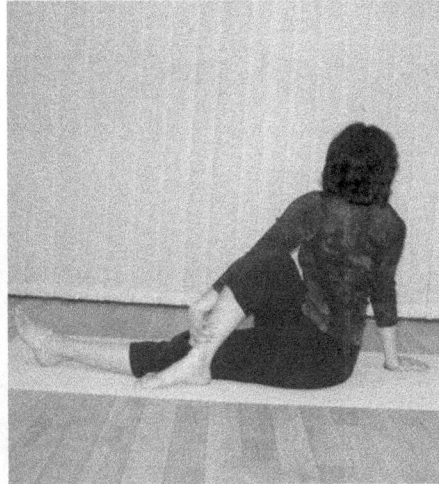

Coming Out of the Pose—Inhale and look straight. Exhale and bring the left hand back to the normal position. Inhale and bring the right hand back to the normal position. Exhale and stretch the right leg back to the normal position. Repeat the same with the left side, using the left leg.

Focus—On steady breathing and twisting the spine.

Breathing Pattern—Ujjayi breathing.

Physical Benefits—Relieves stiffness in the back and hip-joint, strengthens the neck, opens the chest and shoulders. It revitalises the abdominal/vital organs and helps ease bladder, ovarian and uterine problems.

Psychological Benefits—Makes your thinking flexible and brings about a change for the better in your perception and perspective. It also balances the chakra energy by transfering excess energy from one side to the other side of the chakra. Releases tension from the inter-vertebral muscles and keeps the spine healthy and elastic.

Contraindications—Knee or hip injury or inflammation, back or shoulder injury or bursitis.

Value Addition—Today you are going to take things less seriously than usual.

Thought for the Day

Discipline your mind to focus on the positive and avoid seeing everything from the most troubling perspective.

---

10 Suchi-Randhrasan
(The Thread and the Needle Posture)

Aim—To bring ease in the body and peace in the mind spontaneously.

Time Span—Two to three minutes.

Technique—Inhale and kneel down on all fours. Keeping the hands on the floor in front of you, exhale and twisting your torso to the left side, slide your right hand through between your left hand and left knee as if you are threading the needle. Inhale and stretch it as far it goes. Exhale and rest your head and right shoulder on the floor and gently place the left hand on the right hand, with palms together. Look at your hands on the left side and breathe four times.

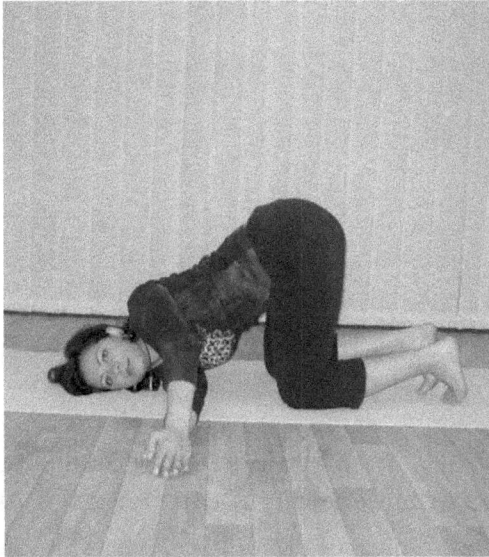

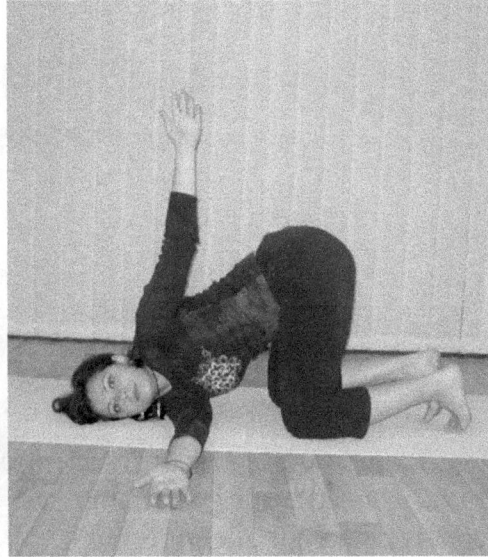

Coming Out of the Pose—Inhale and release your left palm and place it firmly on the floor in front of you. Exhale, slowly bring out your right hand and place the palm on the floor in front of you in the starting position. Inhale and pushing downward with your palms, raise your body. Exhale and come back on all fours.

Repeat with the left hand.

Focus—On easy breathing and resting each side comfortably on the floor.

Breathing Pattern—Normal and easy.

Physical Benefits—This relaxes the whole body and like magic, the tiredness dissolves instantly. This is an excellent pose for loosening up the muscles.

Psychological Benefits—This brings instant relaxation to the body and mind and it brings you into a lighter, easy-going mood.

Contraindications—Nil.

Value Addition—Yoga keeps you physically, mentally and emotionally pure and you can find out how purity can be analysed. Purity can be tested only when it is pitted against impurity.

Thought for the Day

Happiness keeps you sweet
Trials keep you strong
Sorrows keep you human
Failures keep you humble
Success keeps you glowing
But God keeps you going.

11	**Beej Asan**
	(The Seed Posture)

Aim—To maintain the body's equilibrium and to create physical awareness.

Time Span—Two to three minutes.

Technique—Sit on the floor in any comfortable pose, preferably the Easy Pose. Stretch and extend your arms forward by placing your palms on the floor. Breathe gently. Gradually check whether the floor is cold or hot to your palms. Increase the pressure on your hands to perceive the sensation in your palms. Revel in each sensation from the fingertips through the entire palm. You will either draw energy from the floor or drain excessive energy into the floor. If your palms feel colder than the floor, you will draw energy from the floor. If your palms feel warmer than the floor, then you will drain your excess energy into the floor. Breathe normally with your eyes closed. Once you settle down in this pose, offer your respects to Mother Earth—Inhale and slide your arms forward. Exhale and rest your forehead on the floor. This is an intense pose therefore perform it only if possible.

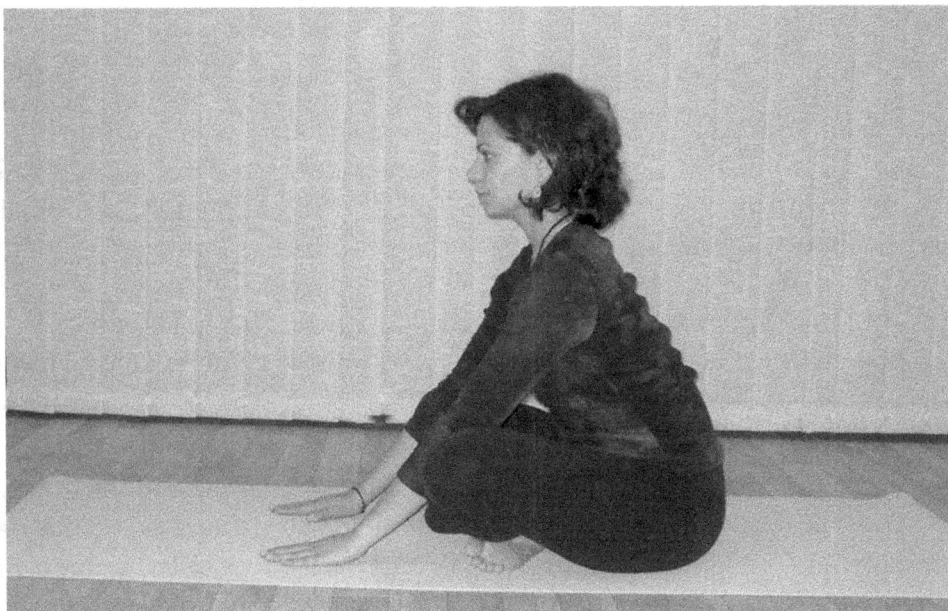

Focus—On reveling in each sensation from the fingertips through the entire palms.

Breathing Pattern—Gentle and steady.

Physical Benefits—If your energy level is too high, the excess energy is released into the floor. If your energy level is too low, your palms will draw the adequate amount of energy from the floor to maintain the body's equilibrium.

Psychological Benefits—When the physical balance is maintained, the mental and emotional equilibrium is easy to come by.

Contraindications—Nil.

Value Addition—Today's yoga homework is associated with Mother Earth—Gardening. First think of all the natural resources and know that they will be used up by man and soon will be wiped off and the earth rendered unfit to sustain life. These natural resources or energies can be used only once but there is one divine entity on this earth which can be used again and again which is in the form of Plant Energy. Plant some herbs like basil (Tulsi), Thyme or Fennel and see how it grows and re-grows. Its perennial potency can be utilised forever.

Thought for the Day

Let's become the trustees of Mother Earth and always remember that this earth is neither yours nor mine. It is a heritage to be passed on to the next generation and generations after that. Let us not be egoistic, greedy and money-minded, fame-crazy and power–hungry and needlessly consume everything possible.

12

Paschimottanasan
(The Forward Spine Stretch)

Aim—To bring flexibility to the upper and lower body.

Time Span—Two to three minutes.

Technique—Sit on the floor with legs outstretched in front, keeping your feet together. Inhale and stretch the arms overhead. Exhale and bend forward from the hips, reaching out towards the feet. Hook the big toes with the index and middle fingers and thumbs and rest the head on the knees. If you find this easy, try to rest your elbows on the floor. Breathe four times. If you find this hard, you can hold the ankles or calves but maintain a firm grip. Do not strain too much at any time.

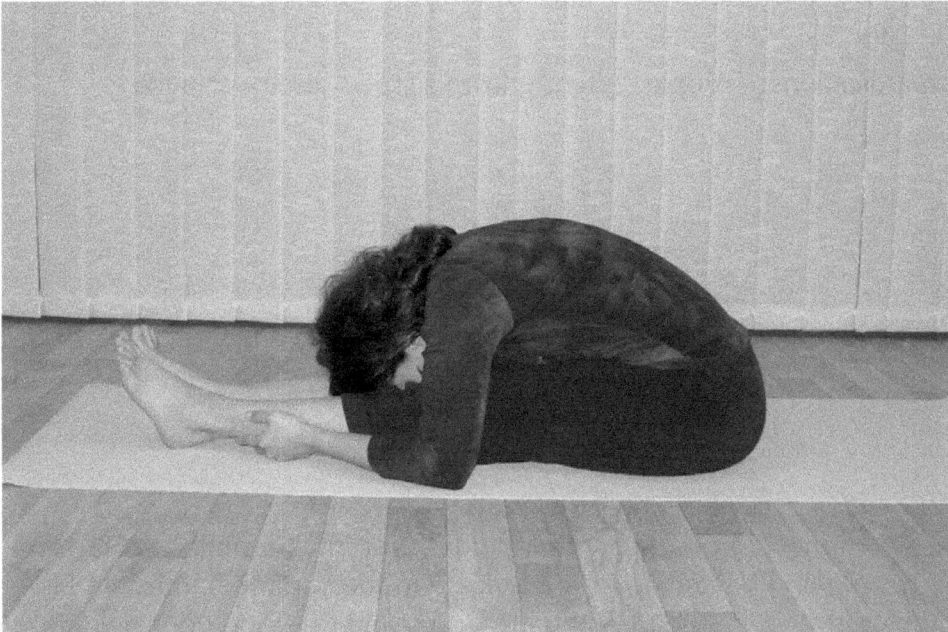

Coming Out of the Pose—Inhale and raise your head to look straight in the front. Exhale and loosen the grip from the legs. Inhale and raise your arms overhead. Exhale and bring the arms back to the normal position.

Focus—On the abdomen and stretching the back muscles without straining too much. Staying well within the natural limits of your flexibility and slowing down on the breathing.

Breathing Pattern—Check the 'Technique'.

Physical Benefits—This pose stretches the spine in the upper part of the body and the hamstrings in the lower part of the body. This also increases the flexibility of the hip joint. It provides a strong stimulus to the bladder meridian and to all the urinary structures and rectifies any complaints or complications. It also massages and tones the entire abdominal region including the liver, pancreas, spleen, kidneys and adrenal glands. Good for diabetes, colitis, menstrual disorders or even bronchitis.

Psychological Benefits—Teaches you to turn inward and to give way to your own second opinion or give way to others' opinions. This pose allows you to take a second opinion about yourself from others. In this pose, as you bend forward, the level of your head comes lower than the heart which promotes your heart to govern temporarily which instils an attitude of gratitude and admiration for life. Otherwise your head usually decides everything when it is above the heart level.

Contraindications—People suffering from slipped disc or sciatica.

Value Addition—Find out how many lives you have touched so far and how many people you have helped to navigate in their spiritual journey. Have you planned your own journey? When are you going to set on your own journey?

Thought for the Day

A pilot's job is to help people cross continents and reach them to their destination from one end of the world to the other but he himself is stuck in a cockpit most of the time in his life. Are you stuck in one place? Where is your spiritual destination?

13

Yog-Mudrasan
(The Divine Posture—Variation)

Aim—To massage the abdominal organs and remove impurities.

Time Span—Five minutes.

Technique—This is a tough posture. If you feel stiffness in the back, begin by stretching the spine sideways and backward to lengthen it before you bend forward. This is done through *three stretches* before you commence the actual posture.

Sit in any cross-legged position. Ideally in the Lotus Pose but The Easy Pose would be more practical.

Stretch (1)—Inhale and twist your torso to face the right side, keeping your hands straight on the floor, on either side of the right knee. Exhale, stretch your torso, reaching out on the right side and place your forehead on the right knee. Breathe four times.

Coming Out of the Pose—Inhale and raise your head and torso. Exhale, release your hands from the floor and bring your head, torso and hands back to the normal position.

Stretch (2)—Repeat the same stretch to the left side.

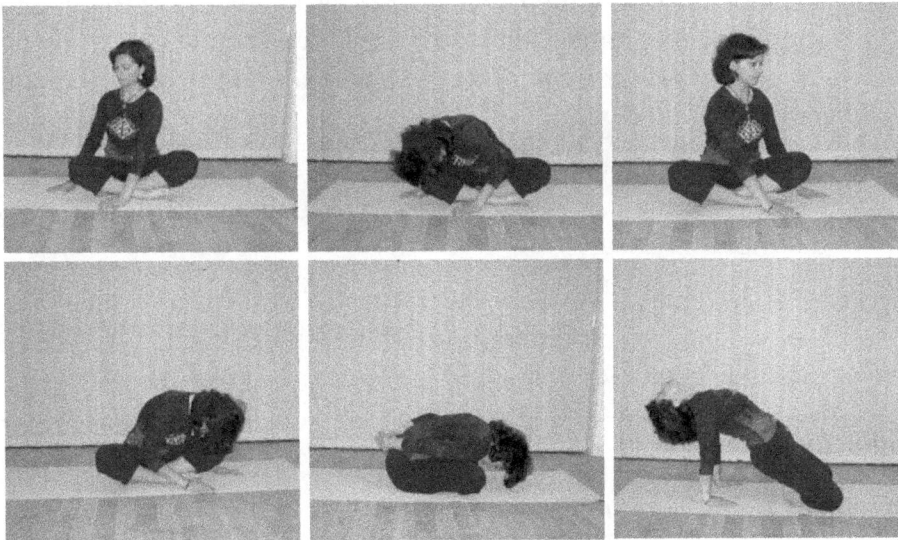

Stretch (3)—Stretch your hands behind your hips, keeping your palms on the floor with fingers pointing backward. Stretch your spine upright. Inhale and open your torso. Exhale and arch your back by pushing the floor with your palms and tilting your head backward, looking at the ceiling. Breathe four times.

Coming Out of the Pose—Inhale, look straight in the front and straighten your torso back to the normal position. Exhale and release your hands from the floor.

Yog-Mudrasan—The final posture—Inhale and stretch the arms sideways at the shoulder level. Exhale, bring your arms down and behind your back, holding the right wrist with your left hand. Inhale, open your torso by stretching your arms. Exhale, reach out in the front with your torso and rest your head on the floor. Breathe four times.

Coming Out of the Pose—Inhale and raise your head and torso back to the normal position. Exhale, release your hands and bring them back to the normal position.

Focus—On stretching the spine firmly from the tail bone and on the abdominal breathing.

Breathing Pattern—Deep breathing.

Physical Benefits—This pose works on the spine, stretching it and gently toning the spinal nerves along with the spiritual (Sushumna Nadi); improves digestion, reduces constipation, reduces menstrual problems and works on prostate gland disorders, works on the pancreas and alleviates diabetes.

Psychological Benefits—Bending on all four sides teaches you to get an overall view of the situation. This gently stimulates the flow of prana/energy through the connective tissue. *Very Important :* It helps to awaken the kundalini shakti or the latent powers within ourselves.

Contraindications—People with serious eye, heart or back conditions and those in the early post-operative or post-delivery, particularly 'C' section condition, should not attempt this pose.

Value Addition—Chalk out a plan for yourself which will make you feel young—Physically, mentally and spiritually.

Thought for the Day

Getting old is natural; Feeling old is optional.

---

14   **Aakarna Dhanurasan (Simplified)**
(The Namaste Posture with
One Leg Held in the Hand)

Aim—To balance and coordinate.

Time Span—Two to three minutes.

Technique—Sit in the cross-legged position. Inhale, lift the right leg and bring it in front of your chest by tucking both hands under the calf. Exhale and join the palms in Namaste position. Breathe four times gently.

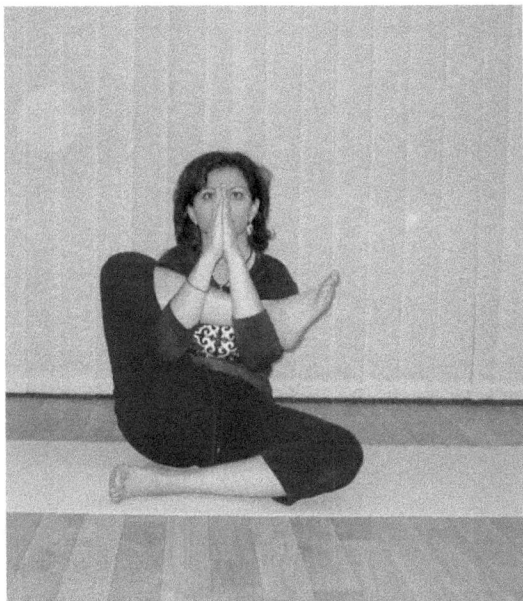

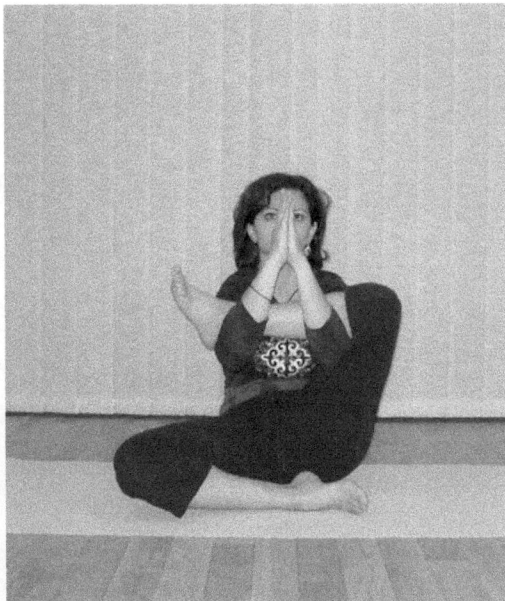

Coming Out of the Pose—Inhale and release the palms/hands. Exhale, lower your leg to the initial position and withdraw the hands. Inhale and exhale.

Repeat the same with the left leg.

Focus—On the grip of your hands and keeping your posture steady.

Breathing Pattern—Normal and steady.

Physical Benefits—Leg muscles become very flexible. The abdominal muscles are contracted which helps to move the bowels. The abdominal organs are toned. Minor defects in the hip joint are rectified.

189

Psychological Benefits—This pose prepares you for the advanced pose or the actual 'Archer's /Bow Pose' or 'Aakarn Dhanurasan'. The energy that you use to perform this pose recharges your mental batteries. Like a real archer you excel in concentration and coordination.

Contraindications—People suffering from any leg ailments should avoid this.

Value Addition—Check whether you have the freedom to make important decisions in life particularly about your own life.

Thought for the Day

If you have no freedom to make decisions, you repeat someone else's karmic goals rather than fulfil your own. In such cases, you don't progress or evolve.

15

Seated Tolasan
(One Arm/Leg Stand)

Aim—To stretch the opposite limbs to maximise the lateral pulls.

Time Span—Two to three minutes.

Technique—Drop your knees and hands on the floor and kneel down on all fours. Inhale and stretch your right leg straight at the back, parallel to your torso. Exhale and stretch your left arm in line with the right leg. Balance on your opposite limbs. Breathe four times.

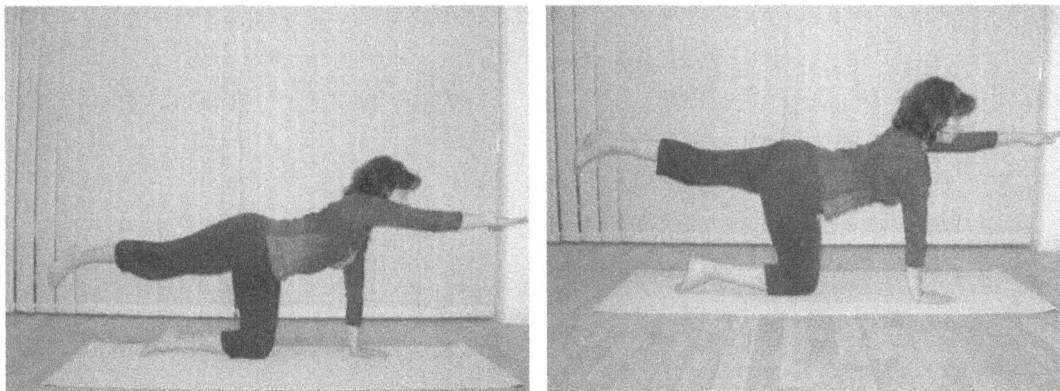

Coming Out of the Pose—Inhale and bring your right leg on the floor. Exhale and bring your left arm on the floor.

Repeat this with the left leg and the right arm.

You can do the same thing with limbs of the same side as well (right hand/right leg and then left hand/left leg).

Focus—On your breathing, stretching and balancing.

Breathing Pattern—Normal and steady.

Physical Benefits—This pose tones the spinal nerves. It relieves sciatica pain by gently stretching and relaxing the sciatic nerves. This stretches and tones abdominal muscles and several internal organs, specially, the reproductive organs. It stimulates blood circulation and promotes digestion. It reduces flab from the hips and thighs.

Psychological Benefits—Balances the brain/cerebral hemispheres and you learn to balance your emotions. Your thought process becomes coherent and your verbal presentation becomes very articulate.

Contraindications—People with weak knees or any inflammatory condition like arthritis or severe osteoporosis in the hip joint.

Value Addition—Define richness in your own words and think about how you would like to be rich.

Thought for the Day

A rich person is not the one who has the most but the one who needs the least.

16

Ardha Ushtrasan
(The Partial Camel Posture—Simplified)

Aim—To loosen up the vertebrae and its connective tissues. To stimulate the spinal nerves, relieving backache, lumbago, rounded back and drooping shoulders.

Time Span—Two to three minutes.

Technique—Sit in the Diamond Pose. Kneel with the arms by your sides, keeping the bridges of the feet flat on the floor. Inhale and stretch the right arm up over the head. Exhale, lean backward toward the left heel and reach back with your left hand to grab the left ankle or the heel. Inhale, stretch and tilt the right arm slightly backward. The head should be tilted slightly backward as well with the eyes focussed on the raised hand. Push the abdomen forward by tilting the pelvis. Hold for four breaths.

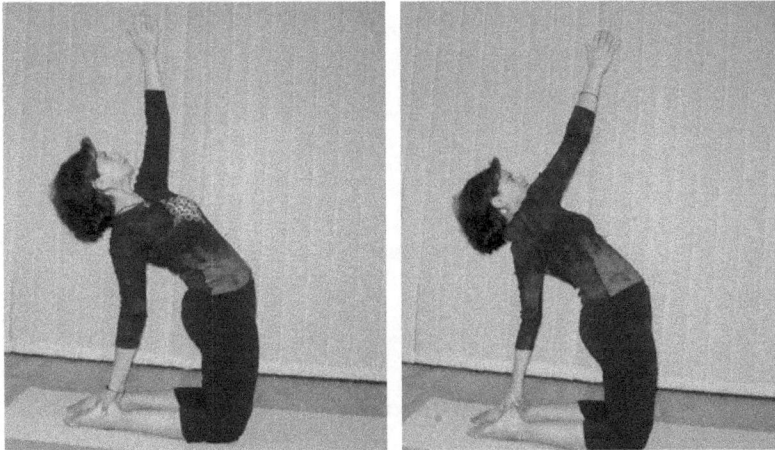

Coming Out of the Pose—Inhale and release the left hand from the left heel or ankle and bring your torso upright to the centre. Exhale and bring the right arm down back to the normal position.

Repeat the same on the other side to complete one round, holding the right heel with the right hand.

Focus—On the stretch in the back and neck and on the normal breath.

Breathing Pattern—Slow and steady.

Physical Benefits—Brings pressure on the spine, shoulders, neck, throat and chest which has a favourable effect on the several chakras. This balances, strengthens and improves the condition of ovaries, thyroid and other endocrinal glands. It strengthens the heart and lungs and cures hunch back condition. It is beneficial for the digestive and reproductive systems. It stretches the stomach and intestines alleviating constipation.

Psychological Benefits—You stop worrying about petty issues as this pose energises and balances the Throat or Vishuddhi chakra which is connected to the 'space' element and corresponds with sinus cavities. Eases constipation and eating disorders, restores your self-esteem and confidence in yourself and in others. You can overcome grief and survival crisis. You can counteract the agitated mind and overcome unrealistic views.

Contraindications—People with severe back ailments such as lumbago or those suffering from an enlarged thyroid, sciatica, high blood pressure, pelvic inflammation or any other abdominal disorder.

Value Addition—Find out whether you can detect when your closest friend lies to you.

Thought for the Day

At a time of universal deceit, telling the truth becomes a revolutionary act.

---

17   Ardha Matsyendrasan–II
(The Spine Twist Posture–II)

Aim—To twist the torso to equalise the energy from both sides of the body.

Time Span—Two to three minutes.

Technique—Stretch your legs in front. Keeping the left leg straight in front of you, inhale, bend and cross your right leg over the left leg, placing the right foot on the floor in front of the left knee. Exhale and place your right hand on the floor at the back, close to your right buttock and sit upright on your left buttock. Inhale and stretch your left arm upward over the head. Exhale, bring the left arm down, across your right knee and hold the outside of your right foot or ankle so that the right knee is close to your left armpit. Inhale and stretch the spine and sit upright. Exhale and twist the torso and head and look over your right shoulder. Keep the right hand on the floor for support. Breathe four times.

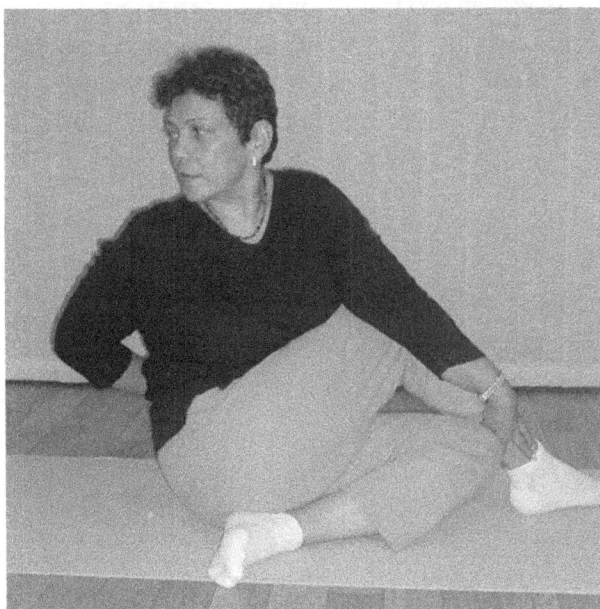

Coming Out of the Pose—Inhale, bring your torso and head to the front looking straight ahead. Exhale and release your left hand. Inhale and release your right hand and bring it back to the normal position. Exhale and stretch your right leg back to the normal position.

Repeat the same with the other side.

Focus—On keeping the spine upright; on the twist of the torso and the movement of the diaphragm while breathing.

Breathing Pattern—Breathe deeply but slowly without any strain in the final position. You can try ujjayi breathing.

Physical Benefits—It makes your spine flexible thus making your thinking flexible. Releases tension in the inter-vertebral muscles, keeps the spine healthy and elastic, relieves backache and hip-joint pain, strengthens the neck and opens the chest and shoulders. Revitalises the abdominal/vital organs, helps with bladder, ovarian and uterine problems. This also helps in diabetes, digestive and urinary disorders.

Psychological Benefits—Brings about a change for the better in your perception and perspective. It also balances the chakra energies, the excess energy being transferred from one side of the chakra to the other side. It brings about a change for the better in your perception and perspective.

Contraindications—Knee or hip injury or inflammation, back or shoulder injury, bursitis, peptic ulcers, hernia, hyper-thyroid, sciatica, slipped disc, pregnancy specially during the second and third trimester. However, when done under expert guidance, it helps alleviate many of the above ailments.

Value Addition—Equalise inhalation and exhalation gently. Soon it leads you to experience peace. Try it at home this evening.

Thought for the Day

There is no substitute for peace.

18

Utkatasan
(The Air Douche Posture)

Aim—To serve like an air douche to the groins and the pelvis plexus area.

Time Span—Two minutes.

Technique—Squat with feet flat on the floor and comfortably apart. Keeping your knees wide apart, place your elbows against the inside of the knees, gently pushing them apart. Join your palms in Namaste position. Breathe gently all throughout.

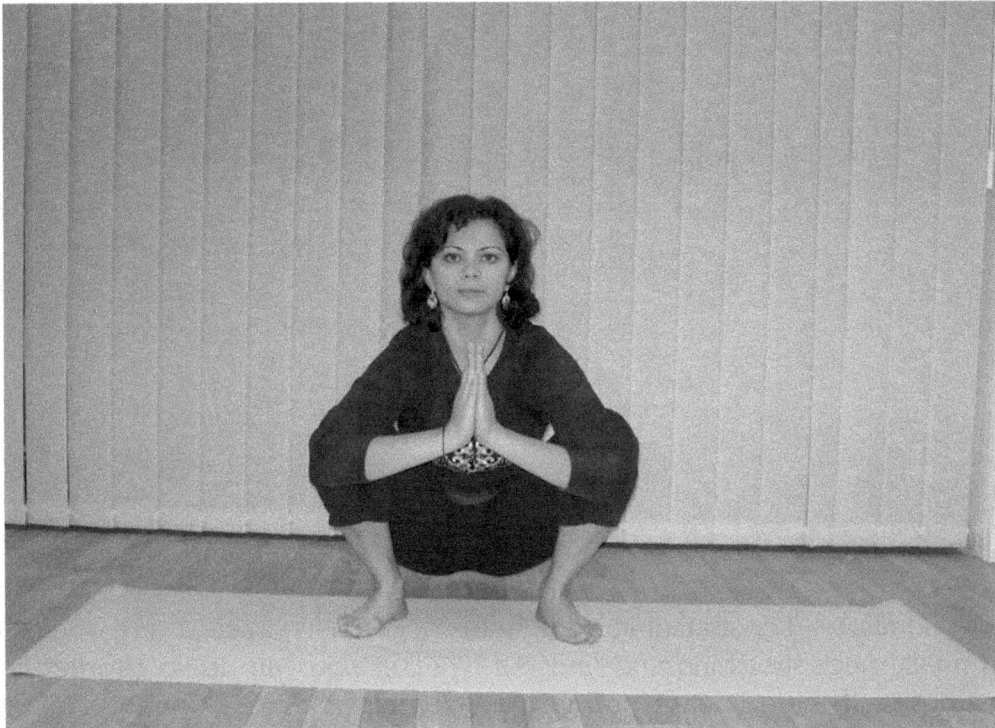

Coming Out of the Pose—Release your hands from the Namaste position and release your knees and sit in a comfortable position.

Focus—On the breath, on keeping the neck, back and torso upright, keeping the feet on the floor and stretching the knees outward with the elbows.

Breathing Pattern—Gentle and steady.

Physical Benefits—This loosens up the pelvic region and tones the pelvic muscles as it brings pressure on the Navel/Manipur chakra (solar plexus) and on the pelvis plexus (swadhishthan chakra). This, therefore, prevents colon problems, indigestion and gastric trouble, etc. If done under expert guidance, pregnant women can practice this to prepare for labour. This pose has a profound effect on the nerves and muscles of the thighs, knees, shoulders, arms and the neck.

Psychological Benefits—Promotes vitality and develops the instinct of knowing (intuition) and the presence of mind.

Contraindications—People suffering from any leg ailment.

Value Addition—Try stretching your hamstrings, then practice arm stretching and finally neck stretching and find out whether you can do so effortlessly in your poses. If there is ease you will experience pleasure. 'Yoga Chitti Vritti Nirodaha'—When there is ease while performing postures, the mind too is at rest.

Thought for the Day

Set yourself free to explore your goals. Practice yoga to innovate and experiment to find the balance in your life.

19

Maha Mudra
(The Head to Knee Posture)

Aim—To strengthen your body to overcome any diseases.

Time Span—Two to three minutes.

Technique—Sit with legs outstretched straight in front of you. Bend the left knee, keeping it flat on the floor and bring the left foot closer to the right inner thigh near the perineum. Keep the right leg stretched out straight in front of you without making any change in its angle to your body. Inhale and stretch your arms overhead, interlocking your fingers. Exhale, bring your arms down forward and cup the right foot with both hands. Lower the head and bring it closer to the torso. Tuck your chin into the notch between the collar bones. Breathe four times keeping the spine upright. Contract your abdominal muscles, diaphragm and anus.

Coming Out of the Pose—Inhale and look straight in the front. Exhale and relax the abdomen, diaphragm and anus. Inhale and release the right foot and keep the arms by your sides. Exhale and straighten your left leg.

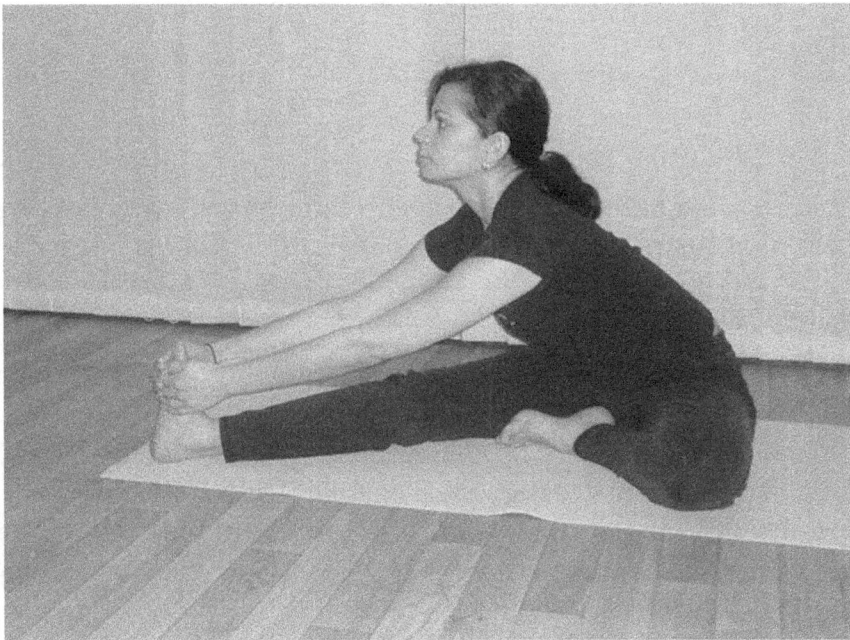

Repeat the same with the other side.

Focus—On contracting the abdominal muscles, diaphragm and anus and keeping the chin tucked into the notch between the collar bones.

Breathing Pattern—Normal and steady.

Physical Benefits—Increases blood flow in and around the spine, relieves backaches, tones the liver and spleen aiding digestion. It is believed that if you practice this pose and even if you swallow poison unwittingly, you will still be out of danger as it gets consumed and digested because of the increased power of your liver. Stretches and massages the abdominal/vital organs, invigorates the nervous system, strengthens kidneys and increases lung power.

Psychological Benefits—This creates a protective shield around you to fight any diseases. When you are physically fit, you automatically feel mentally fit and your mood is very pleasant. This leads you to emotional well-being and later spiritual awakening.

Contraindications—People suffering from hamstring, groin, kidney or shoulder injury, bursitis.

Value Addition—Introspect on the daily events through self-awareness and soon you will know that awareness or consciousness is the master key to well-being.

Thought for the Day

There are four types of illnesses: physical, mental, emotional and spiritual. Physical illness is caused by the accumulation of chemical and biological toxins. Mental illness is caused by the accumulation of mental debris in the form of negative or unnecessary thoughts or mental clutter. Emotional sickness results from the accumulation of emotional rubble which is anger, fear, greed, remorse, jealousy, hatred, lust, ego, attachments and arrogance. Spiritual sickness is due to ignorance.

20

Gomukhasan–I
(The Cow Head Posture—Simplified)

Aim—To improve bone density.

Time Span—Four to five minutes.

Technique—Stretch your legs in front. Inhale and fold your left leg by bringing the left heel under the right leg and close to the right buttock. Exhale, bend your right leg crossing the knee over the left knee and keeping the right heel close to the left buttock. Inhale and keep the feet pointing outward. Exhale and place your right hand on the right foot and left hand on the left foot. Sitting upright, breathe twice. Inhale and stretch your arms over the head in Namaste position. Maintain the position and exhale. Inhale once again. Exhale and bring your right arm downward, bending it at right angle, in front of the torso. Bring the left hand down to entwine the right hand. Breathe twice. Inhale and release the hands. Exhale, bend forward and resting the torso on the thighs, wrap your hands around the knees. Breathe four times and try to bring the weight of the upper body to bear on the lower body.

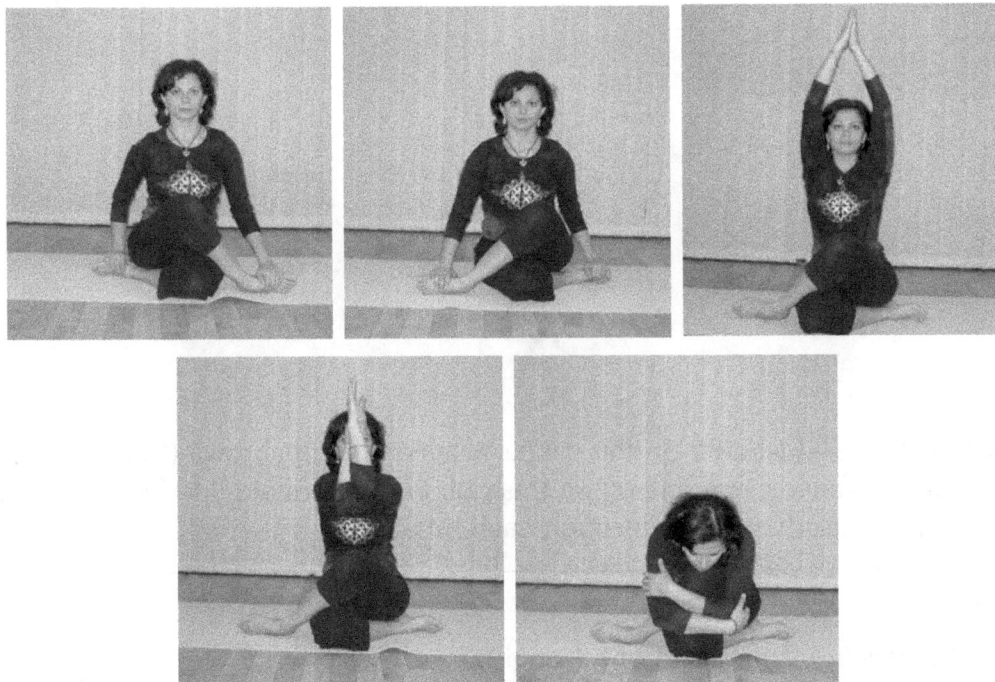

Focus—On steady breathing and different positions in the posture.

Breathing Pattern—Steady and normal.

Physical Benefits—Is extremely good for improving your bone density. It stimulates the kidneys and prevents the onset of diabetes. It relieves backache, sciatica, rheumatism and general stiffness in the upper and lower body. It loosens up the muscles in the neck and shoulders. It relieves cramps in the legs and makes the leg muscles strong and supple.

Psychological Benefits—It alleviates tiredness (physical or mental), tension and anxiety and relaxes the mind. This prepares you for the cow-head pose.

Contraindications—People suffering from any severe leg complaint.

Value Addition—Meditate on the space between the eyebrows (*Bhrumadhya*). Focus your attention and energy on this point and meditate. Meditation can be done in the present moment through each breath.

| **Thought for the Day** |
| Our body is the facsimile of our thoughts. |

21

Gomukhasan–II
(The Cow Head Posture–II)

Aim—To work as a chest opener exercise and to make the knees and legs strong and supple.

Time Span—Two to three minutes.

Technique—Stretch your legs in front. Inhale and fold your left leg by bringing the left heel under the right leg and close to the right buttock. Exhale, bend your right leg crossing the knee over the left knee and keeping the right heel close to the left buttock. Inhale and keep the feet pointing outward.

Inhale and stretch your right arm up and bring it behind your back, keeping your palm between the shoulder-blades. Exhale, stretch your left hand down and bring it behind your back to hold the right palm by interlocking your fingers. Inhale and stretch your right armpit, elbow pointing further up. Exhale and keep your base, the lower body, firmly on the ground. Breathe four times looking upward.

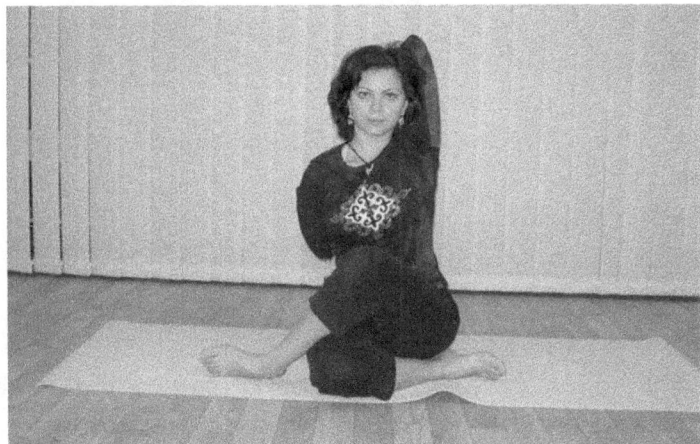

Coming Out of the Pose—Inhale and look straight ahead. Exhale and release your hands and bring them to the normal position. Inhale and release your right leg. Exhale and release your left leg. Stretch your legs in front, back to the normal position.

Repeat the same by folding the right leg first and bringing the left knee over the right.

Focus—On stretching the spine and on the heart centre (Anahata chakra).

Breathing Pattern—Normal and steady or Ujjayi.

Physical Benefits—This stretches the spine and alleviate stiffness, tiredness and tension along the spine and the upper body. It stimulates the kidneys and prevents the onset of diabetes. It relieves backache, stiffness in the neck and shoulder area and alleviates sciatica and rheumatism.

Psychological Benefits—This energises 'the back heart chakra' which fosters the capacity to love and respect yourself. It also teaches you to be sensitive to yourself and become receptive to the love and affection given to you by others. This gives you relief from tension. It also instils peace, serenity, joy, compassion, kindness, gentleness, tenderness, caring, patience and tolerance. This gives a feeling of tranquillity as the back heart chakra is energised. The front heart chakra is 'others-oriented' and the back heart chakra is 'self-oriented'. At times, when the front heart chakra is over-stimulated with loving kindness for others, there are chances of you getting carried away or going overboard. This pose helps you to regain the balance between self-interest and interest for others.

Contraindications—People suffering from any severe leg complaint.

Value Addition—Find out the real meaning of contentment and check what the difference between happiness and contentment is.

(Happiness is sensual i.e. related to our senses and as long as the stimulus lasts the happiness lasts whereas contentment is everlasting.)

Thought for the Day

Contentment (santosh) is a journey and not the final destination. Acceptance of life is being satisfied with what you are and have.

22

Veerasan (Variation)
(The Seated Archer Posture)

Aim—To acquire concentration like an archer.

Time Span—Two to three minutes.

Technique—Sit in the Diamond Pose. Inhale and stretch your right leg out in the front. Exhale and keep the left hand on the floor for support. Inhale, hold and raise the right leg with your right hand. Looking straight ahead, breathe four times and settle down in the pose.

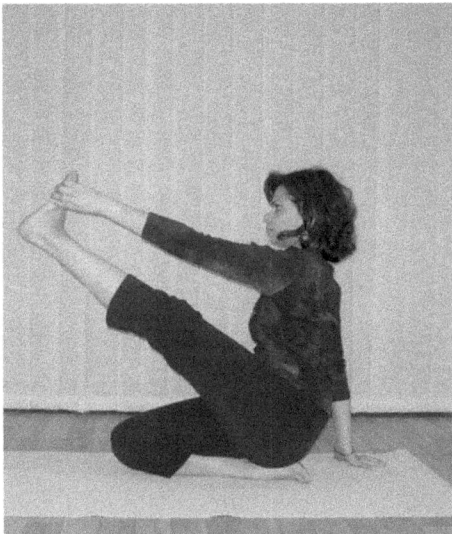

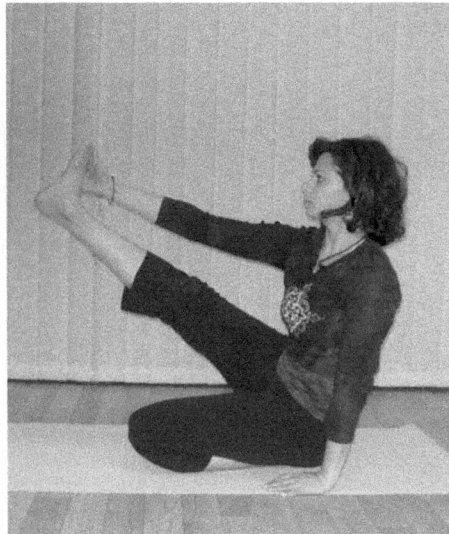

Coming Out of the Pose—Inhale and get ready to come out of the pose. Exhale and release the right leg and keep the right hand and right leg on the floor. Go into the Diamond Pose once again. Breathe gently and reverse the pose using the left side.

Focus—On your steady breathing and maintaining the balance.

Breathing Pattern—Normal and steady.

Physical Benefits—Improves concentration and coordination. It improves muscular and nervous balance. It improves blood circulation in the lower body. The hips and legs muscles are strengthened and toned. It improves eye sight with a steady gaze.

Psychological Benefits—Balances the cerebral hemispheres. Your thought process is coherent and your verbal presentation becomes very articulate.

Contraindications—Any leg or knee pain, slipped disc condition.

.

Value Addition—Celebrate the Life Force Energy through each breath.

Thought for the Day

Patanjali's two distinct yoga projects:
1. Unravelling the causes of negativity.
2. Cultivating true equanimity through self-disciplining.

23

Veerasan–I, II, III, IV
(The Dragon Posture–I, II, III, IV)

Aim—To stimulate different meridians or nadis (energy pathways).

Time Span—Two minutes.

Technique—(I) Kneel down. Step forward with your right leg, keeping the right foot on the floor and holding the right knee in between your palms. Keep your left knee on the floor. Inhale and keep your torso upright and balance. Breathe four times deeply and settle down in the position.

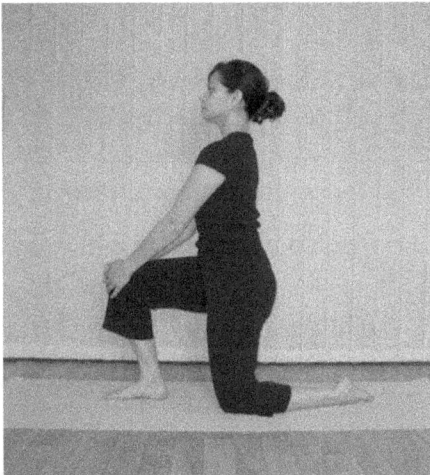

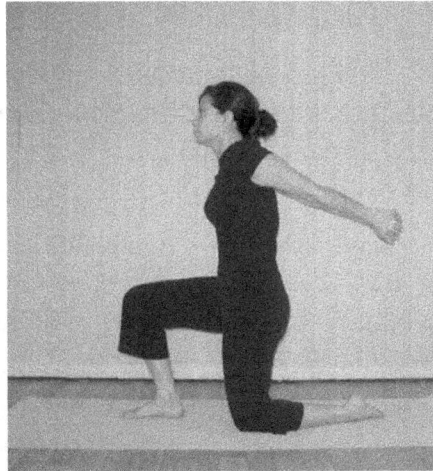

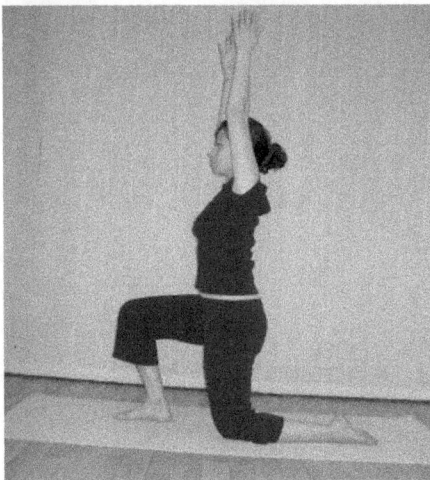

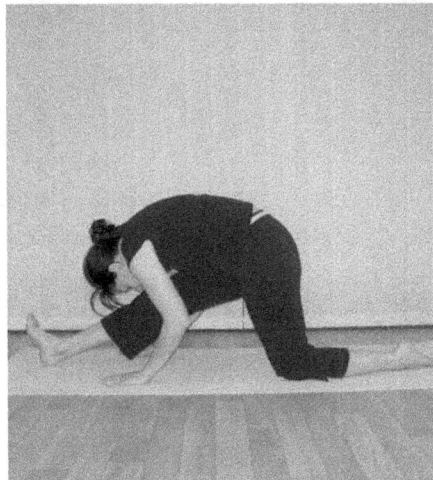

(II) Inhale and stretch your arms sideways. Exhale and bring them together at the back and interlock your fingers. Breathe four times.

(III) Inhale and raise your arms upward. Breathe four times.

(IV) From pose III, continue to pose IV. Inhale and stretch your arms further up and stretch your right leg forward. Exhale, lower your arms bringing them on either side of the right leg and bring your chin closer to your knee. Breathe four times.

Coming Out of the Pose—Inhale and release your hands from the knee. Exhale and drop your right knee on the floor and go back into the starting position. Repeat using the other side.

Focus—On breathing and balancing.

Breathing Pattern—Normal and steady.

Physical Benefits—It stimulates the stomach and spleen meridians. It also stimulates the kidney and liver meridians. It brings fresh energy into stiff knees and helps relieving backache. By stretching the connective tissue of the spine, this pose conditions you to sit longer and more comfortably in meditation.

Psychological Benefits—Teaches balance and poise and the pose II encourages you for higher aspiration and ambition. It gives you better insight in any situation. Instils confidence and makes you assertive about your goal.

Contraindications—Any knee or back problems, high blood pressure, vertigo and pregnancy.

Value Addition—Check whether you are giving your 100% while doing yoga postures, deep breathing and meditation.

Thought for the Day

Tapas in Sanskrit means Ignition. By performing yoga postures, deep breathing techniques and meditation discipline the body and mind and fuel purification.

24

Trikonasan
(The Wind Mill Posture)

Aim—To tone the muscles on the sides of the torso which are not generally used.

Time Span—Two to three minutes.

Technique—Kneel down on the floor. Inhale and stretch your arms sideways at the shoulder level. Exhale, raise your right leg to the right side, making a right angle to the body. Inhale and turn your right foot outward. Exhale and bend to the left side keeping the left palm on the floor. Inhale and stretch the right arm upward. Exhale and look up at the right thumb. Settle down and breathe four times.

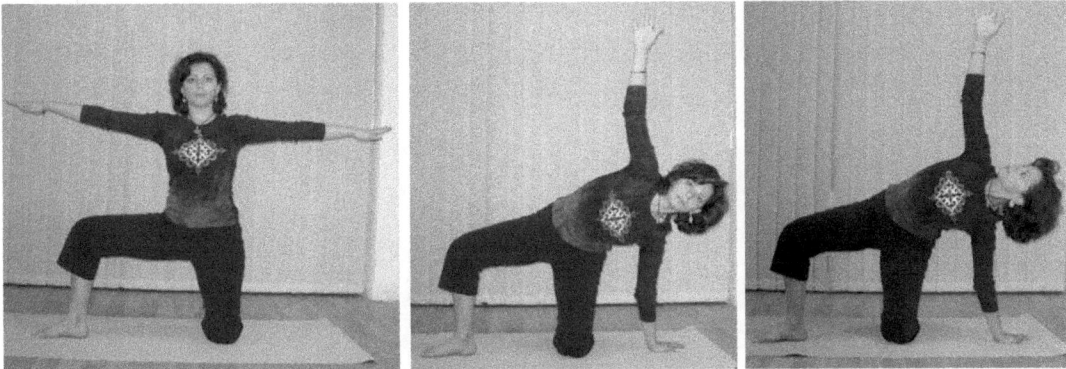

Coming Out of the Pose—Inhale and look straight ahead in the front. Exhale, bring the right arm down and the left arm up, both to the shoulder level simultaneously. Inhale, turn your right foot in and drop the right knee back to the normal position. Exhale and bring the arms down.

Repeat the same pose using the other side.

Focus—On the stretch and coordination of movement and on balancing the body steadily.

Breathing Pattern—Normal and steady.

Physical Benefits—It strengthens the muscles on the sides of the trunk, waist and the back of the legs. It stimulates the nervous system and alleviates nervous depression. It improves digestion, stabilises appetite. It alleviates constipation by activating intestinal peristalsis. It also rejuvenates the pelvic region and removes impurities, tones the reproductive organs and alleviates menstrual complaints. Regular practice helps in reducing flab around the abdomen and waist.

Psychological Benefits—Teaches you that when you take a little extra help from the resting/supporting arm symbolising the society, you can aim for superior goals and greater ambitions with regard to your group, team, community or society. This improves your PR—Public Relations.

Contraindications—Those suffering from back pain, knee joint problems or carpel tunnel syndrome.

Value Addition—Find out more about prana energy on your own.

> ### *Thought for the Day*
>
> There are five prana energies: prana, apana, vyaana, udana and samana. These are known as 'Panch Vayus'. There are also five sub-prana energies known as 'Panch Upavayus' which are Naga, Kurma, Krkara, Devadatta and Dhananjaya.

25

Trikonasan—Intense
(The Seated Triangle Posture)

Aim—To improve the sideways stretch as the knees get a good support from the floor and that makes performing the Standing Triangle pose much easier later on.

Time Span—Two to three minutes.

Technique—As in the Wind Mill Pose, drop your knees on the floor, inhale and stretch your arms sideways at the shoulder level. Exhale, raise your right leg to the right side, making a right angle to the body. Inhale and turn your right foot outward. Exhale and bend to the right side, twist your torso and head to the left and tuck your right arm below and around the right leg/knee. Inhale, stretch your left arm behind you and take it around your waist to hold your right hand. Exhale and interlock the fingers. Inhale, prop up your left shoulder and look upward which allows your hands to be snugly interlocked. Exhale and settle down in the position. Breathe four times.

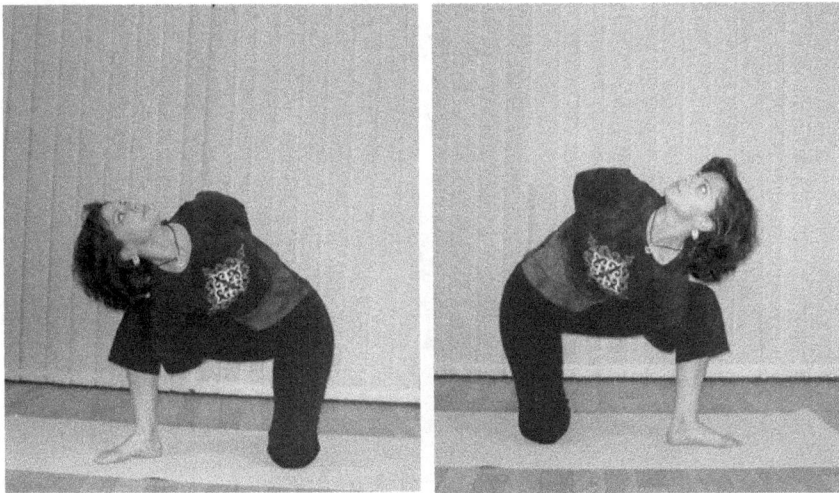

Coming Out of the Pose—Inhale and look straight in the front. Exhale and release your interlocked fingers. Inhale and release your hands and bring them back to the sides by straightening and lifting your torso and head. Exhale, bring your right knee to the front and place it on the floor beside the left knee.

Repeat the same with the left leg.

Focus—On bending and twisting sideways and lifting the shoulder upward.

Breathing Pattern—Deep and rhythmic or ujjayi.

Physical Benefits—This pose is excellent for the muscles on the sides of the trunk, the waist and the back of the legs which are not used often. It stimulates the nervous system and alleviates nervous depression. It improves digestion, activates intestinal peristalsis and alleviates constipation. Strengthens pelvic area and tones the reproductive organs. Also reduces flab from the waistline.

Psychological Benefits—This teaches balance and focus. It makes you realise the importance of Trinity and interdependence. This pose improves your public relations and inter-personal relationships. This also makes you focus correctly when you look upward at the thumb.

Contraindications—People suffering from acute back or knee conditions, neck or shoulder-joint pain, tendency to dislocate the joint and during pregnancy.

Value Addition—Through your yoga practice, from now on try to look deeper inward and trust your instincts.

Thought for the Day

ESP (Extra Sensory Perception) is not a gift for only the chosen few but available to all.

26

Parighasan
(The Cross-Beam Posture)

Aim—To stretch and strengthen the upper as well as the lower body.

Time Span—Two to three minutes.

Technique—Kneel down. Inhale and stretch the right leg sideways. Exhale and keep the right hand on the right knee. Inhale and stretch the left arm upward. Exhale, bend sideways to your right and bring the left hand close to the right foot simultaneously sliding your right hand toward the right foot. Finally, hold the right foot with both hands. Settle down in this position. Breathe four times and in ujjayi if you find the posture strenuous.

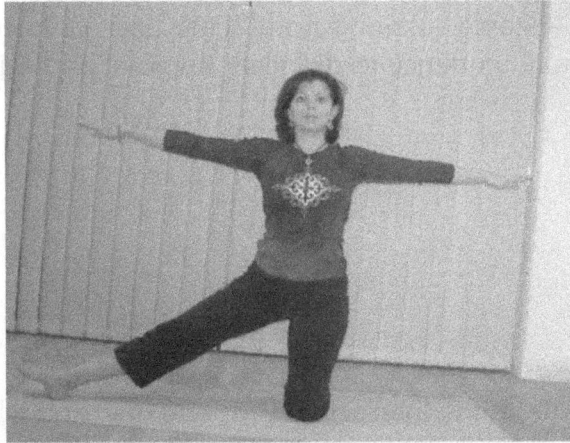

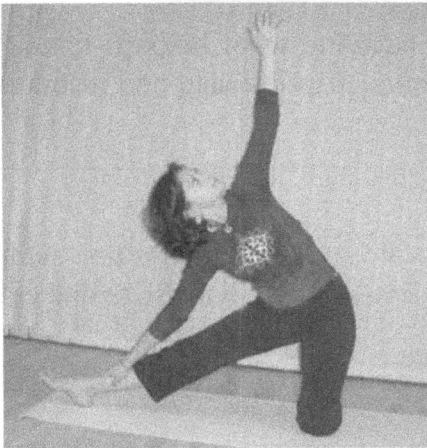

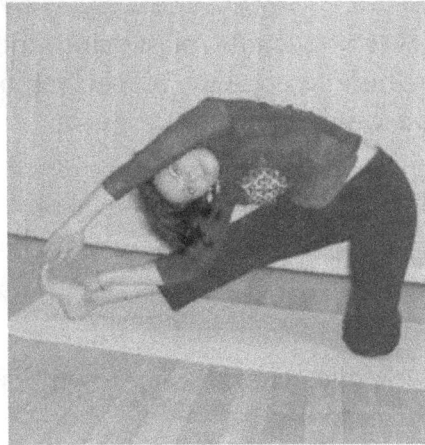

Focus—On the lateral stretch, maintaining the balance and on steady breathing.

Breathing Pattern—Deep and rhythmic or ujjayi.

Physical Benefits—This stretch tones the waist and dissolves excess flab from the waist. It strengthens the abdominal muscles and internal organs, boosts spinal flexibility and breathing capacity. It also improves respiration and thereby alleviates problems like asthma or allergies. It promotes digestion and elimination. Since the pelvic region is stretched on either side, it brings pressure and strengthens the liver in the right side and brings pressure on the spleen and rejuvenates the spleen chakra in the left side.

Psychological Benefits—All reclining poses teach parallel choices and alternative possibilities to certain halted issues. Your unresolved issues get your attention they deserve. The issues that are either stuck or unsolved can be tackled through new solutions.

Contraindications—People suffering from acute back or knee conditions, neck or shoulder-joint pain, tendency to dislocate the joint and during pregnancy.

Value Addition—What is the Intellectual Property Law and why did it come into force?

The answer is because of stealing and coveting what belongs to others. We should adhere to equality, respect for others, responsibility and resourcefulness which are the derivatives of Asteya.

Thought for the Day

The third precept of 'Yama' is 'Asteya' which not only means non-stealing by not taking or coveting what belongs to someone else but also taking credit for someone's achievements or success.

When you take what belongs to others it amounts to using their credit card for your personal use.

27

Tolasan (Variation)
(The Balancing Archer)

Aim—To feel centred and balanced.

Time Span—Two to three minutes.

Technique—Squat on the floor with or without the heels touching the floor. Inhale. Exhale, lift your right foot with the help of your hands and cross it over and place it on the left knee and balance. You can raise the left heel for better balance. Inhale. Exhale and keep the hands on the floor by your sides. Inhale and look straight in front. Exhale and settle down in the pose. Breathe four times.

Ideally you should release the hands from the floor and join them into the Namaste position. However, you can do so only if you balance well.

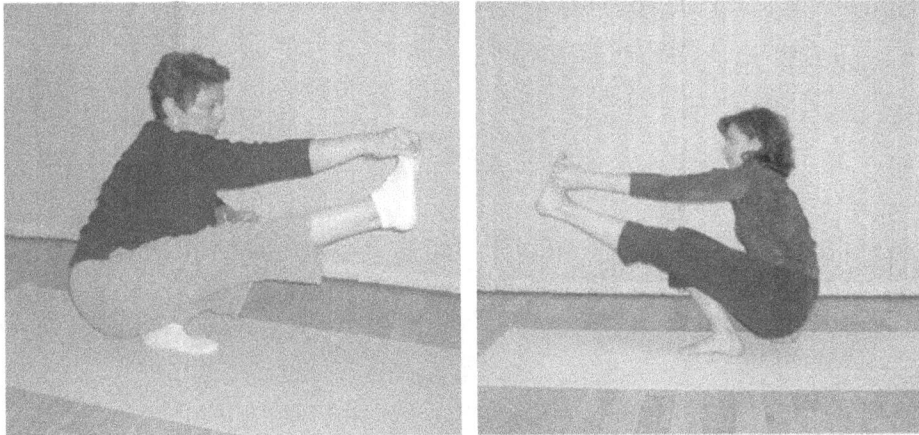

Coming Out of the Pose—Inhale and take your right leg back to the floor. Exhale and return into squatting pose. Breathe gently to bring your heart rate back to normal. Repeat the same using the other side.

Focus—On breathing and maintaining balance.

Breathing Pattern—Ujjayi.

Physical Benefits—Strengthens the abdominal muscles, the ankles, legs and the lower body. It also improves digestion and elimination. It promotes blood circulation in the lower body.

Psychological Benefits—Improves balance and concentration, coordination, mindfulness and attention span. Helps you feel centred.

Contraindications—Ankle pain, hip or spinal injury especially in the lower spine.

Value Addition—Find out what are the other derivatives of Ahimsa? The answer is—Unconditional love, affection, concern, compassion, kindness, altruism, forgiveness.

Thought for the Day

Patanjali's first precept in 'Yama' is 'Ahimsa' which means non-violence and not hurting self and others and being gentle to all living creatures. This includes not only refraining from physical violence but also from harsh words, criticism and being judgemental.

---

28 | Supta Vajrasan–I, II
(The Backward Diamond Posture–I, II)

Aim—To encourage spinal rotation.

Time Span—One or two minutes.

Technique—Inhale and sit in 'Vajrasan' or the 'Diamond Pose'. Exhale and keep your hands on the floor at the back. Inhale, lean backward and rest your elbows on the floor. Exhale and bend backward, very gently and cautiously, resting your head on the floor. Place your hands on the thighs. Arch your back as much as possible and breathe four times. For a more intense pose, rest your upper back on the floor and place your hands on the heels.

If you feel too much strain on your thighs or knees, separate your knees slightly. Breathing should be deep and slow as in Ujjayi.

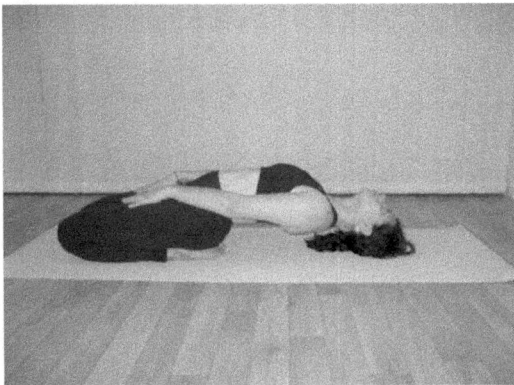

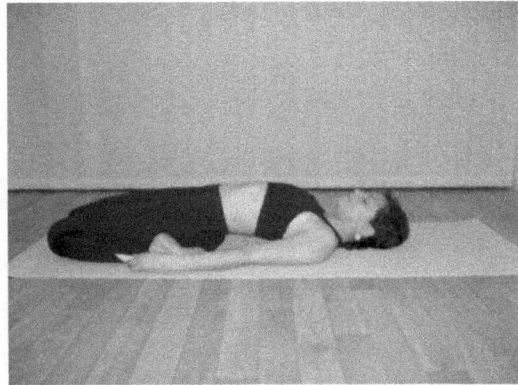

Coming Out of the Pose—Inhale and adjust your head to come out of the position. Exhale and take the support of your elbows and hands to return to the sitting position. Inhale and raise your torso and head to come back into the Diamond Pose. Exhale.

Focus—On the lower back, abdomen or breath.

Breathing Pattern—Deep and slow as in Ujjayi.

Physical Benefits—This stretches the feet, ankles, knees, thighs, sacrum and lumbar spine. It also stimulates the digestive meridians of the stomach, spleen and the gall bladder.

Psychological Benefits—The back chakras and the throat chakras are energised. This develops creativity, intuition and gut feeling from the navel or 'Manipur' chakra.

Contraindications—People suffering from sciatica, slipped disc, sacral ailments or knee complaints.

Value Addition—Find out which hymn from the Bible; which Aya from the Quran or which mantra from the Bhagvat Gita you prefer.

> ### *Thought for the Day*
>
> The man who swims against the flow knows the power of the current as well as his own strength.

29	**Ek Pad Rajkapotasan 1, 2, 3, 4, 5**
	(Royal Dove Posture as a Sequence 1, 2, 3, 4, 5)

Aim—To open the hip joint known as the 'hip opener'.

Time Span—Four minutes.

Technique—Sit in the Diamond Pose.

1. Inhale, keeping your right leg in the Diamond Pose, exhale and stretch your left leg backward so that it remains in line with your right leg.
2. Inhale and keep both your hands on the floor in front of you. Exhale.
3. Inhale and place your hands on the hips. Exhale.
4. Inhale and stretch your arms sideways. Exhale.
5. Inhale. Exhale and bend forward stretching your arms straight out on the floor in front of you. Breathe gently. Finally, exhale and rest your forehead on the floor with the torso on your right knee. Breathe four times.

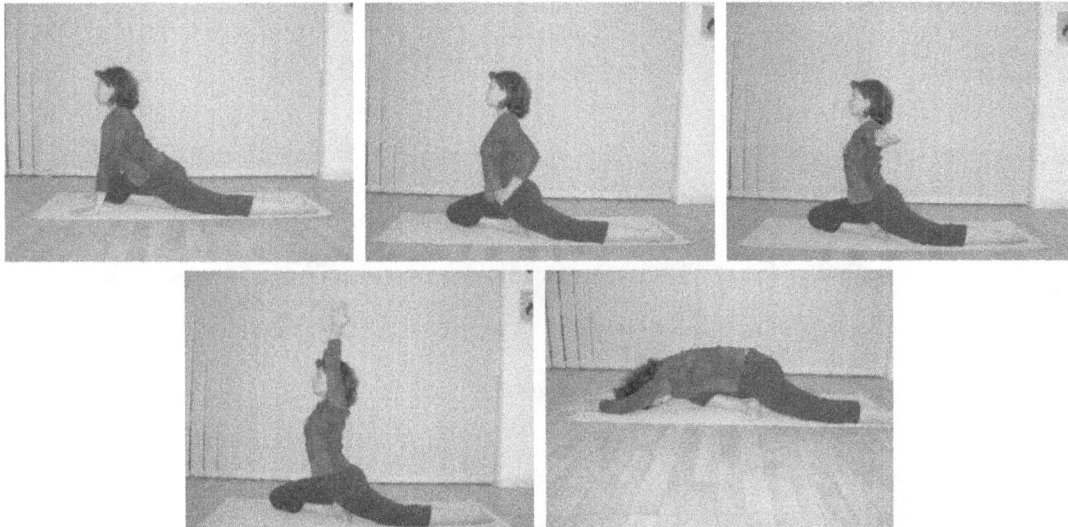

Coming Out of the Pose—Just like going into the pose, you can come out step by step or inhale, raise your head and look straight in the front. Exhale and slowly bring your hands closer to your knees. Inhale, push the floor with your hands and raise your head and torso to the sitting position. Exhale, release the hands and place them on the floor. Then go into the Diamond Pose again to repeat the same pose using the other side.

Focus—On breathing steadily and maintaining the posture.

Breathing Pattern—Slow and steady.

Physical Benefits—It rejuvenates the lower body and improves the blood circulation in the pubic region keeping the lower chakras healthy and the corresponding internal organs free of diseases. This helps in any urinary problem. It brings fresh prana energy to the thyroids, para-thyroids, adrenals and gonads, increasing overall vitality. It also regulates sexual desire (whether it is over or under).

Psychological Benefits—Brings harmony in your life and teaches adaptability. This helps you in quitting certain old and unwanted habits by making your resolution stronger. Your will power gives you strength to quit any addiction effortlessly. It also makes you think about making lifestyle changes for the better. You can overcome emotional turmoil or loneliness. This pose also gives an insight into emotional intimacy. In other words, it teaches more openness in matters of the heart. You can also enjoy sensuality or pleasures of the senses.

Contraindications—People suffering from any hip joint problem, sciatica or pregnancy.

Value Addition—Check whether you see any doves or pigeons around and whether you can feed them some grains or unpoped left-over popcorn?

Thought for the Day

Our bodies and subconscious minds carry the residues of all sorts of cruel words and criticism that we have absorbed. Expel them through deep breathing to feel rejuvenated.

30

Ardha Navasan/Naukasan
(The Anchored Boat Posture—I, II and III)

Aim—To improve attention span, balance and coordination.

Time Span—Two to three minutes.

Technique—(I) Sit with your knees bent and feet on the floor. Lean backward, resting your elbows/forearms on the floor at the back and hands near the hips. Inhale, straighten and raise your legs in line with your head to make the shape of a boat. Exhale and settle down in the pose. Breathe four times.

(II) Continue keeping your knees bent, tuck your hands under your knees. Inhale and point your toes, exhale and flex your toes.

(III) The final position is the continuation of II, but the only difference is that the hands are not used as a support. Instead, the hands are stretched out parallel to the floor, on either side of the legs.

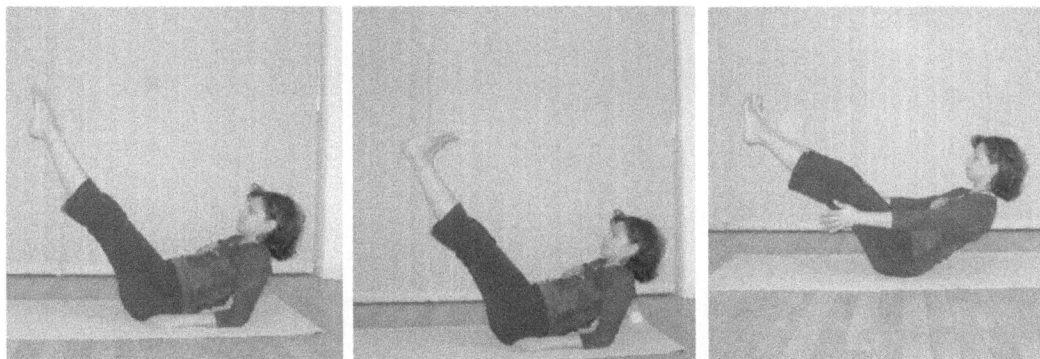

Coming Out of the Pose—Inhale and keep your hands on the floor. Exhale, bend your knees and keep your feet on the floor and sit.

Focus—Maintaining balance by focusing on a fixed point.

Breathing Pattern—Slow and deep as in Ujjayi.

The Physical Benefits—This tones abdominal organs, especially the liver and strengthens the abdominal muscles relieving fatigue in the belly and reduces the strain in the lower back by realigning the spine. This helps to remove intestinal worms and stimulates peristalsis, alleviating constipation. The first two are simplified boat poses which build the necessary strength to move into the full pose–III.

Psychological Benefits—This improves concentration and mindfulness.

Contraindications—People suffering from slipped disc, sciatica, sacral infections, high blood pressure or heart disease.

Value Addition—What are the other virtues which come in this classification?

Ans: Honesty, integrity, forthrightness, reasoning, etc., come under the same classification.

Thought for the Day

The second precept of 'Yama' is 'Satya' or Truthfulness i.e. avoiding all falsehood and fabrications. The yogic practice of truthfulness focuses on carefully and correctly choosing words when they are flowing out of our mouth so that they do the least harm and the most good to us and others.

31

Parivratta Janushirasan
(The Revolved Head to Knee Posture)

Aim—To stimulate blood circulation in the spine and along the chakras.

Time Span—Two to three minutes.

Technique—Sit with your legs stretched 3 feet apart in front of you. Inhale and fold the left leg in such a way that the left foot should touch the left inner thigh and the perineum. Exhale, bend and twist your torso sideways and hold the arch of the right, foot sliding the right hand under the right calf, with the elbow resting on the floor. Breathe gently. Inhale and raise your left arm. Exhale and hold the right foot with the left hand as well. Breathe gently and settle down in the position. You should rest the entire right side of your torso on the right leg, holding your right foot with both hands. Breathe four times.

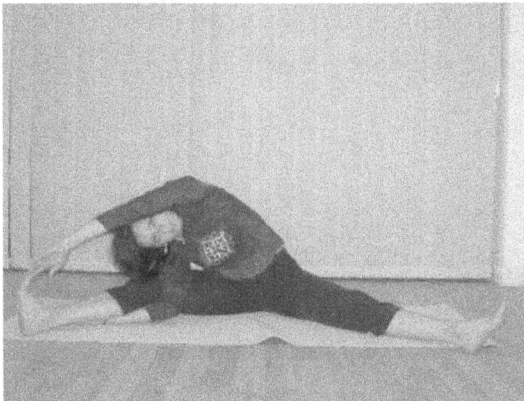

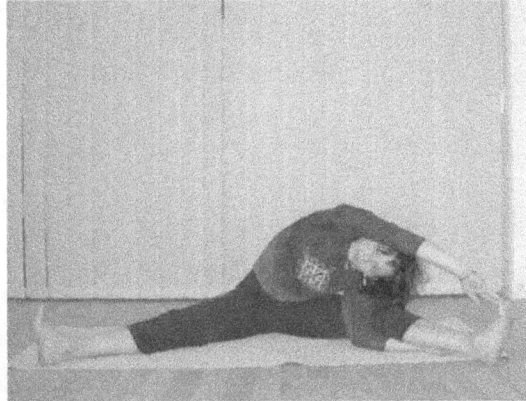

Coming Out of the Pose—Inhale and release your left and right hands from the right foot and raise your head and torso upward. Exhale and come to the normal position. Inhale and stretch your left leg. Exhale and bend the right leg.

Repeat with the left side.

Focus—On maintaining the pose especially twisting the torso fully on one side each time.

Breathing Pattern—Normal and steady; if you need extra strength, try ujjayi breathing.

Physical Benefits—Increases blood flow in and around the spine, relieves backaches, tones the liver and spleen aiding digestion. It is believed that if you practice this pose, and even if you swallow anything toxic unwittingly, you will still be out of danger as it is expelled by the enhanced, powerful capacity of your liver and kidneys. Stretches and massages the abdominal/vital organs, invigorates the nervous system, strengthens kidneys and increases lung power.

Psychological Benefits—Any sideways bending changes the outlook in life. Instead of looking at things from the point of view which you are generally familiar with, you learn to acquire a new approach which helps you understand situations in a better way. This physical twist strethes your mental rigidity and you learn to have an open mind. This also teaches you to get rid of your emotional stiffness. While twisting the torso and if you feel too stiff, it signifies that your emotions are bundled in a tight knot and you need to loosen up. By practicing this pose, you improve your willingness to reach out to more people around you in a very healthy way.

Contraindications—Hamstring, groin, kidney or shoulder injury, bursitis.

Value Addition—Find out how many helpings of your favourite food you wish to take? If the answer is two, that is fine but if it is three, then you need to follow this precept of self-control.

Thought for the Day

The fourth precept of 'Yama' is known as 'Brahamacharya'. Although it is commonly associated with celibacy it means self-control or moderation in its entirety by avoiding excesses in all respects.

32

Tri-Ang Pranam or Ek Pad Karshanasan
(Namaste with Three Limbs or Cradle the Baby Posture)

Aim—To loosen up the hip joint.

Time Span—Two to three minutes.

Technique—Sit with legs together and outstretched in front of you. Inhale, lift and bend the right leg and bring it in front of your chest by tucking both hands under the calf. Exhale and join the palms in Namaste position. Breathe four times gently and steadily.

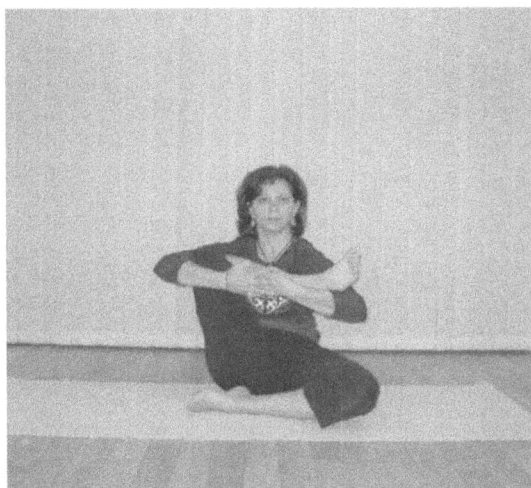

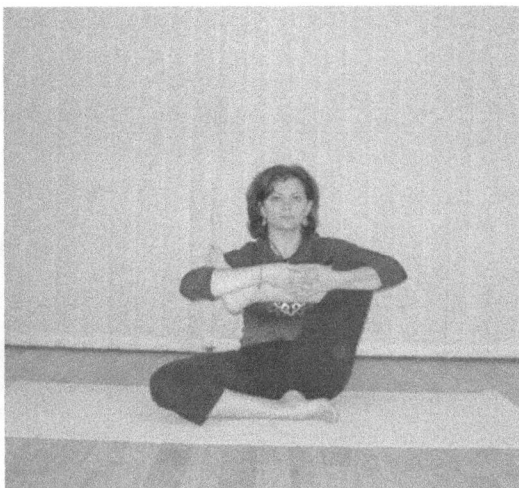

Breathing normally, release your hands from Namaste position and place your right foot snugly on the left inner arm. The right knee should rest on the right inner arm. Once again hold the hands together interlocking the fingers to form a cradle. Breathe four times.

Coming Out of the Pose—Inhale, release your fingers gently and slide your hands apart, holding the knee with your right hand and the foot with your left hand. Exhale, release your right leg down to the floor and bring it back to the normal position.

Repeat the same using the other side.

Focus—On stretching the leg and holding it.

Breathing Pattern—Ujjayi and steady.

Physical Benefits—This strengthens the hamstring muscles, arms and the shoulders and relieves tension from the back and neck. It also helps in loosening up the hip joint. It tones the abdominal organs and eases constipation. This is believed to be a useful treatment in conditions like hydrocele.

Psychological Benefits—Improves attention span, balance and coordination.

Contraindications—Those suffering from slipped disc, sciatica or dislocation of the hip joint.

Value Addition—Patience is the key to Aparigraha. Try Aparigraha once a week to know that you are able to curb your sensual urge.

Thought for the Day

The fifth precept of 'Yama' is 'Aparigraha' which means non-possessiveness by abstaining from greed, hoarding, possessing beyond one's needs or engaging in emotional or sensual over-indulgence which proves to be an empty search for pleasure.

33

Prarthanasan
(The Prayer Posture—A Therapy)

Aim—To achieve contentment, clarity of mind, concentration and compassion.

Time Span—Two to three minutes.

Technique—Sit in the Diamond Pose. Inhale and stretch the arms over the head. Exhale, bend forward and stretch the arms shoulder-width apart on the floor and rest the forehead on the floor. Breathe gently for two to three minutes.

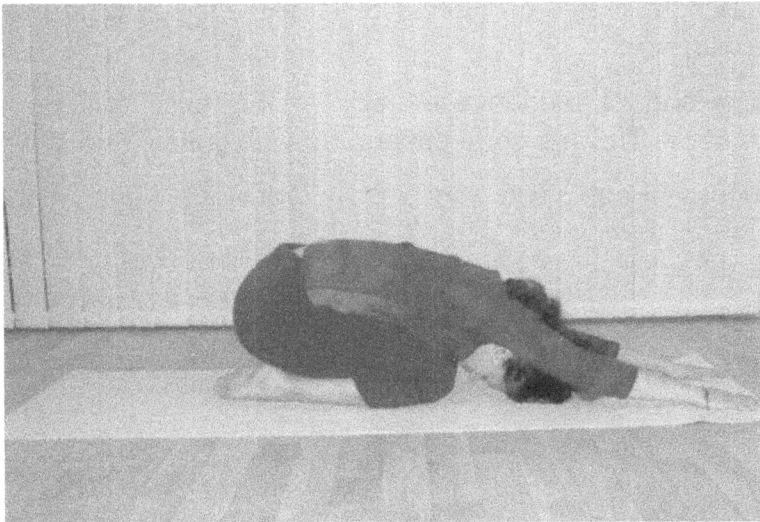

Coming Out of the Pose—Inhale and raise your head, looking straight in the front. Exhale and slide your arms back to your knees. Inhale and raise your head and torso to the sitting position. Exhale.

Focus—On the steady breath. Spiritual : on the Manipura Chakra or 'Solar Plexus', the Adnya Chakra or the 'Third Eye' Chakra and the Sahasrara Chakra or the Crown Centre.

Breathing Pattern—Gentle and steady.

Physical Benefits—This stretches the spine right from the Mooladhar Chakra, (the base chakra) up to the Sahasrara Chakra (the Crown Chakra) and tones the spinal nerves and the connective tissues of the spine. This massages the abdominal organs and removes impurities and ailments from the system.

Psychological Benefits—This is a special pose and a therapy. People gravitate to this pose with ease and peace. This teaches humility and surrender in front of the Almighty—the two main factors for mental clarity and sanity. People are drawn to this pose as it creates a sense of serenity and contentment. This pose releases tension and leads to greater understanding. It inculcates the willingness to surrender to the higher order with utmost faith. You begin to feel that you can safely unburden yourself by putting your mental load on the shoulders of the Almighty. When your personal will does not have the power to change the despairing situation on its own, you turn it over to the higher power. This creates a very calming effect on the mind and a secure feeling. Surrendering instantly gives you back the energy you have been spending in resisting your life, in feeling victimised, frustrated or depressed. This teaches the most profound form of alignment with reality.

There is some sort of hidden symmetry in this pose that appeals to the subconscious mind. This has something to do with gravity and instinct.

Contraindications—People with serious conditions of the eye, heart or back.

Value Addition—Invite your mind to breathe prana or life force energy into every part of the body. Hold a group discussion on 'Faith Healing through Group Prayers'.

Thought for the Day

Being a yogi is having the wisdom to remove anything that stifles your consciousness, through your prayers.

---

34 Vikasita-Kamalasan
(The Blossoming Lotus Posture)

Aim—To open the hip joint and strengthen the spine.

Time Span—Two minutes.

Technique—Start from Baddha Konasan or the Butterfly pose. Inhale, tuck your hands under your calves and lift both feet off the floor. Exhale and keep your heels pressed together. Inhale and join each thumb and index finger together as in Jnan Mudra. Exhale and looking straight ahead, balance on your hip bone and settle down. Keeping your spine upright, lift your heart and take your gaze up with confidence. Breathe four times.

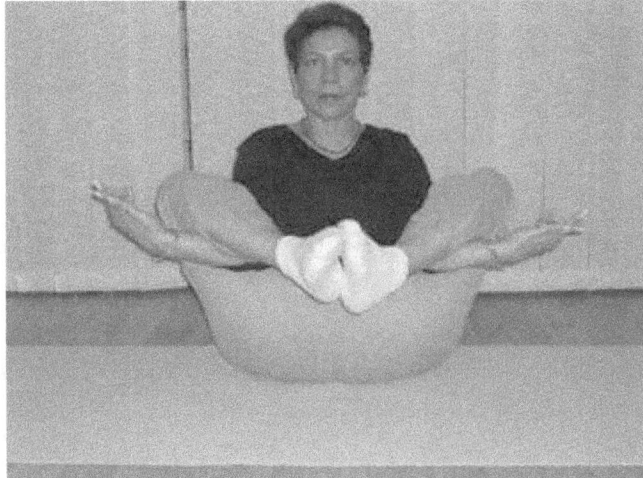

Focus—On balancing yourself on your sit bones.

Breathing Pattern—Normal and steady.

Physical Benefits—This is an excellent pose for ladies to open their pelvis and the hip joint. It is good for conception and improves the functioning of the kidneys, bladder and other urinary structures. This pose can be done during pregnancy for easy and natural delivery. It brings pressure on the pelvis chakra and promotes vaginal elasticity and firmness.

Psychological Benefits—This also teaches balance and concentration, patience, tolerance and perseverance. These virtues are important to stay in control and gain mastery over your emotions. It promotes free, independent and original thinking, self-reliance and taking independent decisions.

Contraindications—Hip joint or knee problems.

Value Addition—Find out what pleases you most and always have a goal in life.

Thought for the Day
Luck and joy awaits those who know the value of things. Forget what is gone, leave what is behind you; look forward to something pleasant.

35

Balasan
(The Foetus/Child's Posture as a Therapy)

This is a very good posture also practiced as an excellent therapy.

Aim—To surrender completely to gravity and to enter into the deeply relaxing pose.

Time Span—Two minutes as a posture and three to four minutes as a therapy.

Technique—From the Prayer Pose, place your hands by your sides or tuck your hands under your thighs. Imagine you are a little baby now and tell yourself this once again and see how you feel. You begin to feel light and happy like a baby. Just breathe gently and surrender yourself to the floor. Put all your physical weight on the floor and feel grounded. If anything is bothering your mind, this is the time to pass on the mental pressure and all those nagging and bugging issues onto the floor and unburden yourself. This floor has a tremendous capacity to absorb your worries or all the unwanted emotional baggage. Just pass it on to the floor and feel very safe and secure. This floor is Mother Earth who is holding you and supporting you right now. She will also comfort you with her graciousness.

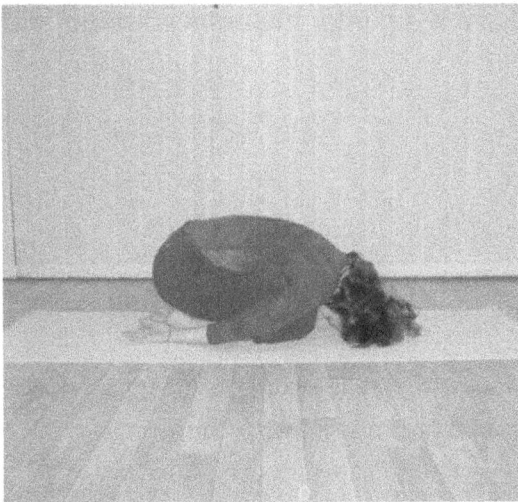

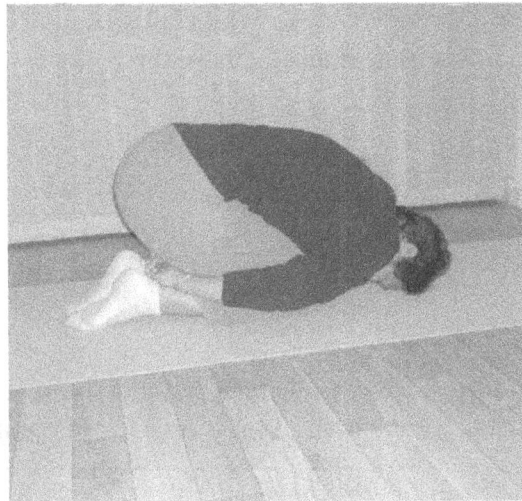

Focus—On total surrender to the floor.

Breathing Pattern—Normal and steady.

Physical Benefits—You begin to feel very light-hearted and happy like a little baby. This pose brings a gentle and healthy pressure on the entire chakra system. The flow of subtle energy (prana) starts moving and ascending upward from the Root chakra (Mooladhar chakra) to the Crown chakra (Sahasrara chakra). This has a stabilising and calming effect on the mind which promotes serenity. This pose is almost addictive as it has a beautiful soothing effect on the body and mind. It eases constipation and prevents eating disorders like 'comfort eating'.

Psychological Benefits—The word 'mother' brings certain tender emotions to your mind and heart which helps in awakening the inner child in you. The word 'mother' will remind you of her unconditional love, tender care, compassion, sacrifice, warmth and a sweet smile, patience and tolerance. You will also think that "Mother Earth has bestowed on me a body that supports an auspicious life through which I am able to progress spiritually. She carried me for nine months although it was making her heavy and hard to move about. She has taken special care to feed me and sustain me till today. Her sense of intimacy is divine". Remain in this thought for a while.

All this has a beautiful impact on your psyche and you begin to feel peaceful and blissful like a baby. This deepens your appreciation for others and increases your capacity to love unconditionally and teaches you the art of forgiveness. This pose restores your self-esteem and confidence in yourself and in others. You can overcome grief and survive crises. You counter the agitated mind and overcome unrealistic views.

Contraindications—Nil.

Value Addition—Check whether you learn and teach yourself how to do those small things in life that may look insignificant but yet are important.

Thought for the Day

If you give a man fish to eat, you can feed him for a day, but if you teach him to fish you feed him for life.

36

Padmasan
(The Partial and Complete Lotus Posture)

Aim—To balance the mental and pranic forces.

Time Span—Two to three minutes.

Technique—The Partial Lotus Posture—Inhale and sit with the legs stretched in front of you. Exhale, gently bend your right leg and lifting it with your hands, place the right foot on top of the left thigh. Inhale and exhale and check whether you feel comfortable with this position.

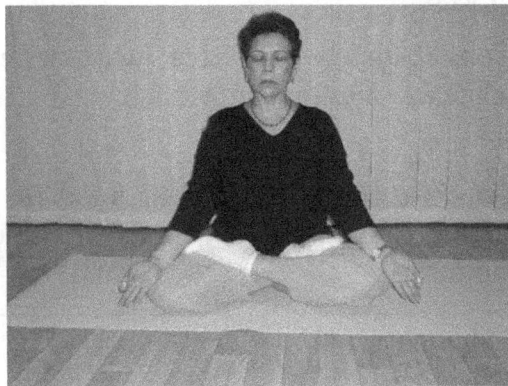

If so, then get ready to perform the Complete Lotus Posture—Inhale and hold the left foot. Exhale and gently bend the left leg, lifting it with your hands, place the left foot on top of the right thigh. Breathe gently. This posture is difficult and may not be perfect on the first attempt. Ideally, the soles should rest on the groins and the heels should be close to the pubic bones. Sit upright so that the spine remains erect. Keep breathing gently. Place the hands on the knees, palms facing upward and join the index fingers of each hand with the thumbs of the respective hands. This is known as Jnana Mudra which enhances your concentration. Perfecting the posture may require a lot of time. You need to make necessary adjustments by moving your legs and torso till you feel aligned without any pain in the legs.

Focus—Once accomplished perfectly, the focus should be on breathing.

Breathing Pattern—Slow and steady.

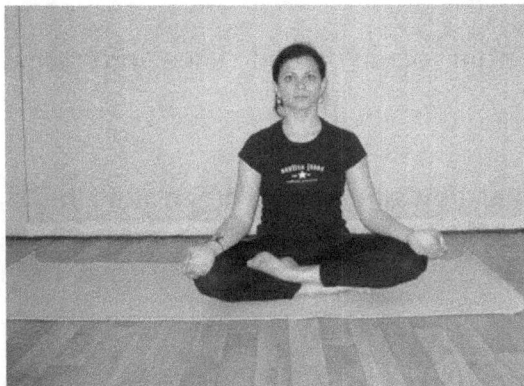

Partial Lotus   Complete Lotus

Physical Benefits—This pose is called the king of the yoga postures because while you are in this posture, you can hold the body steady for an extended period of time with the mind being totally immersed in meditation and without feeling any physical sensation. However, reaching that level of perfection takes hours and hours of practice. Initially there is a lot of discomfort in the thighs and knees. If you can sit in the half lotus pose, continue with it, folding one leg at a time and alternating the leg to encourage the external rotation of the hips. After practising the partial Lotus Posture, you will have some external range of motion in your hips. In order to progress safely to the full lotus pose, you need to further encourage the external rotation without straining the knees which can be done only through regular practice. Each one takes their own time in feeling comfortable in this posture. But once accomplished, this posture directs the flow of prana energy from Mooladhara Chakra in the perineum to the Sahasrara Chakra in the crown of the head, heightening the experience of meditation. This posture has a balancing effect on the body and prana (energy) and thus a calming effect on the mind. In yoga texts, it is often touted as the destroyer of all diseases. It brings about excellent changes in the metabolic structure and brain patterns. It also stimulates the acupuncture meridians of the stomach, gall bladder, spleen, kidneys and the liver. It promotes digestion. This keeps Wind (Vata), Bile (Pitta) and Phlegm (Kapha) in balance. It also tones the sacral and coccygeal nerves by supplying them with an increased blood flow. These are all good reasons to aspire to sit in the full Lotus Pose. However, this pose is often hard to accomplish therefore practice with caution and patience.

Psychological Benefits—This pose is ideal for deep breathing practices (Pranayam) and meditation. It brings tranquillity to the mind. This heightens the awareness, alertness and the ability to have clarity of the mind and thinking process.

Contraindications—Those who suffer from acute/injured knee problems, sciatica or legs that are too stiff.

Value Addition—Keep your mind on what you are doing. When your mind wanders off to work, worries or responsibilities, bring it back to the present moment.

Thought for the Day

Listen to your body; there is an inner teacher within.

| 37 | **Sukhasan**
(The Easy Posture) |

Aim—To establish an inner harmony.

Time Span—Two to three minutes as a posture but you can sit in this posture whenever you cannot sit in difficult postures.

Technique—Sit on the floor with legs stretched forward. Bend the right leg and place the heel under the left thigh. Similarly, bend the left leg and place the left heel under the right thigh. Some people may feel comfortable in placing the right leg over the left and sometimes the left leg over the right. Sit upright. The head, the neck and the torso/back should be in a straight line. The abdomen should be pulled in slightly. Place the hands on the knees with the palms turned downward and covering the knee caps. The arms, the elbows and the hands should be comfortable. Close your eyes and breathe gently. In case you find this posture difficult, you can take a cushion and sit on it which makes you feel more comfortable.

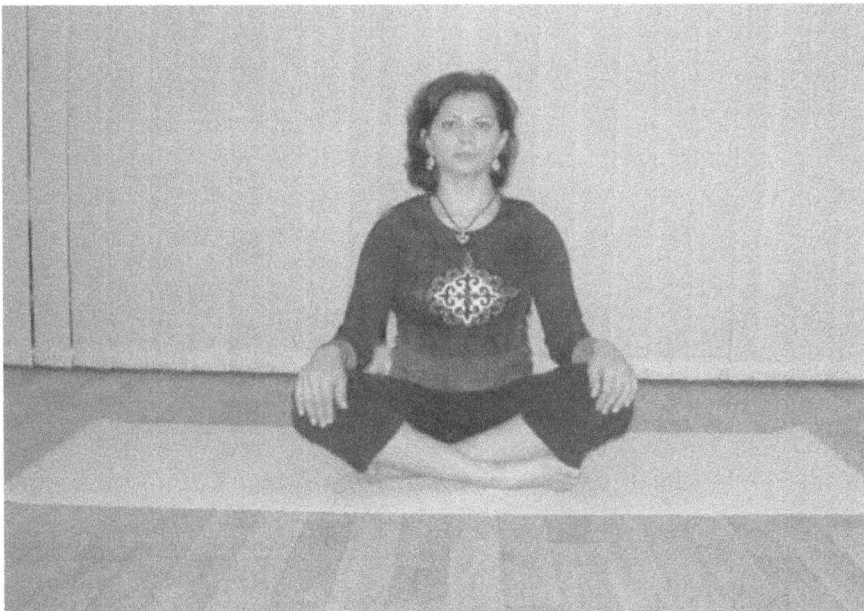

Focus—On keeping the spine erect, abdomen pulled in, arms relaxed and breathing gently.

Breathing Pattern—Slow and steady.

Physical Benefits—This prepares you physically to sit comfortably before you move on to difficult postures. It steadies your nerves or muscular agitation.

Psychological Benefits—This prepares you mentally for certain deep breathing exercises and meditation. This also balances your energy centres or chakras.

Contraindications—If you have injured knees or sprained/fractured ankle, severe varicose veins problem.

Value Addition—Find out which yoga pose is a favourite of yours in standing, sitting and lying postures. Why do you like it?

> ### Thought for the Day
>
> A posture isn't a posture unless you are breathing through it and thus connecting with it.

Supta Pavan Muktasan
(The Wind Release Posture)

Aim—To loosen up the joints of the body without vigorous physical movements and to ward off lethargy and flatulence.

Time Span—Five minutes.

Technique—This pose is done in a series of movements. This is one of my favourite poses as there is good circulation and the entire body feels extremely rejuvenated.

(I) Lie down on your back. Stretch the legs straight out in front of you. Inhale and raise your right leg to 90 degrees. Exhale and bend the right knee. Inhale, interlocking your fingers, grab the right knee/shin. Exhale and as you pull your stomach muscles in, gently and firmly press the knee on the abdomen, especially on the abdominal cavity. Inhale, raise the head, bringing it closer to the knee and if possible rest your forehead on the right knee. Exhale and stretch

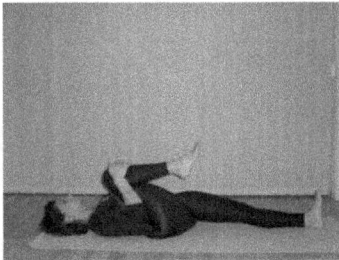

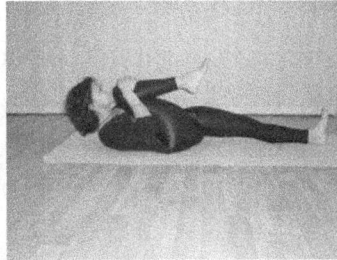

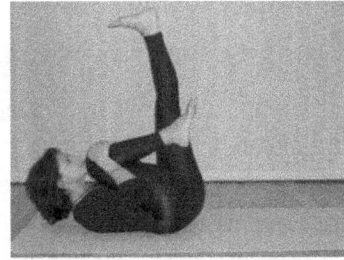

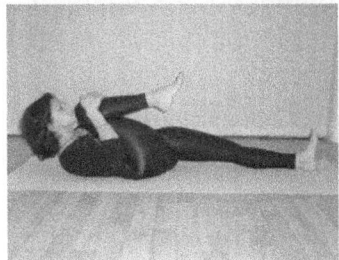

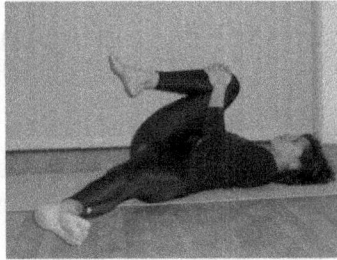

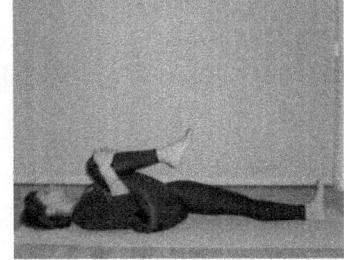

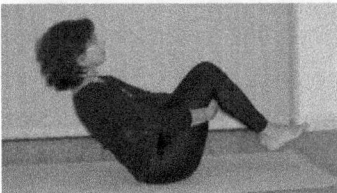

the left leg lifting it slightly above the floor. You can remain in this position for four breaths. In the above position, inhale and raise your left leg 90 degrees. Exhale and bring it down closer to the floor without touching the ground. Repeat four times.

If there is strain on the neck while raising the head, you can also perform this pose by resting the head on the floor.

(II) Rest the head back on the floor. Inhale and stretch the left leg to the left side as much as possible (for instance, from the 12 O' clock position up to the 9 O' clock position). Exhale and bring it back to the centre. Repeat this four times.

Coming Out of the Pose—Inhale and release the right knee and keep the arms back to the natural position by your sides and simultaneously straighten your right leg back to 90 degrees. Exhale, push the floor with your palms and lower the right leg back to the normal position.

Inhale and raise the arms overhead. Exhale and bring the arms back to the normal position which helps in bringing the heat rate back to the normal state.

Focus—Should be on integrated breathing and on various parts of the body which are involved in the pose.

Breathing Pattern—Normal and synchronised as per the 'Technique'.

Physical Benefits—It releases gas or flatulence and eases constipation; it is excellent for rheumatism, arthritis, high blood pressure and heart problems. It eliminates energy blockages in the joints and the prana energy starts flowing freely and evenly.

Psychological Benefits—This works on the pranic and mental bodies whereby it removes obstructions in your thinking and unblocks planning skills which promotes further personal progress with mental clarity, peace, equanimity and single pointedness.

Contraindications—Very high blood pressure, sciatica, slipped disc or pregnancy.

Value Addition—Try some herbal teas which reduce flatulence.

Thought for the Day

Practice of yoga is to pull you out of infatuation from personality to eternity.

---

2   Supta Padangushthasan
(The Toes Touching Posture)

Aim—To work on your limbs for stretching and strengthening them.

Time Span—Two to three minutes.

Technique—Lie on the floor in supine (on your back) position. Inhale and raise your legs upward at 90 degrees angle. Exhale and stretch your legs as much as you can gently. Inhale and raise your arms to touch your toes (if you find it hard to touch your toes, you can bend your knees or increase the distance between the feet). Exhale and make sure your neck/head is in line with the rest of your body. Breathe four times and settle down in the pose.

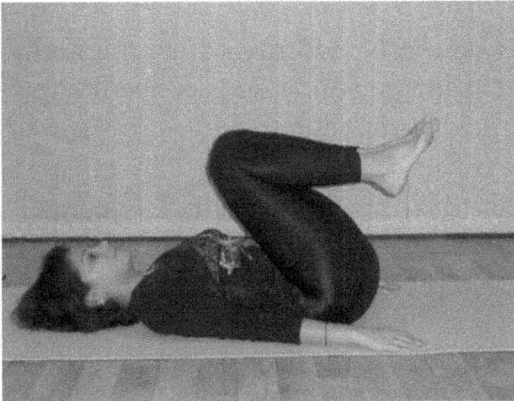

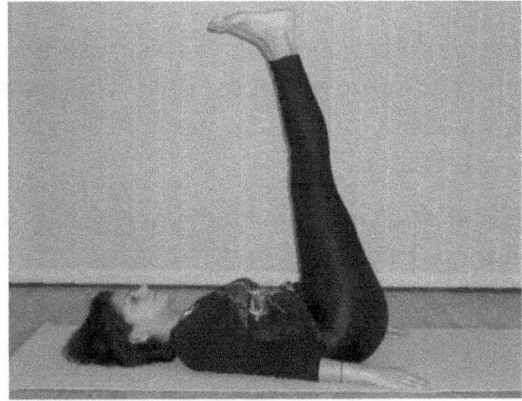

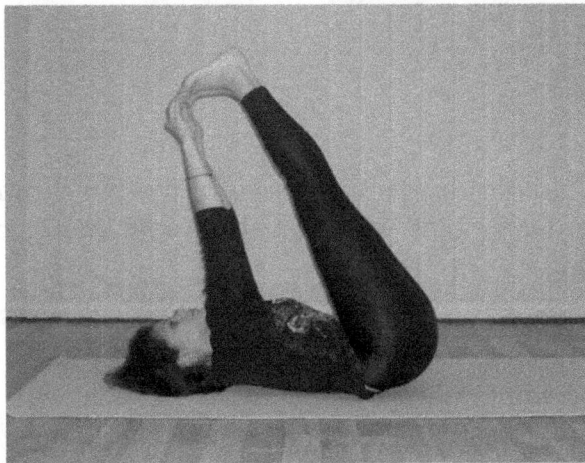

Coming Out of the Pose—Inhale and keep your hands on the floor by your sides. Exhale and lower your legs, back to the normal position.

Focus—Keeping your legs and arms stretched and upright.

Breathing Pattern—Normal and steady.

Physical Benefits—Opens the hamstrings and hip flexors, relieves sciatica, develops power in your abs, increases the length of stride while walking/ running, creates freedom in the hips and mobility of the hip joint and promotes circulation in the thighs, hips and pelvis. This pose relieves muscle tension, improves posture, reduces wear and tear on the lower back and builds hamstring strength in the lengthened position. This pose energises the front and back of your solar plexus which is the 'second brain' of the body. It reduces cholesterol, diabetes, arthritis, high blood pressure and many other ailments. It also strengthens the kidneys, adrenal glands and the body's heating and cooling systems.

Psychological Benefits—This pose teaches you to be assertive, trust the future and not to fret about the past. This pose is challenging and needs concentration. It teaches you take up new challenges in real life situations and improves your concentration.

Contraindications—Hamstring/groin injury, prolapsed uterus, menstruation, during pregnancy.

Value Addition—The third eye is the centre of the Sushumna Channel. Press and release the 'third eye point' which balances your energy centres and serves as a soothing massage.

Thought for the Day

Our eyes are two important sense organs. The right eye is connected to libidinal energy and the left eye is connected to emotional energy.

Salamba-Supta Padangushthasan (The Angle Stretch–I (Simplified), II (The Right Leg to the Right Side Pose and Reverse))

3

Aim—To develop proper strength and stamina in the legs.

Time Span—Two to three minutes.

Technique—I. Lie down on the back and keep both the legs straight on the floor. Inhale and stretch both legs upward to 90 degrees as in the 'Supta Padangushthasan'. Exhale and settle down in the position. Inhale and hook your big toes with your index/middle fingers/thumbs. Exhale and bring the straightened right leg and the right hand down toward the floor on the right side as much as possible.

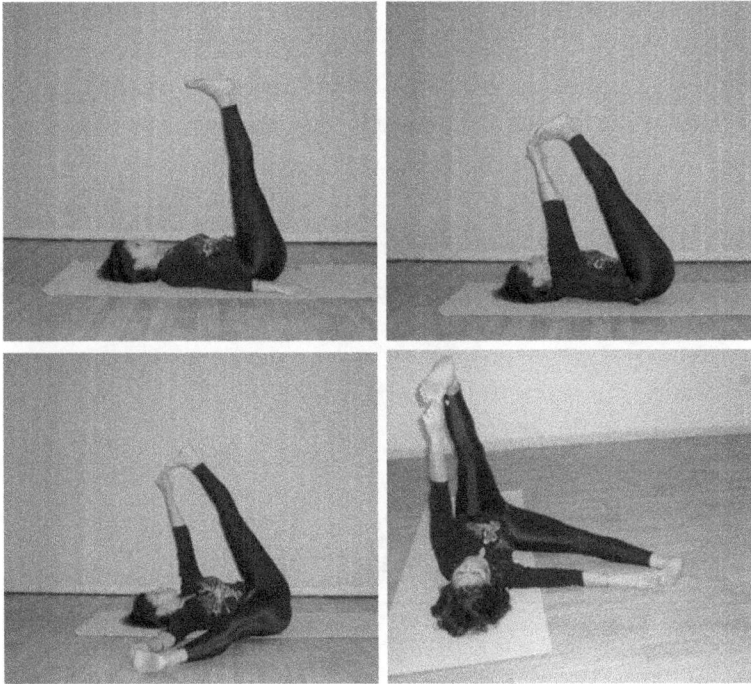

Remain within the limits of your flexibility.

Coming Out of the Pose—Inhale and raise the right leg along with the right hand back to the centre. Exhale, release the right foot and lower the leg/hand back to the normal position.

Repeat the same with the left leg.

II. You can do the same thing without raising the leg at 90 degrees. Keeping your legs stretched, slide each leg sideways to either side, stretching the corresponding hand sideways and see whether you can hold the toes. Breathe four times.

Coming Out of the Pose—Slide the leg back to the centre.

Focus—On breathing and stretching the leg as much as you can and staying well within the natural limits of your flexibility.

Breathing Pattern—Normal and steady.

Physical Benefits—This pose develops good strength and stamina in the leg muscles and the hip joint and promotes blood circulation. It rejuvenates the nervous system, relieves lower back pain and alleviates digestive disorders by which certain digestion-related headaches disappear. This pose strengthens legs and relieves compression in the lower back. If done under expert supervision, people suffering from paralysis (stroke) will receive great benefits. This also removes stiffness in the hip joint and prevents hernia.

Psychological Benefits—Any pain for more than six months is chronic pain which can trigger a cycle of either temporary or permanent disability. In other words, that particular problem area becomes inactive due to the blockage in the energy flow and is unable to function normally. By practicing this yoga pose, one can unblock the energy flow and bounce back to normal life.

Contraindications—Those suffering from sciatica or any severe leg or hip joint pain.

Value Addition—Perform your role with a transparent conscience. Only that will lead you to the path of enlightenment and contentment.

Thought for the Day

There is a method of 'Breath Control' to harmonise the forces of life. With a specific pattern of breathing you begin to realise not to take this life too seriously. When it comes to being 'too serious', our emotions too become intense in every situation unnecessarily and there is really no need to be that serious as this entire life is too transient and nothing but an illusion.

---

4 | Sethu Bandhanasan—Vinyasa I, II, III
(The Bridge Posture—Hip Raise Sequence–I, II[1], III[2])

Aim—To strengthen the neck muscles and prepare for the Shoulder Stand Posture.

Time Span—Six minutes.

Technique—(I) Lie on the floor in supine (face-up position). Inhale and stretch your arms downward closer to your knees. Exhale and bend both the knees by keeping your feet flat on the floor. Inhale and stretch your arms to hold your ankles and raise your hips as much as possible. Exhale and make sure to keep your head in line with your body.

Breathe four times.

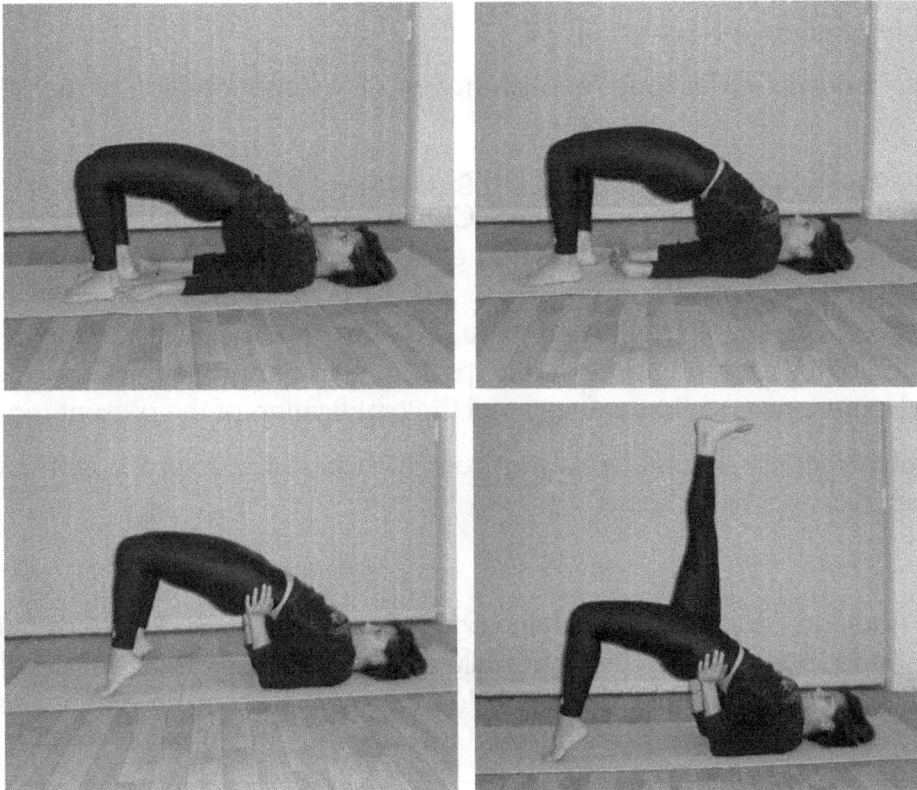

---

[1]With interlocked fingers and hips raised higher.
[2]With hands on the hips and raising one leg.

(II) Release the ankles and stretch the arms on the floor under your hips. Interlock the fingers and raise the hips higher than in the first pose. By interlocking the fingers you can easily raise your hips higher since it provides extra pushing action.

Breathe four times.

(III) In the third pose, release your interlocked fingers, hold the hips and raising your heels, raise one leg upward at 90 degrees. Breathe four times and bring the leg down. Repeat with the other leg.

Coming Out of the Pose—Inhale and release your ankles in the pose-I or release your interlocked fingers in pose-II or your hips in the pose-III and lower your body onto the floor and keep your arms by your sides. Exhale and stretch your legs back to normal position.

Focus—On breathing and raising the lower body.

Breathing Pattern—Deep or ujjayi.

Physical Benefits—This tones and strengthens the lumbar region of the spine. It promotes a healthy nervous system.

Psychological Benefits—This pose brings some amazing results as the energy is transmitted from the 'Swadhishthan Chakra' (Pelvic Plexus) upward to the 'Anahata Chakra' (Heart Centre) and allows you to open the 'Heart Chakra' gently and experience the truth and beauty of your inner and outer worlds. It keeps you from shutting out the reality of your actual needs and enjoying the sensation of the present moment. It helps to free you from the past unwanted or painful experiences so that you can feel the gratification of the present moment.

Contraindications—People suffering from high blood pressure, heart disease, stomach ulcers or weak spine.

Value Addition—Your investment in yoga will give you great dividends in terms of a sound body and mind especially in the old age. It helps develop a transparent conscience by which one loses the capacity to be mean, nasty or negative and in turn never gets affected by them.

Thought for the Day

Future dividends are created in the factories of the present investments.

---

5 | Anantasan
(The Sideways Stretch—Reclining Buddha Posture)

Aim—To stretch muscles not usually used and to reduce flab on the thighs and hips.

Time Span—Four minutes.

Technique—Lie on the left side. Bend and prop up the left elbow, raise and rest your head on the left palm (using the left hand as support). You will be working on the right side of the body first, starting with your right leg. Keep the right palm on the floor, elbow pointing upward in front of you, for support. Inhale and bend the right leg by bringing your right knee closer to the right shoulder. Exhale and hold the right foot with your right hand. Inhale and raise the right leg 90 degrees. Exhale and look straight. Breathe four times.

With each inhalation, send energy to the right leg and with each exhalation, expel impurities or stiffness from the leg. Do not ignore the left leg which is on the floor. Inhale and send energy to the left leg as well, keeping it stretched firmly on the floor.

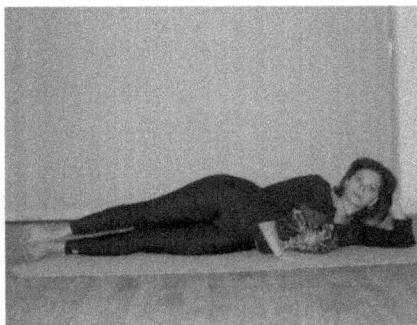

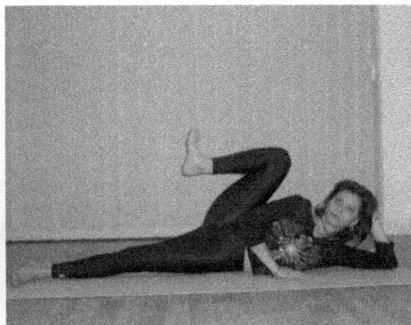

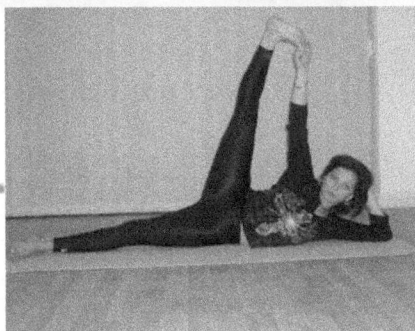

Coming Out of the Pose—Inhale. Exhale and bend the right leg. Inhale, release the right foot, exhale and keep the right hand back in the normal position and straighten the right leg back to the normal position.

Repeat the same with the left leg and lying on the right side.

Focus—On synchronising the movement with the breath, on the stretch in the hip and the raised leg while holding the pose. In case of difficulty in balancing, bend the bottom leg and instead of resting on the elbow, stretch the hand and rest the head on that arm.

Breathing Pattern—Check the 'Technique'.

Physical Benefits—Makes you very flexible, physically and mentally. This pose relaxes the hamstrings, inner thighs and abdominal muscles.

Psychological Benefits—Makes you strong-willed along with a sensible attitude.

Contraindications—Slipped disc, sciatica or cervical spondylitis.

Value Addition—Improve your breathing by lengthening each exhalation more than inhalation.

Thought for the Day

The act of respiration involves inhalation and exhalation. Inhalation is active and requires effort. Exhalation is passive and requires no effort.

6

Bhujangasan
(The Cobra Posture)

Aim—To strengthen the upper back and the spine and its connective tissues.

Time Span—Two to three minutes.

Technique—Inhale and lie on the stomach (prone position) with legs together and the chin resting on the floor. Exhale and place the hands on the floor close to the shoulders, elbows pointing upwards. Inhale and raise the head and the torso up to the navel keeping the elbows slightly bent. Exhale.

Breathe at least three times and remain in the same position.

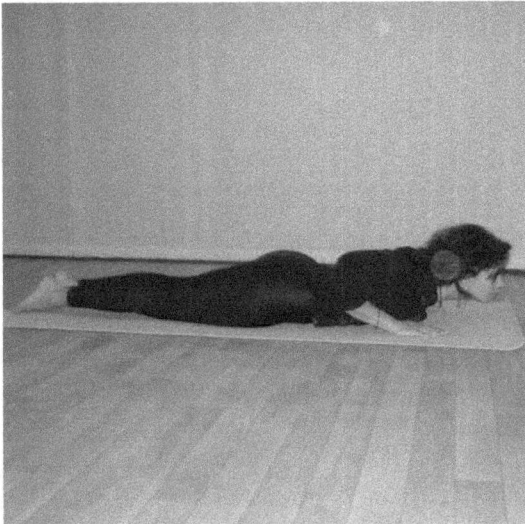

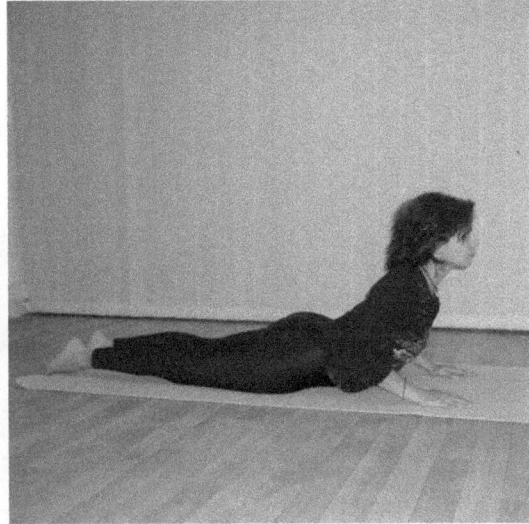

Coming Out of the Pose—Inhale and look straight ahead. Exhale and lower the head and torso back to the normal position. Relax.

Focus—On maintaining the stretch.

Breathing Pattern—Ujjayi or steady.

Physical Benefits—Allows the spine to stretch backward which rejuvenates the entire chakra system. This also relocates slightly displaced discs and removes backache. It improves blood circulation in the spine. This pose also tones the ovaries and uterus and helps alleviate menstrual and other gynaecological disorders and eases constipation. It strengthens the liver and kidneys and adrenal glands.

Psychological Benefits—This is an anti-ageing pose. This brings out your hidden potential and you become wise, watchful and practical just like a cobra with raised hood.

Contraindications—People suffering from peptic ulcer, hernia, intestinal complications and hyperthyroidism should not practice this pose without expert guidance.

Value Addition—Rub the fingernails against each other (except the thumbs). This promotes healthy hair growth.

Thought for the Day

Yoga practice discourages emotional indulgence and encourages spiritual endurance.

Aim—To strengthen the lower back and the spine.

Time Span—Two to three minutes.

Technique—(I) Lie flat on the stomach in the prone position. Keep your legs together and stretched. Make fists of your hands and keep them under your thighs. Rest the chin on the floor. Inhale and raise the right leg as high as possible without bending the knee. Keep the other leg firmly on the floor. Exhale and lower the right leg. Similarly, inhale and raise the left leg, exhale and lower the left leg. Repeat the pose with each leg raised for three breaths.

(II) Repeat the pose with both the legs.

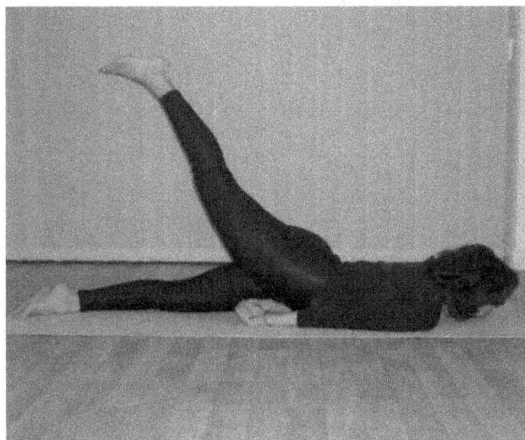

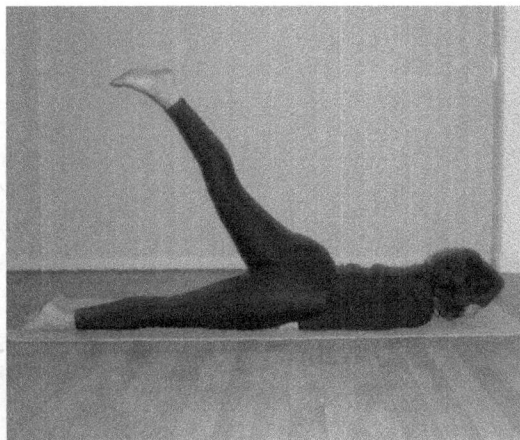

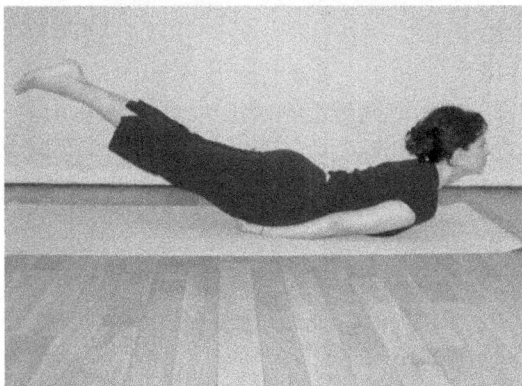

Focus—Raising the leg as high as possible but not to overstretch it.

Breathing Pattern—Normal and steady.

Physical Benefits—Builds core strength and stability, strengthens the buttocks, thighs, shins and feet, tones the muscles of the back, shoulders and arms. It is recommended as a therapy specifically for sciatica and slipped disc problems but under expert guidance. It helps in relieving constipation as it massages the ascending colon of the large intestine. It also helps in peristalsis.

Psychological Benefits—Develops concentration and balance and teaches coordination and alertness.

Contraindications—Knee injury or instability, acute sacroiliac pain or instability, severely strained hamstrings or pregnancy.

Value Addition—Teach this precept to someone you like.

Thought for the Day

The five 'Niyamas' of Patanjali start with 'Saucha' which means self-purification through the Head (mind), Heart and Hands. It is learnt by cleansing the head with positive thoughts, purifying the heart by noble emotions and rinsing the hands with good deeds.

8

Urdhwa Mukha Shvanasan
(The Upward Facing Dog Posture)

Aim—To strengthen the upper body especially the spine and the connective tissues of the spine.

Time Span—Two minutes.

Technique—Inhale and lie on the stomach (prone position) with legs together and the chin resting on the floor. Exhale and place the hands on the floor close to the shoulders, elbows pointing upwards as in the Cobra Posture. Inhale, raise the head and the torso by pushing the floor with your hands and straightening your arms as much as you can to hold the head erect. Raise the entire body off the floor resting only on the palms and the bridges of your feet.

Exhale, look straight ahead and remain in the same position. Breathe four times stretching the spine gently upward and feel the stretch in the gut.

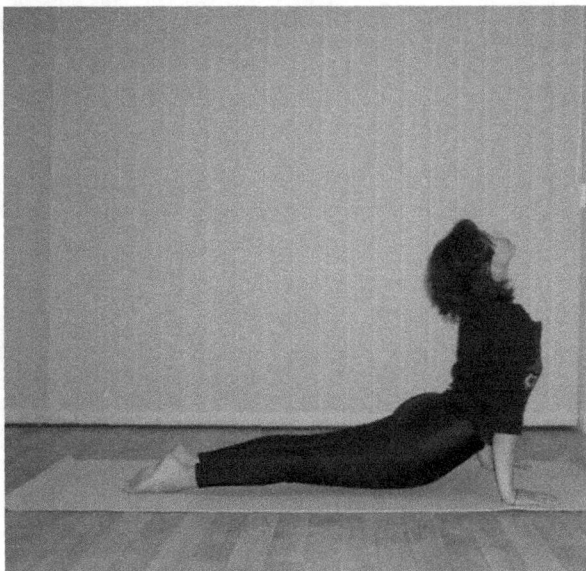

Coming Out of the Pose—On your exhalation, bring the torso and head down on the floor.

Focus—On breathing and stretching the spine.

Breathing Pattern—Ujjayi.

Physical Benefits—Increases the shoulder and spine flexibility, tones the diaphragm, the spinal and abdominal muscles and improves circulation along the spine.

Psychological Benefits—This pose serves like an anti-depressant.

Contraindications—Pregnancy, hypertension, sciatica, back problems, shoulder injury, active asthma or acute respiratory allergies.

Value Addition—Can you find out the difference between happiness and contentment?

Thought for the Day

The second precept of 'Niyama' is 'Santosh' which means being content with what we already have and accepting our life with total satisfaction. Fulfilment of desires is called happiness which is short-lived whereas contentment means looking at the positive things that have already happened in our life and feeling fulfilled.

9

Simplified Santolasan
(The Both Legs Up in Sideways Balancing Posture)

Aim—To learn balance and coordination.

Time Span—Two to three minutes.

Technique—Lie on your right side, rest the upper torso on the right elbow and keep both the palms on the floor in front of you for support, keeping both legs stretched together. Inhale and raise both legs off the floor. Exhale and look straight ahead. Breathe four times.

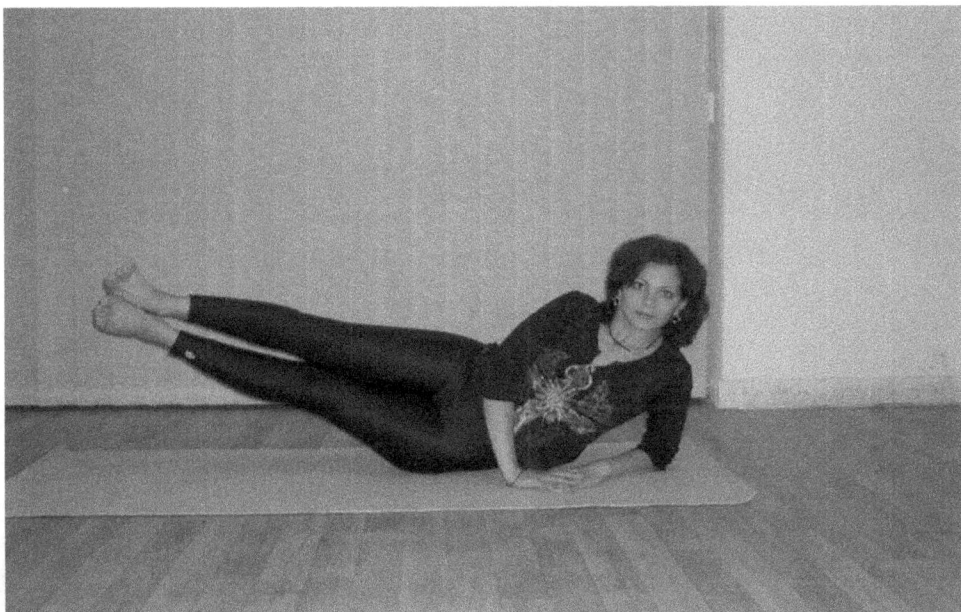

Coming Out of the Pose—Inhale and get ready to come out of the pose. Exhale and lower the legs back to the normal position. Repeat with the left side.

Focus—On breathing and maintaining balance.

Breathing Pattern—Normal and steady.

Physical Benefits—This pose strengthens the muscles of the arms, shoulders, spine and legs which balances the interaction between the dorsal and ventral muscles. It tones the hips and makes the lower back supple. It also reduces flab on the thighs.

Psychological Benefits—This pose improves balance of the nervous system and develops a sense of inner equilibrium and harmony. It teaches you to overcome obstacles and encourages you to face new situations confidently.

Contraindications—Slipped disc, hip joint dislocation or any severe back ailment.

Value Addition—Chant a Mantra of your choice to enhance Tapas.

Thought for the Day

The third precept of 'Niyama' is 'Tapas' meaning fire. However, it also means continuous, determined effort which generates heat or purity and rigorous discipline that brings about any kind of desired change in our thoughts and behaviour.

---

10 Santolasan or Simplified Vasishthasan (The Sideways Torso Stretch)

Aim—To improve balance, concentration and coordination.

Time Span—Two to three minutes.

Technique—Lie on the left side so that you begin with your right leg. Inhale and raise your torso by pushing with your left palm and balancing only on the left hand and foot, with the right palm gently resting on the floor. Exhale and cross your right leg over your left leg. Inhale and place your right hand firmly on the floor for good support. Exhale. Inhale and pushing with both your hands raise your entire body. Exhale, rest your right hand on the right knee and balance your body only on your left hand and both feet. Breathe four times. If you wish to challenge your body a bit further, you can try the 'Advanced Arm Balance' by raising your right arm upward and gazing at your right hand. Breathe four times.

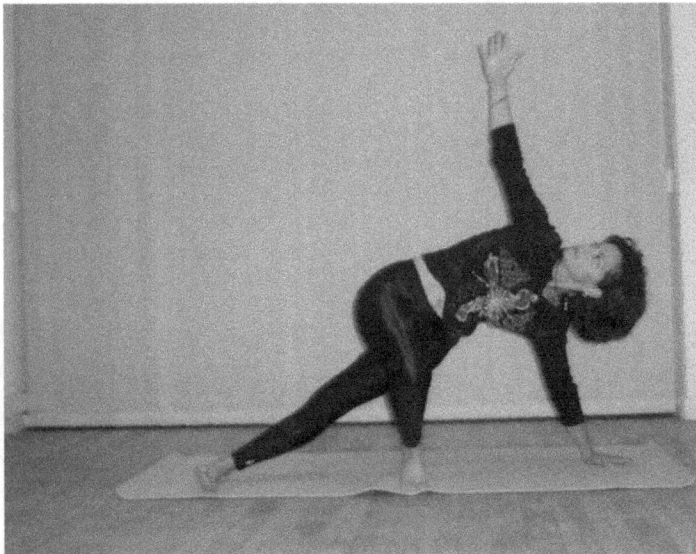

Coming Out of the Pose—Inhale and look straight ahead. Exhale and bring your right hand on the right knee. Inhale, uncross your legs and place your right hand on the floor. Exhale, bend your left hand and lower your torso to rest on the left elbow and come back to the normal position.

Repeat with the other side.

Focus—Steady breathing and maintaining balance.

Breathing Pattern—Deep and rhythmic or ujjayi.

Physical Benefits—This pose strengthens the wrists, exercises the leg muscles and tones the lumbar and coccyx region of the spine.

Psychological Benefits—The Advanced Arm Balance—with one leg crossed over, teaches balance, concentration and coordination. It is believed that the mental strength that you derive from this posture encourages you to overcome obstacles in life and motivates you to face new or unfamiliar situations confidently.

Contraindications—Weak wrists, slipped disc, pregnancy.

Value Addition—This week end monitor all your feelings and activities through Swadhya.

> **Thought for the Day**
>
> The fourth precept of 'Niyama' is 'Swadhyay' which means 'self-study or analysis' through introspection.

11 Supta Pavan Muktasan–II
(The Wind Release Posture Sequence–II)

1. With both legs up 2. Rolling from Side to Side 3. Rocking on the back.

Aim—To tone and strengthen the spine, the back muscles and the connective tissues of the vertebrae.

Time Span—Five to six minutes.

Technique—Just like Pavan Muktasan I (see Floor Postures—1). You can continue with that pose or perform this one separately.

(I) Lie on the floor on your back (supine or face up position) with your arms by your sides. Inhale and raise both legs upward at 90 degrees. Exhale, bend the knees and hug them. Inhale and raise the head and torso to rest your chin in between your knees. If you find this hard, allow your head to rest on the floor as it is very important that you stay within the natural limits of your flexibility and do not bring undue pressure on your neck. Breathe four times in the same position and continue with the other two poses.

(II) Inhale, bend the knees and bring them close to the torso. Exhale and hug your knees. Keeping the head on the floor, inhale and make sure your head and torso are in one line. Exhale and roll to one side, inhale and come back to the centre. Exhale and roll to the other side, inhale and come back to the centre. This way, roll once to the right and then to the left at least four times.

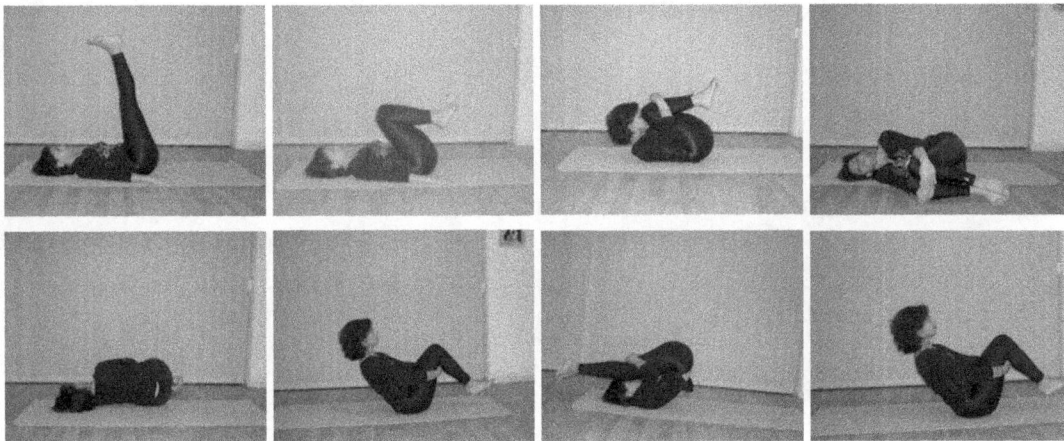

259

(III) From position-2, inhale, tuck your hands under your knees and hold on to the thighs for support. Exhale, lift and bend your torso forward and kick with your feet to begin the rocking movement. Rock on the back for four times. Breathe naturally and go with the flow.

Coming Out of the Pose—Inhale and release your hands, exhale and lie flat on the floor.

Focus—On breathing and bringing pressure on the abdomen.

Breathing Pattern—Normal. Initially if you are not be able to synchronise the breathing with the movement, listen to your body and breathe accordingly.

Physical Benefits—This strengthens the lower back muscles, loosens and aligns the vertebrae, vertically and laterally. It massages the internal organs and helps the digestive system. As the name implies it removes wind, gas or flatulence and alleviates constipation. This helps in massaging the pelvic region and reproductive organs and alleviates any menstrual problem. For men, this pose serves like tonic for their virility and a treatment for impotence, sterility or any prostate gland disorder.

Psychological Benefits—This works on the mental and many other energy centres whereby it removes obstructions in your thinking and unblocks energy for planning good strategies and skills which promote further personal progress. This brings in mental peace, equanimity and single pointedness.

Contraindications—People suffering from very high blood pressure, serious neck or back conditions, severe arthritis or osteoporosis in the spine, sciatica and slipped disc.

Value Addition—Check in what situations you can use your creativity and solve complex problems.

Thought for the Day

Technical skill is the mastery of complexity, while creativity is the master of simplicity.

---

12 Adhomukha Shvanasan (The Downward Facing Dog Posture)

Aim—To strengthen the entire spine right from the neck downward.

Time Span—Two minutes.

Technique—Inhale, kneel on the floor on all fours like an animal, (feet hip-width apart and palms shoulder-width apart). Exhale and stretch your right leg back on the floor, resting it on the ball of the foot. Inhale and look straight in the front. Exhale and similarly stretch your left leg back on the floor. Maintaining hip-width distance between the two feet, rest your heels on the floor. Inhale and look straight in the front. Keeping your palms and feet on the floor, settle down in the pose. Exhale and drop your head between the arms and push your buttocks further up. Breathe four times, stretching your arms in such a way that you can bring your torso and head closer to the floor. Let your heels and palms remain firmly planted on the floor. If possible try to bring your head closer to the floor to the centre point between your legs and arms.

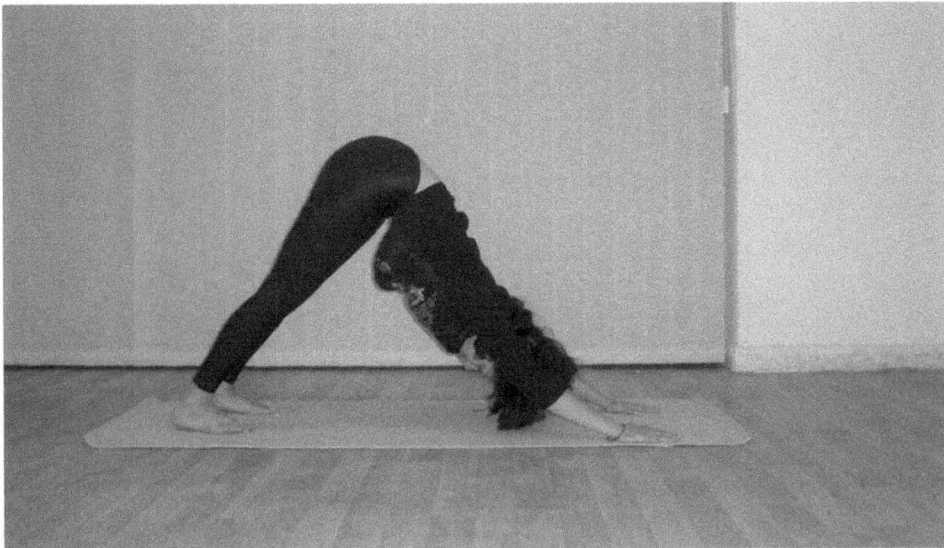

Coming Out of the Pose—Inhale and look straight ahead. Exhale and bring your right and left foot forward alternatively. You will come into the Forward Bending position. Inhale and slowly curl up and come into the standing position. Exhale.

261

Focus—On stretching the hip joint from the back and the shoulders and arms from the front. On keeping your head steady and downward.

Breathing Pattern—Slow and deep or ujjayi.

Physical Benefits—Feel the relaxing stretch in your hamstring muscles and in the upper body as this pose tones the entire spine by massaging and strengthening abdominal organs, arms and legs. This also makes the shoulders more flexible and helps build endurance. It serves like tonic to the nervous system. The blood circulation stimulates the nerves and it strengthens and tones the spinal nerves.

Psychological Benefits—It brings you closer to the floor which instils the attitude of gratitude to the floor or Mother earth. It allows you to succumb to an attitude of appreciation and teaches you to be grateful for even the small mercies in life.

Contraindications—People who have the tendency to dislocate shoulders, chronic shoulder injuries, pregnancy, unmanageable high/low blood pressure, herniated lumbar discs and vertigo.

Value Addition—Today be a messenger of good news. Let it be something pleasant or uplifting. If you look at positive things, your perspective will change for the better.

Thought for the Day
A correct perspective is a potent remedy for a negative attitude.

13

Makarasan
(The Crocodile Posture)

Aim—To activate healing energies in the body.

Time Span—Five minutes.

Technique—Lie flat on the floor on your stomach (prone or face down position). Inhale and cross/fold your hands in the front and rest your forehead or chin or either cheek on your hands. Exhale and stretch your legs 30–36 inches apart. The feet should be turned inward so that your instep rests on the floor.

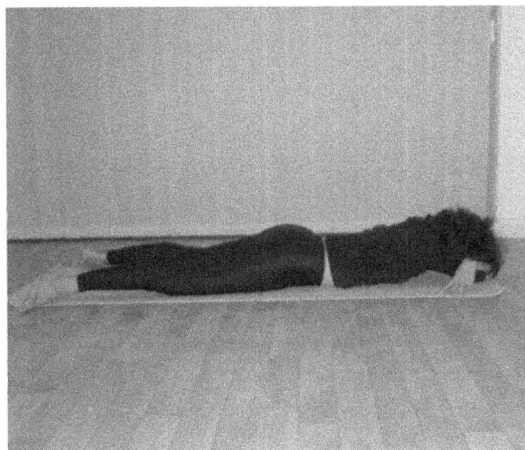

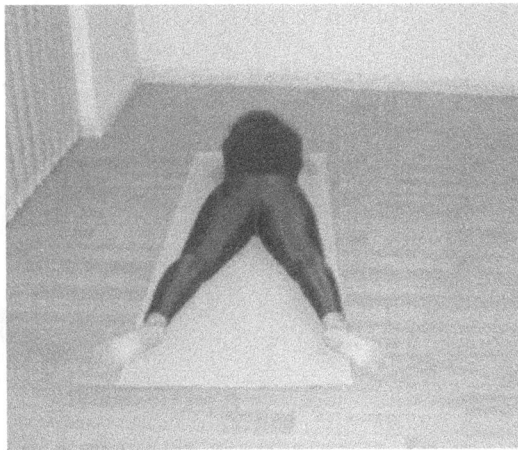

Focus—The feet should be turned inward so that your instep rests on the floor. This is very important to allow your internal organs to rest on the floor for the earthing effect.

Breathing Pattern—Natural and rhythmic.

Physical Benefits—This seemingly simple posture is quite deceptive in terms of benefits. It is a good posture for slipped disc, sciatica, lower back pain. If you remain in this pose for an extended period of time, it rectifies any spinal disorder as it encourages the spine to resume its natural, healthy position by releasing any kind of compression in the spinal nerves. Asthmatic people or people suffering from respiratory or lung ailments should practice this pose with breath awareness as the lungs respond to this pose by taking in more air.

Psychological Benefits—It has an earthing effect on your vital organs. Your soft tissue organs draw energy from the earth and get strengthened. Some organs are under-active and they draw energy from the floor and get energised. Some organs are over-active and they start releasing their excess energy into the floor and get stabilised and all the internal organs remain in balance and in harmony, individually and with one another.

Contraindications—Nil except pregnancy.

Value Addition—Keep a journal of gratitude and write down at least five things you are grateful for. Within a week, you will find that your daily gratitude level will heighten and your anxiety level will be lowered.

Thought for the Day
Think not of big things but of good things.

14

Matsya Kridasan
(The Playful Fish Posture)

Aim—To relax the entire body.

Time Span—Three to four minutes.

Technique—From the Crocodile Pose, switch to this pose. Inhale and interlock your fingers. Exhale, twist and turn your torso sideways resting on your left side on the floor and raising the right side off the floor. Inhale and rest your left cheek and head on the angle formed by the left elbow. Exhale and bend the right leg sideways by bringing the right knee close to the right elbow. The left leg should remain straight. Relax in this position for four breaths. Change and repeat the same with the right side.

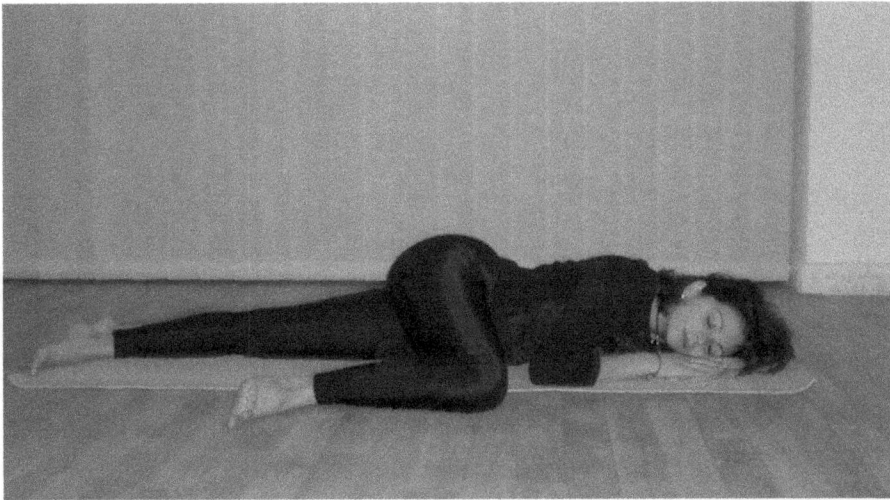

Coming Out of the Pose—Inhale, bring your head and torso to the normal position resting your palms on the floor. Exhale and take the support of the floor. Inhale and slowly come into the sitting position. Exhale.

Focus—On the breath and bringing the elbow and knee close together.

Breathing Pattern—Natural and rhythmic.

Physical Benefits—This pose stimulates digestive peristalsis by stretching the intestines. It eases constipation. It relieves sciatica pain and relaxes the nerves in the legs. It also removes excess flab around the waist and abdomen. Those who cannot bend forward should attempt this with ease. This is specially recommended for women in their advanced pregnancy as they should not lie flat on their backs since it can cause pressure over major veins and may block circulation. It helps in insomnia.

Psychological Benefits—This pose relaxes the body and mind entirely. When the body is relaxed, the mind too responds to relaxation. It encourages positive thinking.

Contraindications—Nil.

Value Addition—Make sure you drink eight glasses of water everyday. Water is a great lubricant and it helps to dissipate stale energy from your system.

Thought for the Day
Hate the sin and not the sinner.

15

Sarvangasan
(The Shoulder Stand Posture)

Aim—To rejuvenate the entire chakra system.

Time Span—Two minutes.

Technique—Lie on the back (supine or face up position). Make sure the head and the spine are aligned properly in the centre. Inhale and stretch the legs and feet straight in front. Exhale and place the hands by the sides. Relax your entire body and mind before you begin. Inhale, bend both the legs and bring the knees closer to your abdomen. Exhale and slide your hands under the hips holding the lower back with both hands. Inhale, straighten and raise your legs to 90 degrees. Exhale and settle down. Inhale and raise your legs further along with your torso, supporting the back on the raised forearms and elbows. Breathe four times and settle down in the position.

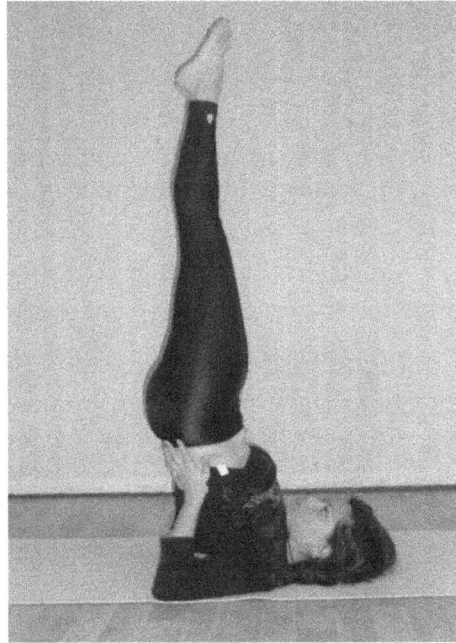

Coming Out of the Pose—Inhale and get ready to come out of the pose. Exhale, bend and bring the knees down towards the torso. Inhale and lower the torso to the floor, keeping the legs bent. Exhale, lower and straighten your legs on the floor. Simultaneously, release the hand support from the back and keep your hands by your sides.

Focus—On breathing, balancing and steadying the body, avoiding jerks.

Breathing Pattern—Slow and deep abdominal breathing.

Physical Benefits—This pose activates the thyroid gland which stimulates the respiratory, nervous, skeletal, digestive, circulatory, reproductive and endocrine systems. The immune system is strengthened by an activated thymus gland. It supplies oxygenated blood supply to the brain which helps in regenerating the brain cells. It relieves emotional stress, mental fatigue and headaches and imparts a tranquilising effect on the mind. It helps in regenerating the bones and prevents premature osteoporosis or calcification. It massages the abdominal organs. It reverses the normal gravitational force on the anal muscles and the internal organs and alleviates haemorrhoids. It strengthens the muscles of the legs, abdomen and reproductive organs, draining them of impure blood and lymphatic fluid. It revitalises our senses and relieves us from any respiratory ailment. It is recommended for diabetes, colitis, constipation, prolapsed uterus, menstrual disorders and impotency. This helps in removing sluggish phlegm from the lungs.

Psychological Benefits—This pose lightens the body and enlightens the mind and is called the 'Queen of Yoga'. (The 'King of Yoga' being the Head Stand Pose). In this pose, the position of the head is lower than the heart and as the heart is raised above the level of your head, it activates your heart centre. This is the first time you allow your heart to express itself and you will be amazed to see how your suppressed or frozen emotions are thawed and you expand your affection towards some truly deserving people in your life.

Contraindications—People suffering from severe medical problems like high or low blood pressure, very weak eyes, slipped disc, enlarged thyroid, liver or spleen, cervical spondylitis, heart disease, glaucoma, during menstruation or pregnancy.

Value Addition—What is your concept of a divine spirit? Set aside some time each day for spiritual practice, prayer or meditation and honour your inner spirit.

Thought for the Day

Unrestricted individualism or total self-indulgence is the law of the jungle and does not belong to a civilised culture.

16

Halasan Vinyasa–I, II, III, IV, V (The Plough Posture—Sequence–I, II, III, IV, V)

Aim—To regenerate the spine and the entire system.

Time Span—Four to five minutes.

Technique—(I) You can continue from the Shoulder Stand Position. Drop your legs over your head and touch the toes on the floor, behind the head. If you are unable to touch your toes on the floor, stretch your legs and lower back as much as possible, within the limits of your flexibility and hold on there. Take a few breaths and settle down in the position. Hold on and continue supporting your back. Breathe at your own pace all throughout the posture. There are four hand positions as follows:

(II) In the same position and once you feel confident, release your hands from the hips and stretch them towards your feet and hold on to your toes.

(III) In the same position, release your toes, bring your hands close to the head and then fold them on the head.

(IV) In the same position slide your hands behind your upperback and interlock your fingers. Stretch your arms further which allows your legs to stretch even further, straightening your back.

(V) Drop your knees near your ears and hug your knees.

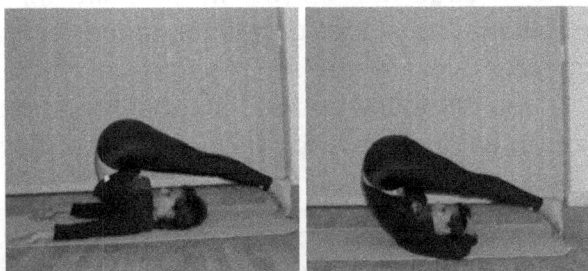

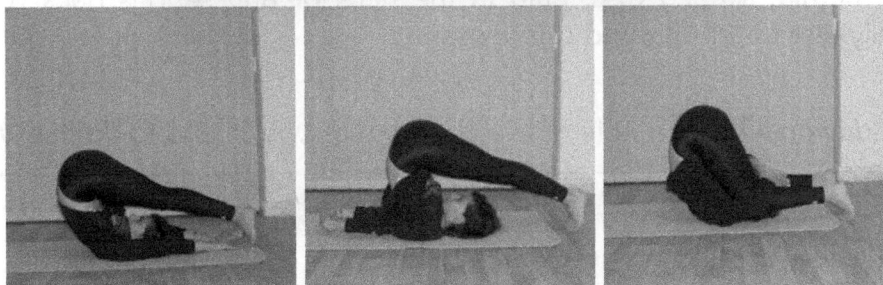

Coming Out of the Pose—Inhale and get ready to come out of the pose. Exhale, bend and bring the knees down towards the torso. Inhale and lower the torso to the floor, keeping the legs bent. Exhale, lower and straighten your legs on the floor. Simultaneously, release the hand support from the back and keep your hands by your sides.

Focus—On the abdomen and rhythmic breathing.

Breathing Pattern—Slow and deep all throughout the practice.

Physical Benefits—The pressure that is put on the diaphragm massages the internal organs. It activates digestion, relieves constipation, revitalises the renal glands, spleen and the pancreas which enhances the production of insulin. This also strengthens the spine, its connective tissues and the back muscles. It tones the spinal nerves and lung meridians. This pose nurtures and rejuvenates the immune system. This also regulates the thyroid gland and balances the body's metabolic rate.

This pose increases circulation in the knees and imparts suppleness and vitality. Releases tension in the neck and throat which alleviates phlegm and mucus in the sinuses and respiratory system. This is a general antidote for allergies, asthma, bronchitis, urinary tract disorders or menstrual problems. It activates the thymus gland and keeps the body's resistance generally high.

Psychological Benefits—This pose helps you plough through your past experiences and allows you to sweep away negative emotions. You begin to break up hard lumps of strife and sorrow in your life through wisdom and dedication. You remove past obstacles or painful memories from the mind. You also do not get bowled over by praise, recognition, success or wealth. By practising it regularly you discipline yourself by analysing your 'self' that serves as manure to your individual growth and soon you flow towards divine inspiration.

Contraindications—People suffering from sciatica, high or low blood pressure, vertigo, hernia, slipped disc, pain in the neck or any serious back problem especially due to arthritis and osteoporosis.

Value Addition—Make a note of five good things you intend to do this week.

Thought for the Day

Doing *well* in life is good but do not forget about doing *good* in life as well.

17

Matsyasan
(The Fish Posture—Simplified)

Aim—To strengthen the entire 'Chakra' system. This is a counter-balancing pose to the Shoulder Stand Pose and therefore should be done soon after the Shoulder Stand or the Plough Pose.

Time Span—Two minutes.

Technique—Sit with legs stretched out together in front of you. Inhale and keep your palms near the hips. Exhale, slowly lean backward and with elbows resting on the floor for support, place the top of your head on the floor. Inhale, push the floor with your hands and gently arch your back. Exhale, rest the back of your head completely on the floor and tuck your hands under the hips. Breathe four times.

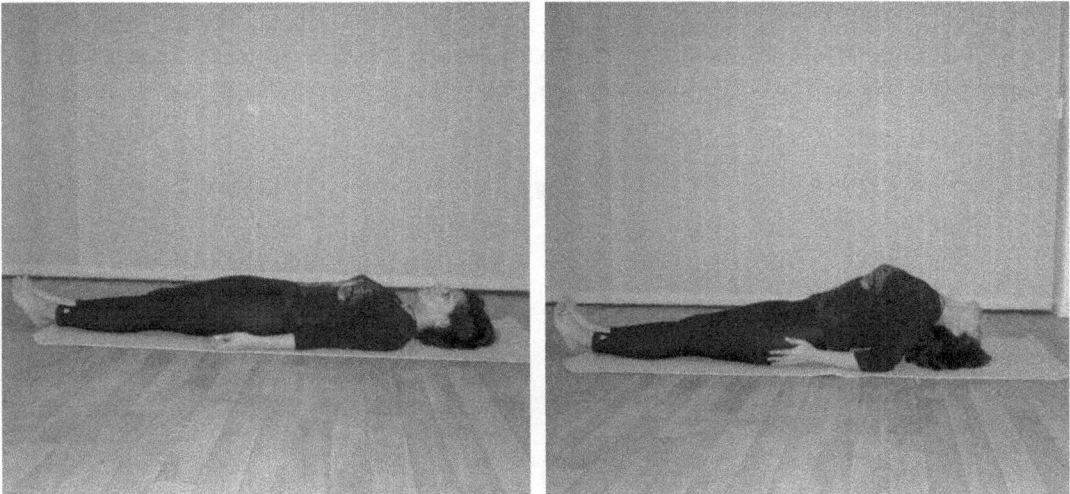

Coming Out of the Pose—Inhale, slowly lower your head and torso on the floor and adjust the head, torso, pelvis and the legs in one line. Exhale and release your hands from the hips and keep them by your sides. Care should be taken to avoid injury of the neck and head. The lowering of the neck and head should be done with utmost care and caution.

Focus—On breathing and on the abdomen and chest.

Breathing Pattern—Normal and steady.

Physical Benefits—It counter-balances the forward bending of the neck with backward bending relieving strain or stiffness in the neck from the earlier postures. There is healthy pressure on the throat which is good for thyroids and para-thyroids. It raises the front and back of the heart centre (chakra) which is good for expansion of the thoracic cavity which stimulates the lungs and the thymus gland boosting the immune system. This pose also stretches the intestines and abdominal organs and is useful for alleviating all kinds of abdominal disorders. It relieves constipation and piles. It encourages deep respiration and helps in asthma and bronchitis. It purifies the stagnant blood in the neck and the back and thus alleviates backache and spondylitis. It regulates the function of the thyroid gland which can combat stress. This also helps in reducing disorders of the reproductive system. It relieves sore throat or tonsillitis. It increases youthfulness and vitality.

Psychological Benefits—This prepares you for new challenges and develops your sixth sense and intuitive power. This also nourishes your spiritual quest.

Contraindications—People suffering from heart disease, peptic ulcer, hernia, severe back problems and during pregnancy.

Value Addition—Why do you need a Guru or a Mentor?

> **Thought for the Day**
>
> The fifth precept of 'Niyama' is 'Ishwar Pranidhaan' meaning the 'total surrender' to the Almighty by surrendering ego-driven activities to the Ultimate Power of this Universe and living constantly with an awareness of the Divine Presence.

18   Supta Vakrasan or Udarkarshanasan (The Spinal Twist Posture)

1. *With both legs on one side on the floor* 2. *With one knee inside the angle of the other knee*

Aim—To twist the spine to relieve pain and stiffness in the spine.

Time Span—Two to three minutes.

Technique—(I) Lie on the back. Make sure your head, torso and legs are in one line. Keep your arms by your sides. Inhale and stretch your arms sideways. Exhale and adjust them to the shoulder level. Inhale, bend and raise your knees, bringing them closer to your abdomen. Exhale, twist the lower torso, dropping both the knees on the right side. Inhale and try to cuddle up and pull your knees towards the right elbow. Exhale and drop your head to the left side. Feel the twist in the spine. Breathe four times in this position.

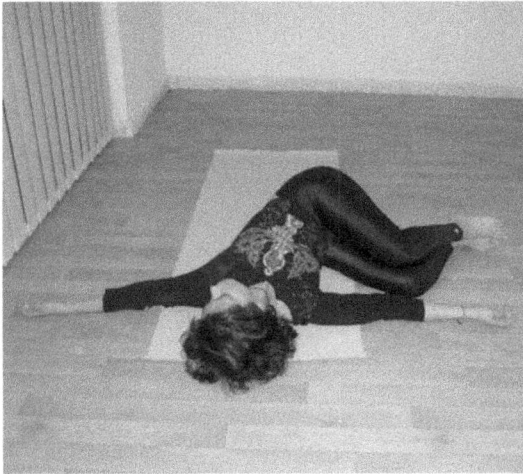

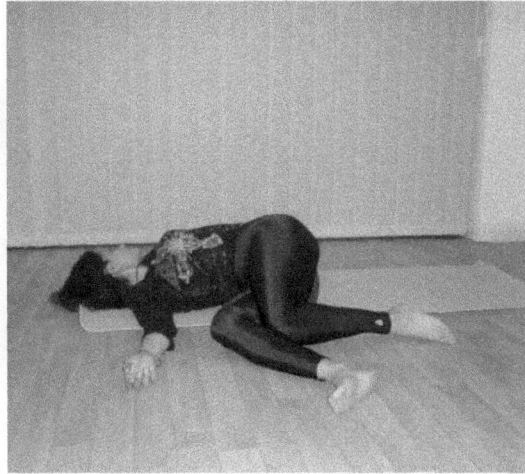

Coming Out of the Pose—Inhale and bring your head in the centre. Exhale and release the knees slowly away from the right elbow. Inhale, raise the knees and twisting back your lower torso, bring the knees close to your abdomen. Exhale and stretch your legs back to the normal position. Inhale and adjust your position in one line. Exhale and bring your arms by your sides in the initial position.

(II) From position–I and before coming out of the pose—Slowly slide down your left knee from your right knee and place it on the floor in the nook of the right knee. Breathe four times. Repeat with the other side.

Focus—On breathing and twisting the spine effectively.

Breathing Pattern—Normal.

Physical Benefits—This twist balances the energy on both sides of the spine and relieves pain and stiffness in the spine. This also tones the abdominal muscles and internal organs and thereby helps digestion and elimination.

Psychological Benefits—The twist teaches re-adjustment in thinking. This makes you more sensitive, more conscious and more aware of your body and mind, your feelings, emotions and your very nature. As sensitivity increases, you can savour each individual moment with awareness and you can taste the unique flavour of each experience or situation. You are prepared to handle life's endless dilemmas elegantly, without feeling overwhelmed or fearful.

Contraindications—People suffering from serious neck or back conditions, severe arthritis or osteoporosis of the spine, sciatica, slipped disc or dislocation in the hip joint.

Value Addition—While chasing your dreams and ambitions, make sure you do not end up perpetually wanting more.

Thought for the Day

Chasing success is like trying to squeeze a handful of water. The tighter you squeeze the lesser the water you get.

---

19   Supta Kati Chakrasan
(The Reclining Side Stretch—
Popularly known as the Banana Posture)

Aim—Is to soften the ribs and the ribcage from each side which helps in more advanced poses.

Time Span—Two to three minutes.

Technique—Inhale and lie on the floor on your back (supine or face up position) with legs apart. Exhale and fold your hands under the nape of the neck. Inhale and cross your left leg over your right ankle. Exhale and slide your legs to the right side as much as you can, simultaneously sliding your torso and head to the right side bringing the elbow downward, pointing toward the right foot. Breathe four times.

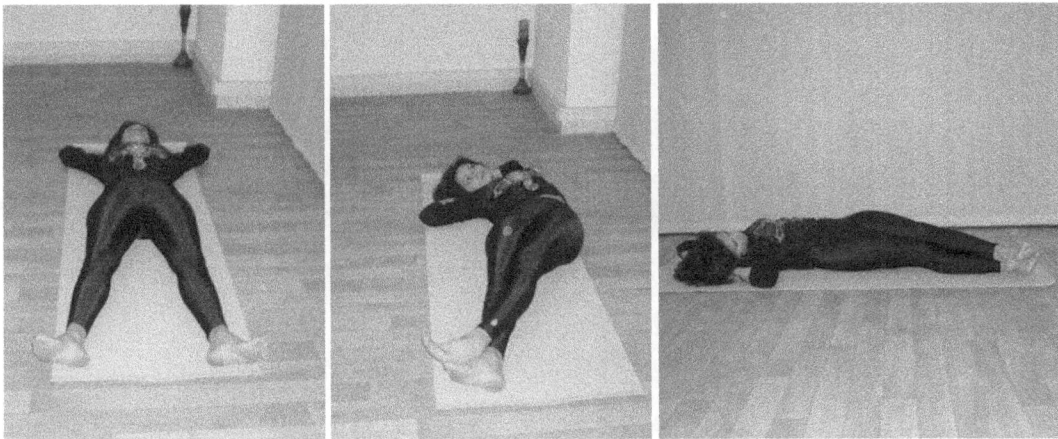

Coming Out of the Pose—Inhale and adjust your head and torso and bring them back to the centre position. Exhale and release your left leg from the right leg keeping your legs apart as in the initial position. Repeat with the other side.

Focus—On breathing and maintaining the sideways stretch.

Breathing Pattern—Normal and steady.

Physical Benefits—This pose softens and strengthens the ribs and the ribcage from each side. There is a lengthening or stretching effect on the ribs bringing in fresh prana energy into the obliques which usually are not used.

Psychological Benefits—This pose has an effect on the mind as it softens and smoothens out the rough edges of the mind or mindset. This improves your capacity to look at the larger picture as you broaden your mental horizon and no longer remain petty minded.

Contraindications—People suffering from any acute hip joint, lower back or spine disorders.

Value Addition—Group discussion on what comes in the way of your courage— Fear or conformity?

Thought for the Day

The antonym of courage is conformity and not cowardice.

Supta Baddha Konasan
(The Sleeping Baby or Butterfly Posture)

Aim—To stretch the spine and to open the hip joint.

Time Span—Two to three minutes.

Technique—Lie on the back (supine or face up position) with legs comfortably apart. Keep your arms by your sides. Inhale, bend your knees with your feet on the floor. Exhale and drop your knees sideways bringing the soles of your feet together (heel to heel and sole to sole). Inhale and keep your palms on either side of your navel. Exhale. Breathe four times. Inhale and stretch your arms overhead and fold your hands under the nape of the neck and feel the stretch in the spine.

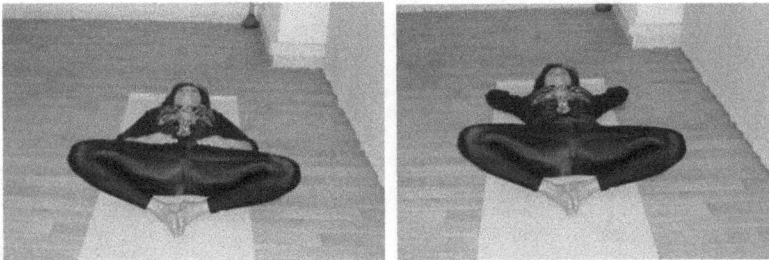

Focus—On breathing normally and relaxing the body.

Breathing Pattern—Normal and steady.

Physical Benefits—This is a very gentle form of relaxation. It opens all the chakra systems and brings in fresh prana energy.

Psychological Benefits—It calms you down. You begin to feel feather-light like a butterfly and calm like a baby.

Contraindications—Generally nil but if you are in doubt, refrain from doing it.

Value Addition—For one week from now, watch everyone who enters into your life and check whether he/she comes with a cause or a purpose and then learn to apply that significance to your life.

Thought for the Day

View everyone who comes into your life as a teacher or a divine messenger.

Supta Konasan
(The Wide Angle Triangle Posture)

Aim—To learn body balance and coordination.

Time Span—Two to three minutes.

Technique—From Halasan or the Plough Pose, inhale and stretch your legs apart. Exhale and release the hands supporting your back. Inhale and stretch your arms wide at the shoulder level and then slide them slightly upward to grab each foot. Breathe four times in this position and settle down. Keep the head on the floor all throughout. Do not bring pressure on your neck. Try to switch your weight towards your legs which will ease the pressure on your neck.

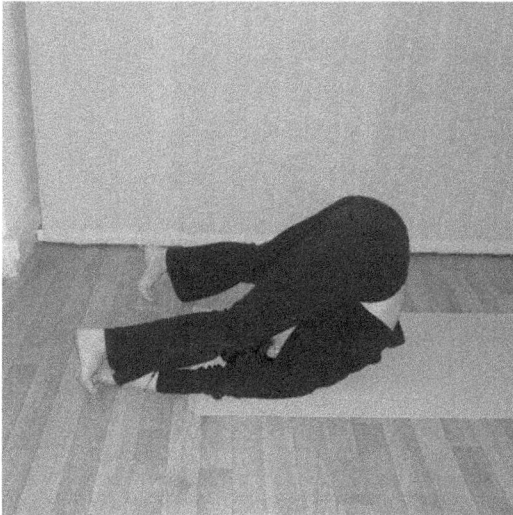

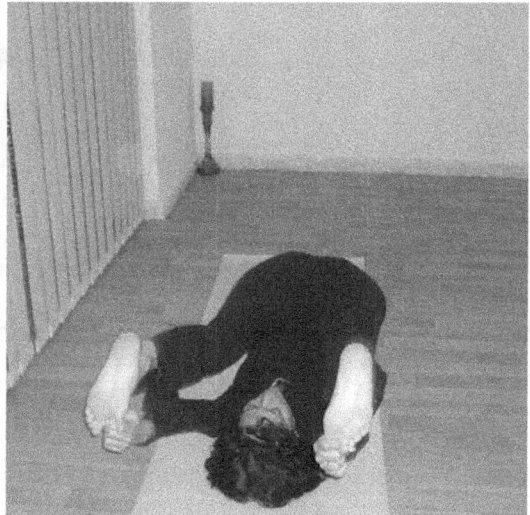

Coming Out of the Pose—Inhale and free your hands releasing your feet and slide your arms downward to support your back. Exhale and bring your feet together in the Halasan or the Plough pose. Inhale and get ready to come out of the pose. Exhale, bend and bring the knees down towards the torso. Inhale and lower the torso to the floor, keeping the legs bent. Exhale, lower and straighten your legs on the floor. Simultaneously, release the hand support from the back and keep your hands by your sides.

Focus—On relaxing the neck and back muscles and shifting the entire body weight towards the legs and feet.

Breathing Pattern—Normal and steady.

Physical Benefits—The pressure that is put on the diaphragm massages the internal organs. It activates digestion, relieves constipation, revitalises the renal glands, spleen and the pancreas which enhances the production of insulin. This also strengthens the spine, its connective tissues and the back muscles. It tones the spinal nerves and also lung meridians. This pose nurtures and rejuvenates the immune system. This also regulates the thyroid gland and balances the body's metabolic rate.

This pose increases circulation in the knees and imparts suppleness and vitality. Releases tension in the neck and throat which alleviates phlegm and mucus in the sinuses and respiratory system. This is a general antidote for allergies, asthma, bronchitis, urinary tract disorders or menstrual problems. It activates the thymus gland and keeps the body's resistance generally high.

Psychological Benefits—This pose helps you plough through your past experiences and allows you to sweep away negative emotions. You begin to break up hard lumps of strife and sorrow in your life through wisdom and dedication. You remove past obstacles or painful memories from the mind. You also do not get bowled over by praise, recognition, success or wealth. By practising it regularly you discipline yourself by analysing your 'self' that serves as manure to your individual growth and soon you flow towards divine inspiration.

Contraindications—People suffering from hernia, slipped disc, sciatica, high blood pressure, vertigo, or any serious back problem especially arthritis or osteoporosis.

Value Addition—When you find that yoga has transformed you physically and mentally, you are moving towards higher awareness.

Thought for the Day
If you are stumbling along in the dark, light your path with the flame from your inner cadle of yoga.

22

Supta Janushirasan
(Assessing the Strength of Your Legs)

Aim—To assess and use the strength of one leg to push the other leg.

Time Span—Two to three minutes.

Technique—Lie on the floor with your legs stretched out together. Make sure your head, torso and the legs are in one line on the floor. Inhale, bend the right leg keeping the right foot on the floor. Exhale and bend the left leg keeping the left foot on the right knee. Keep your arms on the floor by your sides. Inhale, raise and press with your right knee, bringing your left foot closer to the torso using the strength of your right leg. Exhale and lower your right foot taking your left foot away from your torso.

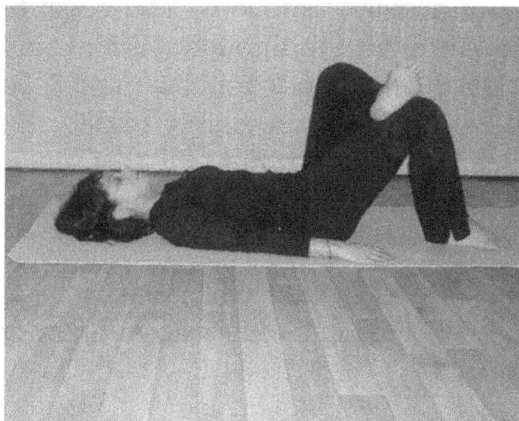

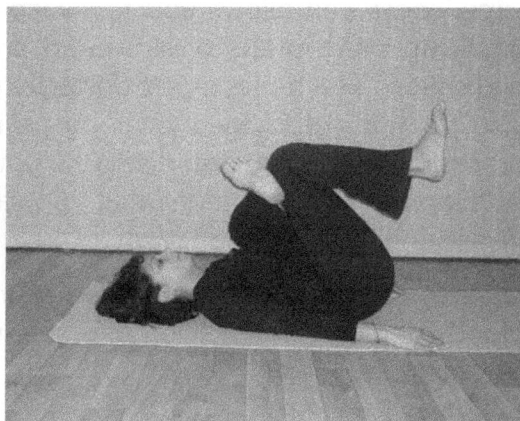

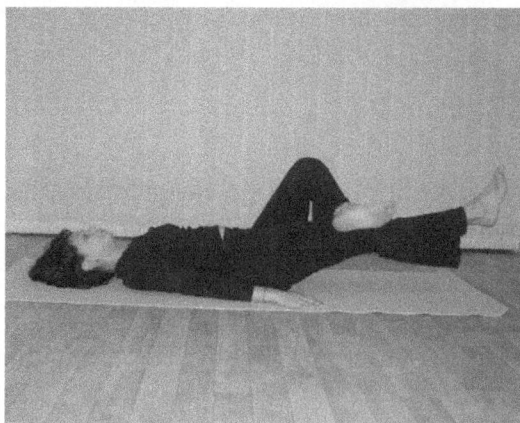

If you wish to challenge your body further, inhale and raise your head and bring it closer to the right foot. Exhale and lower your left leg and stretch it all the way, parallel to the floor.

Coming Out of the Pose—Inhale and lower your right leg and rest your right foot on the floor. Exhale and release your left foot from the right knee and place your left foot on the floor. Inhale. Exhale and stretch both legs back to the normal position.

Repeat with the other side.

Focus—On breathing and synchronising the leg movement.

Breathing Pattern—Rhythmic.

Physical Benefits—Crossing each leg brings equal pressure on either side of the abdomen and the colon and relieves constipation. It brings fresh prana energy which stimulates the spleen on the left side and the liver on the right side which start functioning better. It activates the energy around the knees and makes the knees strong and flexible. The lower part of the spine (lumbar region) also gets rejuvenated. The legs become strong and you feel energetic at once.

Psychological Benefits—It is believed that it has a favourable effect on 'sense-withdrawal' (pratyahara) which leads you to better health and harmony, peace and prosperity.

Contraindications—People suffering from acute backache or knee problems, pregnancy.

Value Addition—From now on change your attitude: check similarities between you and others, instead of comparing yourself with others and trying to find out what is common. That will give you tremendous peace of mind.

> ### *Thought for the Day*
> You are in a partnership with all other human beings and not in a contest to be judged better than some and worse than others.

23 Suchirandhrasan
(The Thread and The Needle Hip Stretch)

Aim—To bring fresh prana energy to your knees for better protection.

Time Span—Two to three minutes.

Technique—This is an extension of the 'Supta Janushirasan Pose.'

Lie on the floor with your legs stretched out together. Make sure your head, torso and the legs are in one line on the floor. Inhale, bend the right leg keeping the right foot on the floor. Exhale and bend the left leg keeping the left foot on the right knee. Keep your arms on the floor by your sides. Inhale, raise and press with your right knee, bringing your left foot closer to the torso using the strength of your right leg. Inhale and insert your right hand through the space between your legs interlocking fingers with your left hand folded around the left leg. Exhale and clasp the back of your left thigh with both hands and pull the left thigh towards your torso. At the same time, inhale and raising your head, use your right elbow to lightly press your right thigh away from yourself and bring your left foot closer to your forehead. Exhale and hold the pose for four breaths.

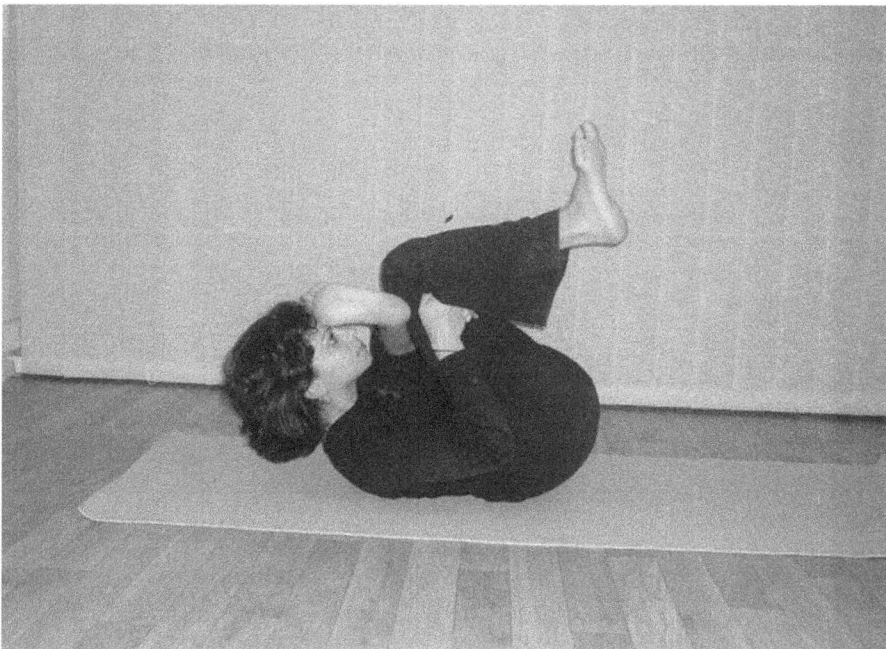

Coming Out of the Pose—Inhale, release your hands and place them by your sides. Exhale and lower your right leg, resting your right foot on the floor. Inhale and uncross your left leg, placing your left foot on the floor. Exhale and stretch both legs back to the normal position.

Repeat with the other side.

Focus—On breathing steadily and opening the hip area for the external rotation.

Breathing Pattern—Normal and steady.

Physical Benefits—This hip-opener pose energises the hip area, pelvic plexus and the knees. Crossing each leg brings equal pressure on either side of the abdomen and the colon and relieves constipation. It also relieves pressure on the knees and repairs their wear and tear. It brings fresh prana energy to the spleen on the left side and the liver on the right side stimulating them to function better. It activates the energy around the knees and makes the knees strong and flexible. The lower part of the spine (lumbar region) also gets rejuvenated. The legs become strong and you feel energetic at once. It alleviates urinary disorders by strengthening the urinary structures. It opens the hip joint, relieving pressure on the knees. Your thighs and hip remain slim and firm.

Psychological Benefits—Since this pose brings pressure on the pelvis plexus and the solar plexus it removes eating disorders.

Contraindications—People suffering from acute backache or knee problems, pregnancy.

Value Addition—Exercise the concept of 'forget and forgive' for one week and see whether you feel triumphant.

Thought for the Day

Forgiveness is the most powerful thing you can do for yourself. If you cannot learn to forgive, you can forget about achieving true success in your life.

24

Chaturanga Dandasan
(The Lying Staff Posture—Yogic Push-ups)

Aim—To strengthen your wrists, the spine and the abdominal organs.

Time Span—Two to three minutes.

Technique—Begin as in the Bhujangasan or the Cobra Pose by lying on the floor in prone (face down) position. The only difference is that you cross your right ankle over your left ankle. Inhale and raise your head and torso. Lock your elbows and let your hands take the weight of your body. Raise your entire upper body up to your knees. (The knees should be on the floor but your crossed legs should be raised upward). Exhale and lower the upper body in the initial position. Repeat this for four times and relax for one breath (inhalation and exhalation). Repeat the same by crossing your left ankle over the right ankle.

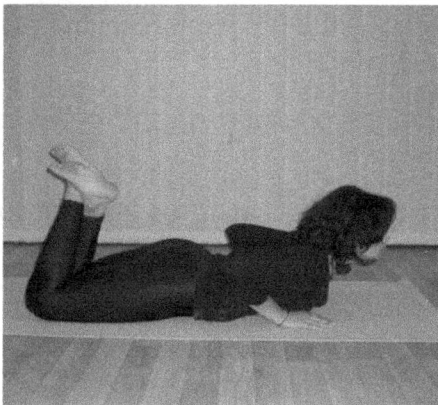

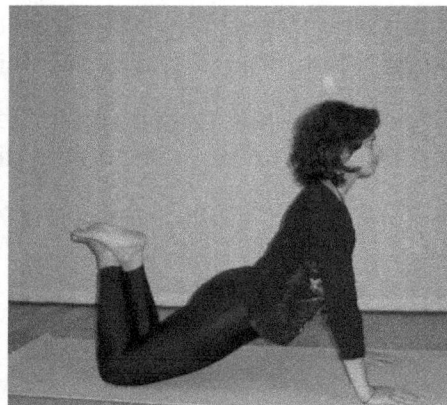

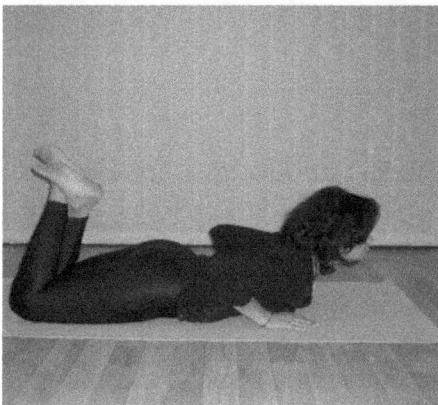

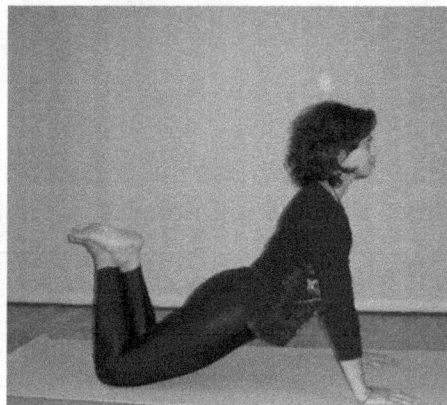

Coming Out of the Pose—Inhale and uncross ankles. Exhale and bring the whole body back into the normal (prone) position like in the Cobra Pose. Inhale and keep the arms by your sides and exhale and rest on the forehead or by turning your head to one side.

Focus—On synchronising your breath with each movement.

Breathing Pattern—Ujjayi breathing.

Physical Benefits—It strengthens and tones the abdominal muscles. When your abdominal muscles become strong, it relieves you off backaches. It also helps to develop flexible and powerful wrists and arms. It rejuvenates the entire body and makes you feel fit and light.

Psychological Benefits—This rids you off inertia. It also helps in relieving anxiety and mental fatigue and boosts your confidence level.

Contraindications—Sprained wrists or ankles, severe neck or back problems, pregnancy.

Value Addition—Be in the 'Present Moment' and 'Today' you can love, dream, work and rest and above all experience joy and peace.

Thought for the Day

Do you know that there are two days in your life that you can do nothing about: one is 'Yesterday' and the other is 'Tomorrow.'

25

Supta Meru Vakrasan
(Lying Spine Twist)

Aim—To make your spine strong and supple.

Time Span—Two to three minutes on each side.

Technique—Lie on the floor in supine or face up position with legs stretched straight in the centre. Inhale and stretch your arms sideways on the floor at shoulder level. Exhale and bend the knees keeping the feet on the floor. Inhale and cross your right leg completely over your left leg/knee. Exhale and drop your knees onto the floor to the right side. Inhale and turn your head to the opposite side i.e. to the left. Exhale and remain in the pose for four breaths. Inhale and bring the head back to the centre. Exhale and swing your crossed legs to the right side on the floor. Inhale and turn your head to the opposite side i.e. to the left side. Exhale and remain in the pose for four breaths.

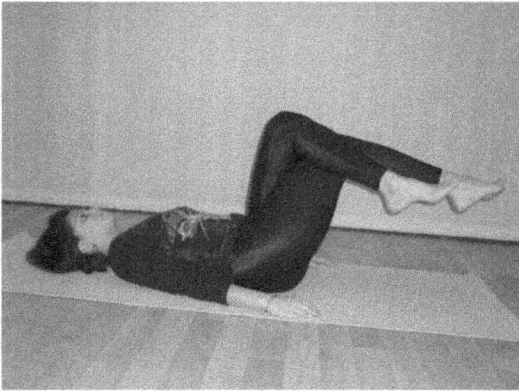

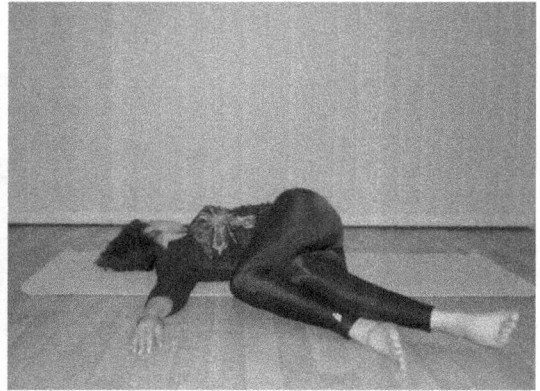

Coming Out of the Pose—Inhale and first bring your head to the centre. Exhale and uncross your legs and keep the feet on the floor. Inhale and bring the arms into the normal position by your sides. Exhale, straighten and stretch your legs back as in the starting position.

Repeat the same steps by crossing your left leg over the right.

Focus—On breathing and gently twisting the spine as much as you can.

Breathing Pattern—Slow and steady.

Physical Benefits—It makes your spine flexible which in turn makes your thinking flexible. Releases tension in the inter-vertebral muscles and keeps the spine healthy and elastic, relieves backache and hip-joint pain, strengthens the neck, opens the chest and shoulders. Revitalises the abdominal/vital organs and helps in alleviating the bladder, ovarian and uterine problems. It helps in diabetes, digestive and urinary disorders.

Psychological Benefits—Brings a change for the better in your perception and perspective. It also balances the chakra energy, the excess energy being redistributed to the other side of the chakra.

Contraindications—Acute knee pain or unstable knees, hip joint pain, hip injury or inflammation, lower back pain or shoulder injury, bursitis, peptic ulcers, hernia, hyperthyroid, sciatica, slipped disc, pregnancy (specially during the second and third trimesters). However, when done under expert guidance, it in fact helps with many of the above ailments.

Value Addition—Think about how many times you considered yourself lucky or unlucky and how you can change it now.

Thought for the Day

Lucky people do not necessarily have the best of everything; they are the ones who make the most of whatever life throws at them and swing it to their advantage.

26

Supta Garudasan
(The Eagle Posture)

Aim—To prepare for the standing version of Garudasan.

Time Span—Two to three minutes.

Technique—Begin as in the Lying Spine Twist or Meru Vakrasan. Inhale, bend your knees and keep your feet on the floor. Exhale, cross your right leg over the left and tuck your right foot under your left knee/calf. Inhale and bring your arms closer to your torso by joining your palms in Namaste position. Exhale, wrap your right hand around your left, once again in Namaste position. Breathe four times keeping the head, torso and the legs in one line.

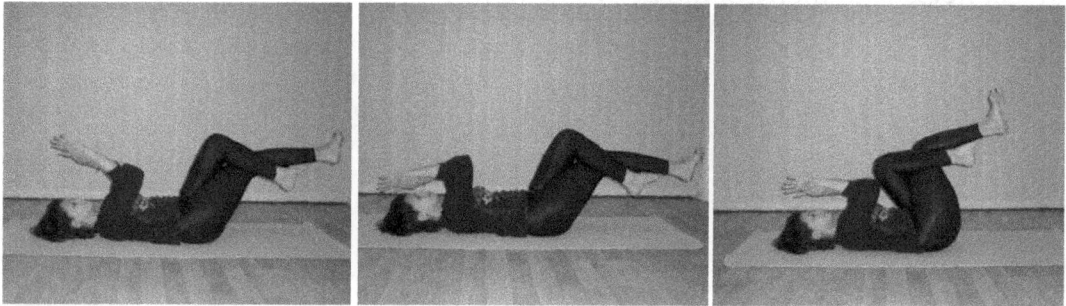

Coming Out of the Pose—Inhale and unwrap your hands. Exhale and keep the arms down on the floor by your sides. Inhale and uncross your legs. Exhale and keep the feet on the floor with knees bent. Repeat the same steps using the opposite limbs.

Focus—On intertwining the legs and the arms.

Breathing Pattern—Normal and steady.

Physical Benefits—This lengthens the deep hip rotators and the illotibial band (at the outside of the thigh), relieving stress on the outer knee. Putting pressure on any one limb is one of the best ways to strengthen the limbs.

Psychological Benefits—Like the eagle's eye, your mental vision becomes sharp by bringing a change for the better in your perception and perspective. It also balances the chakra energies.

Contraindications—Acute knee pain or unstable knees, hip joint pain, hip injury or inflammation, lower back pain or shoulder injury, bursitis, peptic ulcers, hernia, hyper thyroid, sciatica, slipped disc, pregnancy (specially during second and third trimesters). However, when done under expert guidance, it in fact helps with many of the above ailments.

Value Addition—Check whether you can learn from every experience and every person that you meet.

Thought for the Day
If you want peace, work for justice.

Ardha Dhanurasan–I, II and Dhanurasan (The One Legged Bow Posture–I, II and The Simple Bow Posture)

27

Aim—To prepare yourself for the more advanced postures.

Time Span—Two to three minutes for each posture.

Technique—(I) Lie on the floor in prone (face-down) position and keep your feet together. Inhale and fold your left elbow in front of you on the floor. Exhale and fold the right leg resting your foot on the right hip. Inhale, stretch your right hand behind you and hold the right ankle. Exhale and keeping your left leg straight on the floor, raise the body supported by the left elbow and palm. Inhale and raise the torso still further. Exhale and settle down in the pose. Breathe four times. This is the milder version for those with stiff or weak backs. Repeat the steps with the other side.

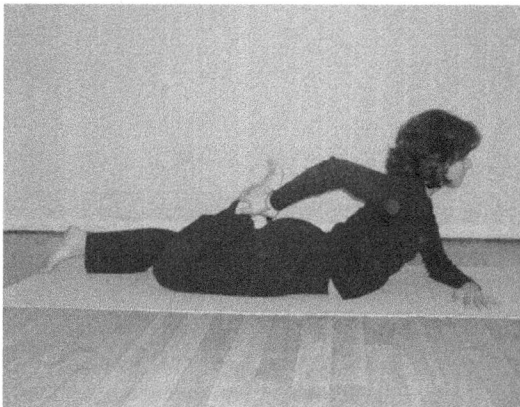

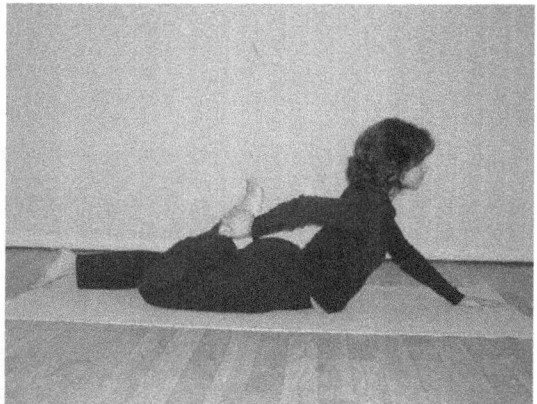

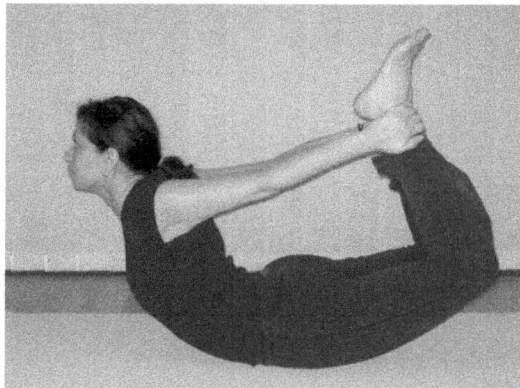

(II) The next version is to straighten the supporting hand, locking the elbow and pushing against the floor to raise the torso. Raise the torso as in the 'Upward Facing Dog' pose. Breathe four times. Repeat the steps with the other side.

(III) In the actual Bow pose, both legs are lifted and held by the corresponding hands, arching the body inversely. Breathe four times in this position.

Coming Out of the Pose—Inhale, release and lower the ankles onto the floor and keep the hands by your side. Exhale and lower the torso back onto the floor.

Focus—On breathing and lifting the leg by the ankle.

Breathing Pattern—Slow and deep.

Physical Benefits—This is a recommended therapy for lower back pain due to slipped disc or cervical spondylitis but should be done under expert guidance or supervision. This pose tones the heart and lungs and is beneficial for all respiratory disorders. The liver, abdominal organs, pancreas, kidneys and adrenal glands are toned and massaged and their secretion is regulated. This is an excellent therapy for diabetes, dyspepsia, chronic constipation, colitis, menstrual disorders and incontinence.

Psychological Benefits—This is excellent for improving your balance, concentration, coordination, confidence, reflexes and your mood.

Pose-II and III are very intense and powerful poses to open the heart centre whereby your emotions are generously expressed especially to the deserving people in your life. Also, certain negative emotions are regulated in such a way that you express them discreetly without hurting anyone but at the same time conveying your feelings. Since it energises the thymus gland, your improved immune system gives a great feeling of confidence and vigour to take up new challenges.

Contraindications—People suffering from heart ailments, high blood pressure, hernia, colitis, peptic or duodenal ulcers. It should not be done before going to bed as it stimulates the adrenal glands and sympathetic nervous system.

Value Addition—Keep a dream diary and write down all the dreams and see whether you can interpret them on the basis of situations in your life.

Thought for the Day

Confession of an error is like vacuuming away dust and dirt from the mental frame.

---

28 Supta-Tadasan and Vrikshasan (The Sleeping Palm Tree and Tree Posture)

Aim—To strengthen the muscles and bones of the limbs which makes balancing poses easier to perform.

Time Span—Two to three minutes on each side.

Technique—This is like the Palm Tree Pose or Tadasan but the only difference is that it is done in the lying down (supine or face up) position. Keep your legs stretched together and the arms by your sides. Inhale, point your toes and simultaneously raise your arms upward on the floor over the head. Exhale and bring the arms down by your side and flex your toes. Repeat this four times.

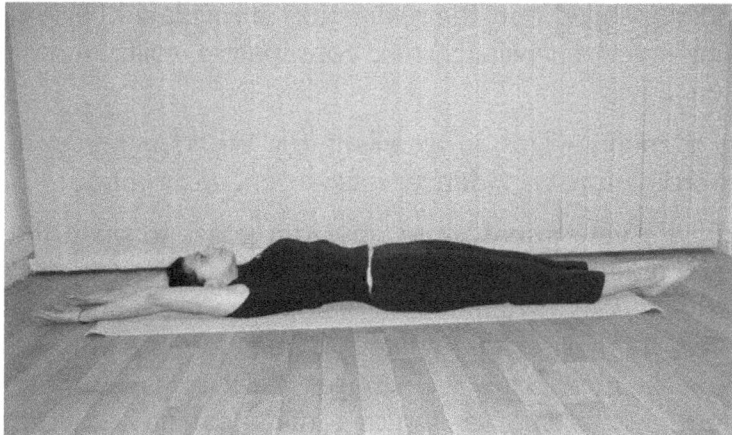

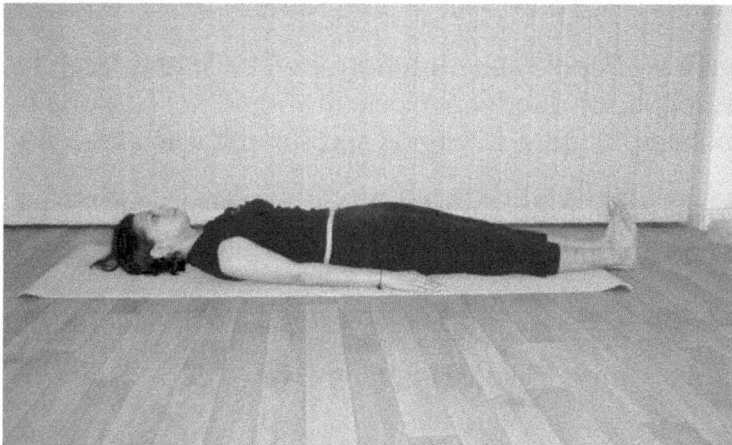

Coming Out of the Pose—Inhale and relax your toes and exhale and bring your arms back to the normal position.

Focus—On proper synchronisation of breath with the specific movement.

Breathing Pattern—Normal and steady.

Physical Benefits—To stimulate digestion and to remove constipation. It improves blood circulation and strengthens the muscles and the bones of the limbs which helps improve balance.

Psychological Benefits—Improves your ability to take independent or the right decisions quickly. When mastered this pose will help you to be self-reliant.

Contraindications—People with sciatica, slipped disc, hernia, very weak legs or high blood pressure and pregnancy.

Value Addition—Think of all the good things people have done for you so far.

Thought for the Day
If at any moment you think that you are unlucky, be assured that whatever 'bad' you received, is a discounted punishment from God.

Jeevan Chakrasan (Forward) and Kaal Chakrasan (Sideways) (The Complete Circle of Life—Forward and The Daily Cycle of Day and Night—Sideways)

29

Aim—To strengthen all the muscles and bones in the lower body and especially the hip joint.

Time Span—Four to five minutes.

Technique—(Forward Circle)—Lie on the floor with legs and feet together in the supine or face up position. Keep your arms by your sides or your hands under the hips for support. Bend your knees and bring them on to your torso. Inhale and raise your legs at 90 degrees angle. Exhale, lower the legs without touching the floor, then bend and bring the knees back on to the torso, drawing a circle with your legs or slow-cycling with both legs simultaneously. Repeat this cycle for four times.

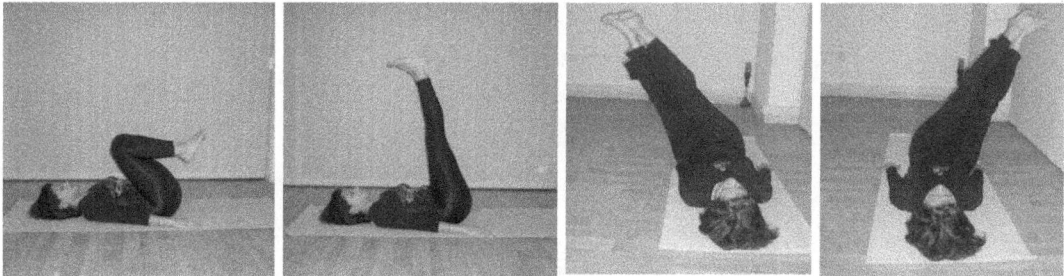

(Sideways Circle)—Continue with the supine position. Imagine your legs are the hands of the clock and you begin with 6 O' clock. Keeping your legs straight, inhale and raising both the legs together, move them clockwise upward up to 12 O'clock (at 90 degrees). Exhale and bring them down from the right side up to 6 O'clock. Without touching the floor, draw this circle four times with your feet. Repeat the same in counter-clockwise circles i.e. inhale and raise your feet from the right side upward at 90 degrees and exhale and bring them down from the left side. Repeat this cycle for four times and finally keep the legs down in the starting position.

Coming Out of the Pose—Inhale, straighten and raise your legs. Exhale and lower your legs on the floor.

Focus—On breathing and making each round of vertical and horizontal circles (clockwise and counter-clockwise).

Breathing Pattern—Slow and steady.

Physical Benefits—This is excellent for the hip joint, reducing obesity around the abdomen and thighs. It tones the abdominal and spinal muscles which relieves lower backaches. This improves the condition of the knees and the hamstring muscles which have the habit of contracting with age or stress. By stretching them fully, they remain strong and supple.

Psychological Benefits—The vertical cycle gives you an insight into the circle of life and its four phases, starting from the childhood phase in the form of bending the knees, adulthood in the form of straightening the legs at 90 degrees, the midlife phase in the form of the downward or descending movement of the legs and the old age in the form of legs coming closer to the floor but not touching the feet to the floor as it is an ongoing process of life.

The horizontal cycle is the daily cycle of day and night which enlightens you with the fact of life that the day and night are the two sides of the same coin which balance our inner force with solar energy and lunar energy and that both are equally important for our existence.

Contraindications—Stomach cramps, hip joint dislocation, severe knee ailments, pregnancy.

Value Addition—While standing or sitting, roll a tennis ball under the soles of the feet. This is very effective in massaging the sensitive 'soles' and sensitive 'souls'.

Thought for the Day

No amount of negativity can ever succeed against unconditional love, honesty and truth.

Viparita Karani
(The Inverted Seal Posture)

Aim—To strengthen and relax the entire body.

Time Span—Two to three minutes.

Technique—This inverted, restorative pose is a milder form of the Shoulder Stand or the Plough Pose with a difference as it can be done with or without the support of a wall and the chin is not pressed on the chest. The legs are stretched up at 90 degrees but the torso is at an angle of 45 degrees to the floor. When you perform this pose with the support of the wall, it can be done as a relaxing therapy with a specific technique. Sit with one side of the body touching and making a right angle to the wall i.e. in such a way that your right hip touches the wall and then swing your legs up the wall, i.e. Swivel, raise and move your legs along the wall and lie on the floor perpendicular to the wall, with head firmly rested on the floor. Keep your arms by your sides or on either side of the navel.

Breathe four times.

Without the support of the wall: Lie flat on the floor in a supine or face-up position. Keep your legs stretched straight, in line with your head and torso. Keep your arms by your sides. Inhale and hold the lower back with your hands. Exhale and relax the body. Inhale and raise both legs along with the hips and the lower back with the help of your hand support. Exhale and roll the spine in such a way that the shoulders should take the entire body weight. Keeping the elbows on the floor let the torso remain at the 45 degrees angle and the legs at 90 degrees angle from the floor. Breathe four times.

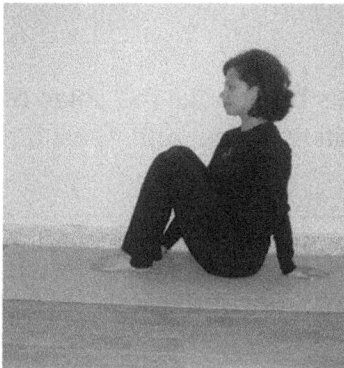

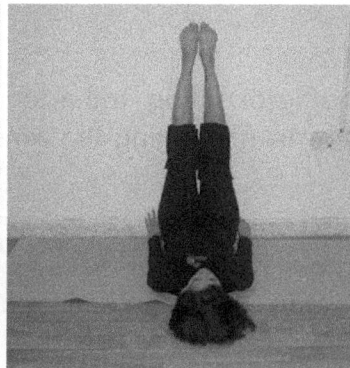

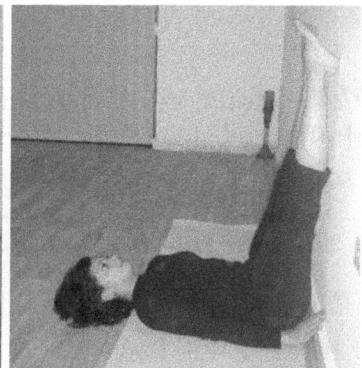

Coming Out of the Pose—Inhale and get ready to come out of the pose. Exhale, bend your knees and lower the legs. Inhale once more. Exhale and rest the hips and the lower back on the floor. Inhale and release the hands from the hips/lower back. Exhale and stretch the legs back to the normal position.

Focus—Keeping the legs up and relaxing the body.

Breathing Pattern—Normal and steady.

Physical Benefits—Since this pose is a milder version of the Shoulder Stand Pose or the Plough Pose, most of the benefits are similar. This pose stimulates the thyroid gland and promotes the circulatory, digestive, reproductive, nervous and endocrine systems. It also stimulates the thymus gland and boosts the immune system. It supplies oxygenated blood to the brain. It has a tranquilising effect on the mind. It relieves you from emotional stress, mental fatigue, fear and headaches. It regenerates bones and prevents premature calcification. It massages the abdominal organs. It releases the normal gravitational force from the anal muscles, giving relief from haemorrhoids. It tones the muscles of the legs, abdomen and reproductive organs, draining the stagnant blood and fluid. It revitalises the ears, eyes and relieves any throat or nose ailments. It is recommended for asthma, diabetes, colitis, impotency, hydrocele, prolapsed uterus, menopause, menstrual disorders, common cold, cough and flu.

Psychological Benefits—This pose lightens the body and enlightens the mind.

In this pose, the level of the head is lowered below the level of the heart which activates your heart centre. This is the first time you allow your heart to express itself and you will be amazed to see that sometimes your suppressed or frozen emotions are thawed and you expand your affection towards some truly deserving people in your life.

Contraindications—People suffering from enlarged thyroid, liver or spleen, cervical spondylitis, slipped disc, high blood pressure, heart disease, nervous problem, very weak eyes, glaucoma, during menstruation or pregnancy.

Value Addition—Have you tried to understand your body language any time? Body language has a lot to do with your expressions and emotions. Try to recognise your emotional map through your body language.

Thought for the Day

All your issues are in your body tissues.

297

31

Urdhwa Naukasan
(Namaste in the Boat Posture)

Aim—To work on the entire spine.

Time Span—Two to three minutes.

Technique—Lie on the back in the supine position with the arms by your sides. Inhale and raise your legs to a 45 degrees angle and the head at a 20 degrees angle, off the floor. Exhale and bring the legs in the centre. Inhale and join the palms firmly in Namaste position. Breathe four times.

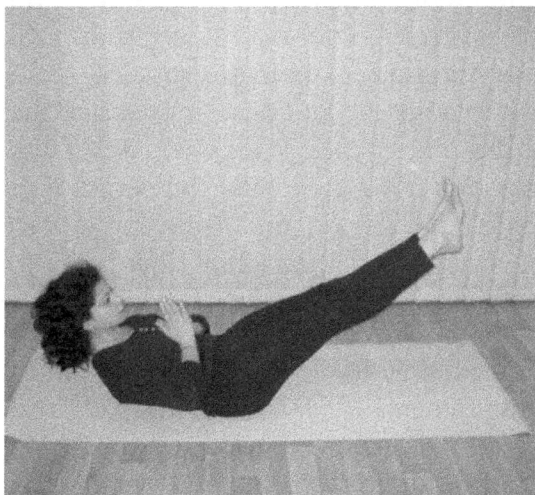

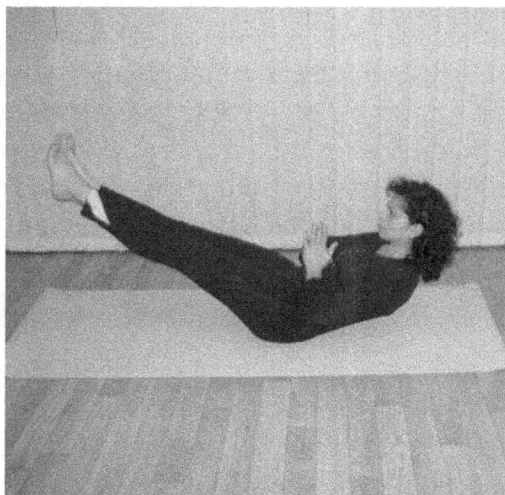

Coming Out of the Pose—Inhale and release the palms and keep your hands/arms by your sides in the normal position. Exhale and lower your legs and head to rest them on the floor as in the initial position.

Focus—On ujjayi breathing and maintaining the pose.

Breathing Pattern—Ujjayi breathing.

Physical Benefits—This pose stimulates the muscular, digestive, circulatory, nervous and endocrine systems, tones all the organs and activates all the energy centres by eliminating energy blockages. This has a positive effect on the pelvic plexus (groins) and the solar plexus (abdomen) and improves the functions especially for regulating the menstrual cycle.

Psychological Benefits—It removes lethargy, nervous tension, induces good sleep at night and relaxation. If done just before the Shavasan Pose, it instils deep relaxation. If done soon after waking up, it keeps you fresh and active throughout the day.

Contraindications—People suffering from any acute neck, shoulder, back or hip joint disorders and during pregnancy but can be performed as a post-natal exercise.

Value Addition—Check your own potential and resourcefulness in order to determine your happiness and success in life.

Thought for the Day

Enjoy everything that happens in your life, but never allow your happiness and success, solely depend on any person, place or thing.

32

Anand-Balasan
(Blissful Baby Posture)

Aim—To make your entire body flexible, especially the spine and the limbs.

Time Span—One to two minutes.

Technique—Lie in supine (face up) position. Inhale and bend the knees and bring them closer to the torso. Exhale, hold your feet with both hands and with feet touching each other, turn the knees outward. This position resembles 'Sleeping Baby or Butterfly Pose'. Inhale, raise your head and legs slightly higher and tuck your hands through the legs and around your ankles. Exhale, and gently pull your legs over the head. This is not an easy pose, requiring great flexibility therefore caution should be taken to remain well within the limit of your flexibility.

Focus—On holding the ankles over the head.

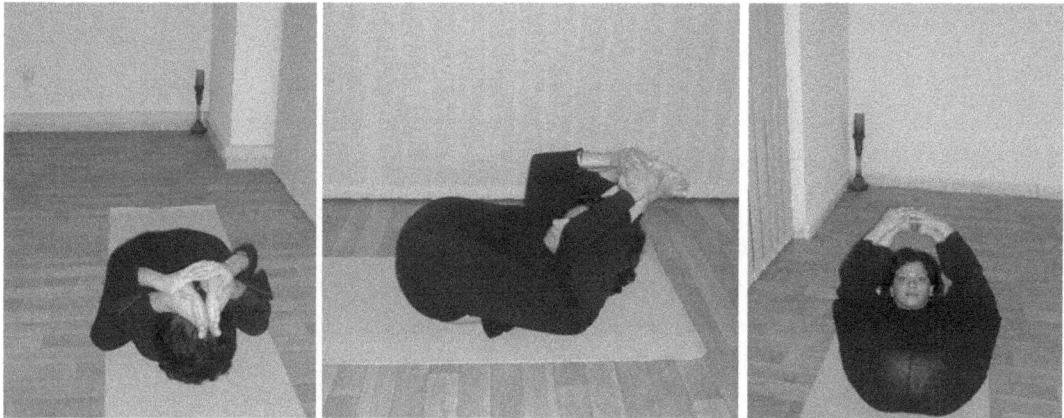

Breathing Pattern—Ujjayi.

Physical Benefits—This strengthens your body's core muscles and emphasises spinal articulation and control that helps you perceive and correct your body's alignment. In this posture, the legs are pulled up right over the head and this stretch helps in contracting the abdominal organs. This improves the circulation in the abdominal organ and has a great impact on the colon which helps in relieving flatulence and constipation. This pose makes the spine extremely flexible. This promotes a sense of balance and creates symmetry between the right and left side of the body. This allows you to compare the strength of both sides and work on them equally.

Psychological Benefits—Usually babies do this all the time when they are growing and they seem very happy as they get good exercise as well as internal massage. This posture teaches balance and coordination and with regular practice calms you down and you begin to feel feather-light like a butterfly and happy like a baby.

Contraindications—Weak knees, neck injury, backache, slipped-disc, pregnancy.

Value Addition—Start a project for children in your neighbourhood.

> ### *Thought for the Day*
>
> There are two ways to slide easily through life: to believe everything or doubt everything; both ways save us from thinking.

33

Ardha-Padmasan
(The Partial Lotus Posture)

Aim—On unwinding and relaxing the stretch of your body.

Time Span—Two to three minutes or more since it is a restorative pose.

Technique—Soon after the Blissful Baby pose, you are required to perform this pose to ease the severe pull on the various body parts. Lie in supine position. Inhale and bend your right knee, bringing it closer to the torso. Exhale and hold the right foot with the left hand and turn the right knee outward, closer to the floor. Inhale and place the right foot on the left thigh or groin. Exhale and turn your head to the left side and simultaneously keeping the right hand stretched out slightly away from your right side. Breathe four times.

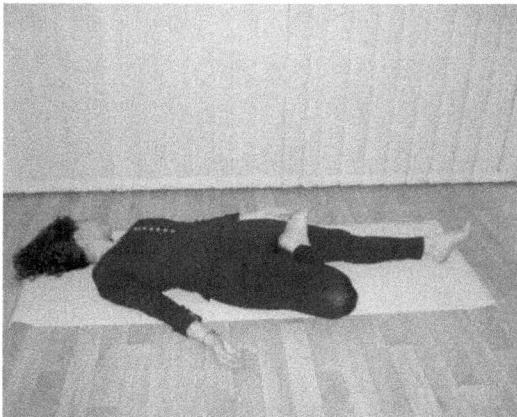

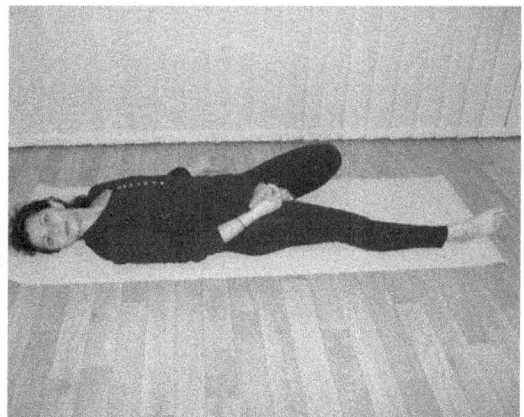

Coming Out of the Pose—Inhale and bring the head back to the centre and simultaneously the right hand back in line with your torso. Exhale and release the right foot and keep the left hand back in the normal position. Inhale and bring the right knee closer to the torso. Exhale and stretch it back to the normal position. Repeat the pose starting with the other leg.

Focus—On opening the hip joint by stretching the knee outward.

Breathing Pattern—Normal and steady.

Physical Benefits—It steadies your nerves from muscular agitation or an intense stretch from the Blissful Baby pose. Since it is done in the lying down position and one leg at a time, it also prepares you physically before you move on to difficult posture like The Lotus Pose. It maintains the flexibility of the bones and bone-density and prevents them from becoming rigid due to old age.

Psychological Benefits—It brings tranquillity to the mind. This heightens the awareness, alertness and the ability to have clarity of the mind and thinking process.

Contraindications—Injured knees or sprained/fractured ankle, slipped disc, severe varicose veins problem.

Value Addition—Plan a schedule for your weekend activities which include personal, social, mental and physical activities and check whether you can stick to it.

> ### Thought for the Day
> When you fail to plan, you plan to fail.

34 Shavasan
(The Pose of Tranquillity—The Corpse Posture)

Each yoga session ought to be concluded with the Classic Corpse Posture (Shavasan). Traditionally, in yogic philosophy it is meant for everyone to be reminded of 'the fact of life' (death) and also realistic about the concept of 'death' which is an inevitable phenomenon of life. "Death is the temporary end of a temporary phenomenon." Death is not the complete annihilation of a being. Death in one place means a birth in another place just like the day in one place means the night in another place. This reminder of death on a daily basis was considered too harsh especially when already depressed yoga practitioners joined yoga with the intention of forgetting certain stressful incidents in their lives. They did not wish to throw themselves back into 'stress mode' soon after the relaxing practice of yoga. The very word or the concept of death is enough to instil fear in them all over again and the purpose of relaxation would be totally defeated. The name 'Corpse Posture', therefore, may be modified into the 'Relaxed Posture' or the 'Pose of Tranquillity'.

Death is a fact of life in classic yoga philosophy and has a different connotation. In 'Shavasan' we symbolically pass on our old ways of thinking and actions to start something new and fresh. The normally perceived boundaries of body image begin to dissolve. We go much beyond the mere word 'death' or shavasan or the dead body pose to look at our body objectively and enter into a state of blissful neutrality. This does total justice to the present by being in the moment. This helps stop our mind from oscillating between the past and future and anchors it in the present.

When you lie down in the relaxed posture for about 5 minutes, deep changes occur at the conscious and subconscious levels. There is a tremendous amount of serenity and inner freedom. The Heart Rate drops to the Resting Heart Rate. Recent studies at many western medical centres have shown clearly that the Relaxation Posture induces marked physiological and psychological changes associated with rest and relaxation of a transforming quality.

The Relaxation Posture done for more than 5 minutes reduces the breathing rate considerably. It also reduces stress, the metabolic rate, oxygen consumption, the concentration of lactic acid in the blood and stabilises blood pressure. Also, Electro Encephalo Graph (EEG) charts show that the Relaxation Posture produces orderly brain patterns of beta and theta waves that are distinct from the patterns that are observed during drowsiness, sleep or sometimes even hypnosis. These effects are associated with very deep rest. You will need to bring yourself back to the ground reality physically, part by part. This can be done by turning to the left or right side and pressing the alternate palm on the floor which serves like earthing and props the body up.

Aim—To relax as well as recharge the whole body, mind and spirit.

Time Span—Five minutes.

Technique—Lie flat on the back with arms and legs stretched out. Keep the arms about 6–8 inches away from either side of your body, palms half closed and facing upward. The feet should be 8–10 inches away from each other. If you feel comfortable increasing the distance between your legs slightly more, you may do so as the length of the legs will determine the distance between each other. However, the legs should not be too wide apart. The head and the torso should be in the centre. Feel comfortable in this position. If not, adjust in such a way that you should be able to sink in that position with ease. Close your eyes and relax. Become aware of your breath and let it follow its own rhythm. Do not force inhalation or exhalation. Just go with the flow. Just focus your attention on your breath and relax the entire body, part by part starting from the feet, heels, soles, ankle joints, calves, shins, knees, thighs, pelvis, hips, lower back, abdomen, waist, torso, upper back, shoulders, arms, hands, wrists, palms, fingers, neck and to the head. Feel each part sinking into the floor and merging with Mother Earth. Feel grounded. Try not to move any part of the body as the slightest movement can cause muscular tension. Now, lie for at least five minutes in this position.

Coming of the Pose—Gently roll your neck from side to side. Wiggle your toes and move your fingers. Fold your right leg and keep the right foot on the floor.

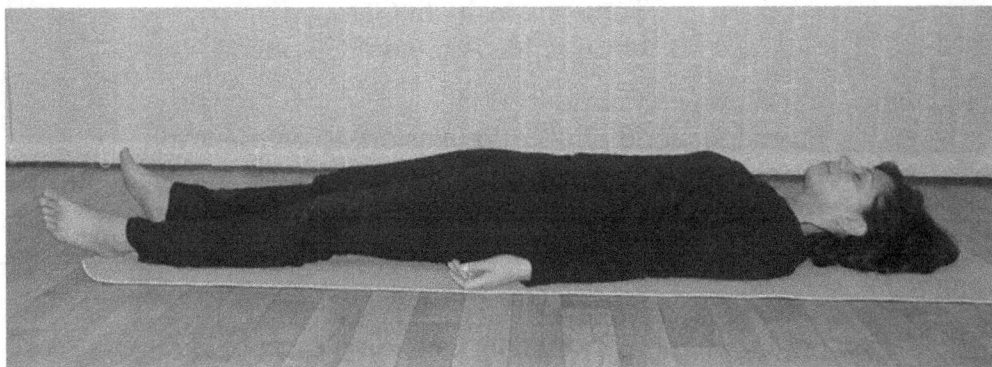

Fold your left leg and keep the left foot on the floor. Bring your knees together. Lift your buttocks slightly and drop your knees to the left side. Turn your torso and head to the left side. Stretch your left arm upward so that you can rest your head on it. Place your right hand on the right hip. Breathe gently for a few seconds. Now, bring your right hand in front of you close to your torso and place your right palm on the floor. Feel the floor with your right palm. Lie in this pose for a few seconds. Press your right palm on the floor for support and push to lift yourself to the sitting position. Sit quietly for a few seconds.

Rub your palms over the head in the energy field of the Crown Chakra (Sahasrara chakra). When you feel your palms warm enough, place them on your closed eyes. Your eyes will absorb this energy from the warmth of your palms which will make you feel relaxed and recharged. You feel revived and renewed. You feel light and happy, strong and healthy. You feel peaceful and blissful.

Focus—On relaxing the entire body and unwinding the mind. On slow and steady breathing.

Breathing Pattern—Slow and steady or natural and rhythmic.

Physical Benefits—This pose is the ultimate in relaxation as the entire psycho-physiological system experiences a sense of tranquillity. This can be performed in between strenuous postures or after a hard day's work. This instils sleep and alleviates insomnia. The relaxation helps develop body and mind awareness and helps you to connect with your pristine inner self (*Antar-atma*) which is devoid of negativity.

Psychological Benefits—This pose instils peace and bliss. Your ego forgets your 'self' and surrenders to the divine.

Contraindications—Nil.

Value Addition—Chant this: Asato Ma Sat Gamaya
Tamaso Ma Jyotir Gamaya
Mrutyor Ma Amrutam Gamaya !

The Meaning—Oh Almighy! Please lead us
From the world of untruth (illusion) to eternal truth
From the darkness of ignorance to the light of enlightenment
From the cycle of life and death to liberation (nirvana).

Thought for the Day

Death is a temporary phenomenon in an unending cycle of life.

The Relaxed Posture/The Corpse Posture

Many students wonder why we turn sideways to the left where the heart is, to come out of the Relaxed Posture; aren't we bringing pressure on the heart by doing so?

Is it OK to get up from our right side? Which is correct and why?

There are two schools of thoughts in yoga philosophy which are influenced by their individual reasoning on whether to turn to the right or left. Both are customary and therefore one may use their own discretion.

Turning to the Left

When we turn to the left, the pressure of the body comes on the heart and serves as a gentle reminder to the heart to regain its normal heart rate and begin normal respiration.

Turning to the Right

Yoga practices in the West typically follow the practice of turning to the right which is also customary in certain yoga practices. The practice of rolling to the right has a symbolic as well as a physiological basis. In India, it is considered more auspicious to enter a holy place with the right foot and in many parts of the world, we extend our right hand in greeting. The right side also represents the East—the place of the rising sun which symbolises an appeal for blessings, grace and bliss.

Physiologically, when we roll to the right to come out of the Shavasan or The Pose of Tranquillity, the heart remains clear and free of pressure. Rolling to the right also keeps the Ida Nadi or the left nostril active. The Ida nadi is one of the main channels of prana or the life force corresponding to the cooling energy which helps keep our body in a state of calmness as we come into the sitting position.

You may pick any option that you like. Listen to your body and decide whether you prefer turning sideways to the left or right. The choice is yours. Your choice may depend on the level of your relaxed state and that will depend on the length of time you lie in the pose and the surrounding factors.

Section—VI
Various Yogic Techniques

(A) Breathing
- Importance of Yogic Breathing
- Step by Step Approach to Yogic Breathing
- Different Techniques in Yogic Breathing

(B) Concentration—Dharana
- Concentration through Breathing—Pran Dharana
- Concentration through the Eyes

(C) Meditation—Dhyana
- Dhyana and its Importance
- Different Meditation Techniques

(D) Relaxation
- What is Relaxation?
- How Does Relaxation Function?
- Different Relaxation Techniques

(A) Breathing

I. Importance of Yogic Breathing

Anything (positive or negative) that occurs around you, affects your breathing.
Your breathing rules your thoughts.
Your thoughts influence your mind.
Your mind governs your mood.
Your mood rules your actions and your actions impact your health.
So, rule your breathing through Yoga and promote your health.

Breathing techniques are as important in yoga as postures and some schools of yoga even believe that breathing exercises are more important than the postures. There are several, different breathing exercises and techniques. Yoga breathing is done by sitting in the cross-legged poses like the Easy Pose (Sukhasan), Adept Pose (Siddhasan), the Lotus Pose (Padmasan) or the Diamond Pose (Vajrasan), where both the legs are positioned in such a way that the Mooladhar Chakra is close to the floor. This has an earthing effect on the internal energy system that steadies the mind.

The other aspect is that around the Mooladhar Chakra at the base of the spine, we have a tremendous amount of primal energy and with regulated breathing this basic energy gets converted into subtle energy and revolves upward in our body through a spiral motion, revitalising and balancing the other chakras.

In our day to day life, our activities reflect on our breathing and our body is in a state of continuous change. Some of the activities that we face are confronting, confusing, pleasing or puzzling and accordingly change our biochemistry and lower the immunity which makes us succumb to various diseases. At times, some disturbing thought patterns challenge our normal, steady breathing turning it into irregular or unsteady breathing that indicates the turbulence. Yoga breathing helps us to remain unperturbed even in the most undesirable situations. This type of breathing prepares our mind to deal with the situation very efficiently and intelligently by finding the right solutions whereby we are least affected.

Whenever we notice any change in our breathing, we can quickly regulate it to a slow and steady pace. Soon we notice a surprising effect on our total existence. We feel that we are in total control of the situation instead of the situation controlling us. Our chemistry also returns to a balanced mental and emotional state.

It is best to practice breathing techniques with a proper understanding. The secret is breathing slowly and steadily. Inhale slowly and let the exhalation leave naturally. Later when this feels comfortable, pause after each inhalation and exhalation. This restful pause complements the natural forces in the body and helps the nervous system to recover, boosting the immune system. Existing diseases or disorders of the body or mind disappear helping achieve a disease-free body and stress-free mind.

The position of the hands and fingers is important for gaining quick concentration. Place the hands, palms upward, on your lap. Join the index finger and the thumb to form an 'O' is called the 'Gyan Mudra'.

The position of the head is also important for stabilising the breathing. It is tilted slightly down to make the chin parallel to the floor.

Beginners may regulate the number of breaths upto 20 times in one breathing session. The duration of each inhalation or exhalation is also kept constant, for instance 4–5 seconds. Steady breathing revives every cell and tissue of the body. Each inhalation brings oxygenated blood supply and each exhalation expels used-up, stale or toxic air from the body.

Deep Breathing or 'D' (Diaphragmatic) Breathing

Our health depends on proper breathing. Everyone wants good physical health and happiness and our entire life revolves around the pursuit of achieving happiness. The ability to feel happy and relaxed depends on how we use our lungs. Therefore, it is essential to study and practice the Science of Breath and its effects on our body and mind.

The manner in which we breathe has an immediate and direct influence on our thoughts. Most people breathe incorrectly using only a small part of their lung capacity and the body and the brain are unnecessarily starved of oxygen. On an average, people breathe 15 to 20 times a minute. In Deep Breathing, we reduce the number of breaths per minute by controlling our breath. Gradually we follow a pattern in which the breathing is slow, deep and rhythmic. This kind of breathing slows down the flow of thoughts and creates a quietening effect on the mind. When we learn to control the breath, we learn to control the mind as well.

It is believed in yogic philosophy that the rate of respiration is directly related to the life span and that each person is allocated a fixed number of breaths. Lengthening each breath prolongs not only the life span, but helps one also gain more vitality. This is evident from Nature around us. Dogs and sparrows, which have faster respiration rates, have correspondingly shorter life spans whereas elephants and giraffes have slower respiration rates leading to longer life spans. The regular practice of deep breathing adds not only quantity to your life but quality as well.

Yoga firmly states that when the breath is flowing through the right nostril—known as the Sun Channel (Pingala), it has a heating and activating effect on the mind-body mechanism. When it is flowing through the left nostril—known as the Moon Channel (Ida), it has a cooling and relaxing effect on the mind-body mechanism. Alternate breathing equalises the effect of the right and left nostrils creating a balance in the metabolism. It harmonises the breathing and biorhythms and promotes tranquillity, peace and alertness of mind, lightness of body, proper digestion and sound sleep. It has the effect of purifying the nerve channels, soothing the nervous system and calming the mind which will be apparent even after a little practice. Above all, yoga breathing develops equanimity of the mind where success and failure and happiness and sadness do not affect the mind much.

The regular practice of deep breathing develops the capacity to recognise the main two layers of our mind, the *Conscious* and the *Subconscious*.

We operate from our conscious state all the time. Whatever exchange of thoughts or emotions that take place in the society get registered in this layer. The negative ones however, cannot be displayed and are passed on and absorbed at the subconscious level. Here they remain since there is a big gap between our social behaviour and inner feelings. This means there is a difference from the image of ourselves that we project to the society and what we really are. If this condition persists, the negative feelings accumulate and these two mental layers go out of alignment. Accumulation of negative feelings causes tremendous stress which over a period of time, can lead to physical ailments and mental disorders. Yoga has a simple answer to rectify this. There are certain breathing techniques which can bridge the gap between our *conscious* and *subconscious* level by bringing transparency and clarity of mind. This means we need not display our negative reactions but just be aware of them. Just by breathing gently and deeply we can gradually sublimate negativity into developing tolerance at the conscious level preventing us from reacting negatively or getting stressed. Ultimately this simple deep breathing practice allows us to experience light-heartedness lighting the way to enter into our *Conscience* where there is nothing but a fountain of happiness, innocence,

313

peace and bliss. Once we get addicted to this divine experience of a feather-light conscience we just cannot tolerate any negativity weighing on our conscience as it feels like putting on extra, unhealthy weight and we wish to shed it quickly by simply breathing gently and deeply.

II. Step by Step Approach to Yogic Breathing

Deep Breathing—Voluntary Breathing—Pranayam

Prana—Bio-Energy (Life-Force)
Ayam—Control/Restraint

Easy to remember about—PRANAYAM: (PRANA – I – AM)

1. Involuntary/Spontaneous Breathing

Normally, in one minute we breathe 10–15 times. Check out what is involuntary breathing by just observing your own breath. Soon you will become aware of your own breathing pattern and understand the distinct difference between inhalation and exhalation. When you inhale, you draw in air from the outside into your body and when you exhale you blow out air from your body into the atmosphere. This is an ongoing process till you breathe your last. This is involuntary or spontaneous breathing which is not consciously controlled by you.

2. Types of Involuntary Breathing

Breathing varies from person to person. Breathing can be slow, fast, shallow, laboured, hasty, irregular, deep or rhythmic. When you observe your own spontaneous breathing, you will know which of the above mentioned category your breathing pattern falls into. When you are angry, depressed, joyful or in pain, your breathing has a different rhythm.

3. Voluntary/Conscious Breathing

When you are aware of your breathing and begin to inhale fully and exhale completely, you become aware of inhalation and exhalation and realise that this type of breathing is different from your involuntary breathing. This is voluntary or conscious breathing.

4. Difference between Voluntary and Deep Yogic Voluntary Breathing

If you decide to become aware of your breathing it may be termed as a voluntary and conscious breathing in which the inhalation and expansion of the lungs is helped by the contraction of the diaphragm and stomach and vice versa during exhalation. The lungs are inflated by pulling in the diaphragm and contracting the stomach. During exhalation, the lungs are deflated by pushing out the diaphragm and expanding the stomach. As opposed to this, in yogic breathing, the stomach and the diaphragm will expand along with the lungs during inhalation and contract during exhalation. When you inhale slowly and deeply inflating your lungs, you lengthen the inhalation by allowing the lungs to expand further by pushing the diaphragm out and expanding the stomach. Similarly, when you exhale slowly and deeply you lengthen the exhalation by deflating the lungs and the diaphragm is pushed up by pulling in the stomach. You will now become aware that yogic breathing involves the lengthening of each inhalation and exhalation as much as you can, while remaining well within the limits of the lung and the diaphragm capacity. In other words in deep yogic breathing when you inhale you will feel that the air is first filling your nostrils, then the lungs and finally the abdomen; while reversely when you exhale, you will feel that the air is expelled completely, first from the abdomen, then from the lungs and finally from the nostrils. It helps to close your eyes in this type of conscious yogic breathing as it will help you realise that the other senses too become sharper. The sense of hearing becomes acute, the sense of smell becomes intense, the sense of touch is heightened and the skin responds to the subtle external changes and the sense of taste too, becomes alive. Overall, closing the eyes help in fine-tuning the senses.

5. *Four Unit Yogic Breathing*

There are four units in yogic breathing. They are—Inhalation—(Purak), Retention—(Kumbhak), Exhalation—(Rechak) and Suspension—(Shunyak) *also known as Bahya or Bahir Kumbhak*. Four unit yogic breathing is begun by observing your spontaneous breath without attempting to control it in any way. Let it be absolutely natural and involuntary. Continue observing your breath for about two to three minutes. Now, inhale gently but fully for three to four seconds. This is Inhalation (Purak). Hold and retain the breath for three to four seconds. This is Retention (Kumbhak). Exhale slowly and completely for three to four seconds. This is Exhalation (Rechak) and finally you will become aware of the pause between the exhalation and inhalation. Hold the pause for three to four seconds. This is Suspension (Shunyak). Once you are aware of these four parts of the breath, it is easy to breathe with total mindfulness in the efficient yogic way.

How is 'four-unit breathing' more beneficial than the two-unit one i.e. inhalation and exhalation alone?

When you inhale fully (purak) and then hold the breath (kumbhak), you allow enough time for all the cells to fully absorb the oxygen. Next you exhale (Rechak) and then when you remain in the pause (shunyak), you allow enough time for all the cells to expel all the used-up air depriving them of oxygen momentarily. This in turn maximises the capacity of the cells and increases their appetite to soak up more oxygen. This subtle aspect of breathing brings about a new awareness in the breathing pattern which otherwise is mostly taken for granted. This helps you improve your breathing pattern and learn new techniques in deep breathing or 'Pranayam' which are used to maximise your capacity to inhale and exhale. This helps you to gain control of the breath, thereby correcting poor or wrong breathing habits, increasing the oxygen intake and absorption and expulsion of impure air thus promoting and enhancing the entire metabolism and mechanism of our body. This especially helps during stressful conditions in calming the nerves. *One point to be noted is that it may not be possible for everyone to continually practice this kind of breathing and besides it may not be absolutely necessary to do so.* Awareness of the breathing process itself is sufficient to calm you down and establish a more relaxed respiratory rate. With regular practice you begin to move your focus from the outer turbulence to the inner calm within you. This experience is very pleasant and satisfying as you log on to the inner respiratory rhythm.

III. Different Techniques in Yogic Breathing

1. *Single Nostril Breathing*

Air is the same everywhere and the nose is the main instrument in breathing. In yoga, the two nostrils are perceived as two channels, each nostril being seen as a separate channel. This is because each nostril has a precise function to convert air into either warm or cool air depending on the inherent property of that nostril which results in two different effects i.e. warmth or coolness to the body. Sometimes our inner energy system becomes imbalanced due to several factors and whenever this happens our immunity is lowered making us susceptible to diseases and disorders. Therefore, to remain in balance and to prevent the lowering of our immunity, we need to use the single nostril breathing technique which enhances the desired warm or cool effect in the body as per the bodily requirement.

(a) *'Moon-Line' (Ida)—Left Nostril Breathing:* The left nostril is known as 'Ida' or the Moon Line. You can breathe through the left nostril by blocking the right nostril in order to activate the left nostril and bring the necessary coolness to the body. Breathe gently without any force.

(b) *'Sun-Line' (Pingala)—Right Nostril Breathing:* The right nostril is known as 'Pingala' or the Sun Line. To bring the necessary warmth to the body, you can activate the right nostril by breathing through it while blocking the left nostril. Breathe gently without any force.

2. *Alternate Nostril Breathing—Anuloma-Viloma*

'Nostril to Nostril' breathing is practised to bring and maintain balance in the energy system by purifying and cleansing the breathing channels. You need to use the Praan Mudra, (Life-force, hand gesture) which is formed by folding your index and the middle fingers of the right hand. Use your right thumb to block your right nostril and inhale gently and completely through your left nostril. Hold your breath for 3–4 seconds. Close your left nostril with your ring and the little fingers and release your thumb from the right nostril. Exhale gently and completely through the right nostril. Pause for 3–4 seconds and inhale through your right nostril. Hold your breath for 3–4 seconds. This is one round. Practice 10 rounds. In this breathing, you need not restrict holding your breath for 4 seconds but can stretch it longer within comfortable limits. Since this is deep breathing, you need to use your breathing span to its full capacity but while doing so utmost care should be taken to avoid hyper ventilation. Always breathe gently but deeply in long and easy breaths.When you start this kind of breathing, you will notice that any one of your nostrils may be blocked sometimes. Do not breathe forcefully to open the nostril. With continuous breathing this blockage opens up and you begin to notice the change as more oxygen comes in and passes through your system. You should not feel any strain while breathing. In fact the more gentle you are, the more effective is your breathing in opening up your nostril. This breathing technique creates an ozone-like, fresh effect in the body in killing any kind of bacteria or free radicals and therefore serves like taking anti-oxidants. With this practice you feel rejuvenated and active and start feeling energetic throughout the day. You can practice this either in the morning or evening, i.e. before lunch or dinner on an empty stomach so that the effect is felt almost immediately.

Benefits of Alternate Nostril Breathing
- Cleanses the entire biological system
- Creates balance in the metabolism
- Harmonises the breathing and biorhythm
- Promotes serenity and tranquillity
- Instils sound sleep
- Eases digestion
- Encourages alertness of the mind and lightness of the body
- Purifies the nerve channels
- Soothes the nervous system
- Calms the mind.

3. Inhaling and Holding the Breath in Antar Kumbhaka Mode for Stamina and Breath Control

Inhale and hold the breath. Check how long you can hold it without feeling much discomfort. This is very helpful in strengthening the lungs, heart and the entire respiratory system. This works wonders while swimming underwater or in any other aerobic activity.

4. Exhaling and Remaining in Pause-Shunyaka Mode or Bhaayya Pranayam to Detect the Tolerance of the Body without Oxygen

Exhale and remain in the pause mode. Check how long you can remain in the pause mode without feeling much discomfort. This is very helpful in emergencies like in oxygen-deficient or polluted atmospheres.

5. Agni Saar

'Agni' means fire and 'Saar' means essence and as the name implies, the 'Agnisaar' breathing technique is mainly for strengthening prana energy.

Inhale completely and exhale, forcefully expelling the air by sucking and deeply pulling in the stomach. Repeat 5–10 times.

Benefits: Many practitioners have felt that practicing the agnisaar kriya resembled having a shot of warm herbal tea (Kashaayam) as it creates instant warmth or heat in the stomach. The inner digestive fire is always present inside the stomach. 'Agnisaar' gives momentum to this fire by fanning it which is helpful to those suffering from constipation, indigestion and eating disorders like mock

318

hunger or loss of appetite. People with a 'middle-aged spread' will notice the excessive flab around the midriff disappearing quickly and almost instantly. It overcomes lethargy and inertia. It strengthens the skeletal, muscular, nervous, respiratory, digestive, circulatory, endocrine and reproductive systems. It rectifies the 'tridoshas' like vata, pitta or kapha. It works on the abdominal muscles, intestines, ovaries, fallopian tubes, uterus, spleen, kidneys, gall bladder, diaphragm and the lower back. Agnisaar should be practiced either in the morning after clearing the bowels or in the evening before having dinner. When you practice this you might feel a slight dizziness due to the expelling of a lot of impure and used-up air from the system. Generally, since the body mechanism is not used to this kind of rapid and intensive cleansing, the brain fails to send the usual messages to the body, resulting in a temporary dizziness. If it continues, then take a short break and try again. Once you are used to this practice, the brain understands the phenomenon and you stop feeling dizzy. Since this pranayam can cause hyper-ventilation or at times even a heat syndrome if done excessively, follow up with ten rounds of 'Sheetali Pranayam.'

Contraindication: People suffering from an acute ear, nose, throat or eye infection or who have undergone stomach surgeries, should not practice Agnisaar Pranayam.

6. *The Dental Breath With 'Cee' Sound-Sheetakari or Sadant Pranayam*

'Sa' – 'with', 'Dant' – 'dental or teeth'

Hold the front teeth together and press the tip of the tongue on the inside of the front teeth. Keep the mouth wide open, inhale through the teeth making the sound 'Cee' and exhale through the nose. Make at least 5–10 rounds.

This is extremely beneficial for strengthening the gums and the teeth and overall dental health and oral hygiene.

7. *Forming an 'O' with the Lips and Curling the Tongue–Sheetali Pranayam*

Stick your tongue out and roll it into a tube like a drinking straw. This is done by curling the edges of the tongue inward, inhaling and sucking air through it and exhaling through the nose. Practice at least 5–10 rounds and in summer continue up to 20–30 rounds. Observe the coolness on the tongue and later the cooling sensation throughout the body.

319

Benefits: This cools the entire system, particularly certain brain centres which regulate the biorhythm, body temperature and mental equilibrium, promoting overall serenity and tranquility. When done regularly it prevents eating disorders and reduces excessive blood pressure and stomach acids. It also soothes the tongue when one feels extremely thirsty and gives a temporary feeling of wetting the tongue with an icy-cool effect.

Contraindications: People suffering from chronic constipation, low blood pressure, severe respiratory ailments, acute heart diseases.

8. *Abdominal or Diaphragmatic Breathing*

Practice slow and deep breathing by enhancing the action of the diaphragm and minimising the action of the ribcage.

Benefits: This action serves like taking anti-oxidants and brings similar benefits like those from the alternate nostril breathing. It slows down your heart rate and brings your blood pressure to normalcy, clears the minds and relaxes all the muscles. It offsets stress in any form—physical or mental. You can perform it even in Shavasan if you wish. This forms the basis for Bhastrika Pranayam or Kapalbhati Pranayam.

9. *The Cranium or Forehead Cleansing Breath—Kapalbhati*

'Kapal' means forehead and 'Bhati' means shining since its practice brings about a state of clarity to the frontal region of the brain imparting light or natural radiance to the forehead. It involves rapid, forceful exhalation and passive, gentle inhalation. It is very much like *sneezing* and *not sniffing.* Inhale completely and exhale, forcefully expelling the air by sucking in and deeply pulling in the stomach. Repeat 5–10 times. This may make you feel light-headed initially and that is because the body normally is not used to and does not know how to expel carbon dioxide completely. However, as and when you continue the practice, this feeling diminishes and the body responds favourably to this intense expelling of carbon dioxide from every cell.

Benefits: This purifies the Ida and Pingala nadis (left and right nostrils) supplying 'prana' or pure life energy to the brain and removing blood impurities and even mental clutter, thereby improving the memory. It has a very powerful cleansing effect on the lungs by clearing toxic and stale air from the system. It cures catarrh, sinusitis, bronchitis, tuberculosis and allergy. It balances the nervous system and tones the digestive system. It purifies the entire system, generates the necessary warmth in the body, improves stamina, removes phlegm and cures respiratory problems. It promotes blood circulation, strengthens the immune system, fans the gastric fire which helps in digestion, improves complexion and the skin texture and for spiritual seekers this practice arrests unwanted thoughts and increases thinking power.

10. *The Bellows Breathing—Bhastrika*

This can be done through the left, right and both the nostrils. However, initially a single nostril is used to clear each nostril. Begin by closing the right nostril with the right thumb. Through the left nostril, inhale and exhale forcefully but without straining, for 10 times. Then breathe through the right nostril keeping the left nostril closed with the little and ring finger and breathe 10 times.

Count each breath mentally, consciously expanding and contracting the abdomen rhythmically. This pumping action should be performed by the abdomen alone without expanding the chest or raising the shoulders. The body should not jerk. There should be a sniffing sound in the nose but no sound should come from the throat or the chest. After completing single nostril breathing, breathe through both the nostrils. Inhaling and exhaling forcefully for 10 times without straining.

Benefits: As in Kapalbhati, it:
- Purifies the entire system
- Generates the necessary warmth in the body
- Improves stamina
- Removes phlegm and also cures respiratory problems
- Promotes blood circulation
- Quickly stimulates the entire body and strengthens the immune system
- Fans the gastric fire which helps in digestion
- Improves complexion and the skin texture
- Increases thinking power.

The Difference between Kapalbhati and Bhastrika Techniques: Though both types seem similar, there are important differences. Bhastrika uses *force on both inhalation and exhalation,* which results in the expanding and contracting of the lungs above and below the level of their resting or basic volume. Kapalbhati on the other hand, involves *forced exhalation* with *passive inhalation.* The exhalation reduces the volume of air in the lungs below the resting level and the inhalation brings the level of air in the lungs back to the basic volume only.

321

11. *The Victorious Breathing—Ujjayi*

Breathing audibly by constricting the throat passage (glottis). The breath sounds like a prolonged audible whisper. The Ujjayi breathing is particularly useful to build up your stamina when practicing difficult postures.

Technique—To begin the practice of ujjayi, breathe through the mouth. Keeping the mouth open, inhale and let the air come in audibly by making a sound resembling a prolonged wind-gushing effect. Similarly, exhale and let the air go out audibly through the mouth. Once you become familiar with this practice, *continue with your mouth closed*. This can be done for 15–20 minutes and performed in any position standing, sitting or lying down. Many people contort their facial muscles while practicing Ujjayi and ought to relax their face as much as possible. Do not contract the throat too intensely. The contraction should be slight and applied continuously throughout the practice.

This breathing sound should resemble the steady and an unending sound of the ocean. It promotes good balance in the body as it acts like a tranquilliser as well as an energiser and has a profound relaxing effect at the psychic level. Ujjayi breathing also increases the internal energy and gives vitality to each and every internal organ, muscle, nerve and blood vein. Ujjayi alleviates fluid retention in the body and removes disorders of the *dhatu* which form the 7 constituents of the body: blood, bones, marrow, fat, semen, skin and flesh.

Benefits:
- Cleanses and purifies the entire system
- Alleviates fluid retention
- Brings the necessary equillibrium to the body
- Improves blood circulation, stamina and vitality
- Removes phlegm and cures respiratory problems
- Promotes internalisation of the senses.
- Stimulates the entire body quickly and strengthens the immune system
- Fans the gastric fire which helps digestion
- Improves complexion and skin texture
- Increases internal energy and thinking power.

Contraindication: Those suffering from a slipped disc or vertebral spondylitis may practice in the Diamond Pose or the Crocodile Pose. Those suffering from acute heart conditions should not perform 'Ujjayi Breathing'.

12. *The Bumble-Bee Sound—(Humming Breath)—Naadh Yoga*

BHRAMAR (sound made by the male bumble bee—deep/low sound)
BHRAAMARI (sound made by the female bumble bee—loud, nasal and shrill sound)

The Bumble Bee Sound Vibrations are powerful and done in two ways. When it is performed in a lower pitch, it resembles the deep, male bumble bee sound 'Bhramar Sound Vibrations' and when done in a shrill, high pitch, it resembles the female bumble bee sound 'Bhraamari Sound Vibrations'. It is also known as Naadh Yoga, 'Naadh' meaning sound vibrations. The universe is believed to be the source, associated with the primordial sound or vibration known as 'Naadh'. When done by plugging your ears with your thumbs, you can hear only your own sound vibrations which may take you through several manifestations of the sounds of a divine and psychic nature.

Technique—Sit in any comfortable pose. Breathe gently. Adjust the fingers and gently place the index fingers of the right and left hands on the forehead on either side of the third eye, the middle fingers on the eyes, the ring fingers close to the flare of the nostrils, the little fingers on the edges of the mouth and the thumbs placed on the ears, plugging them gently but firmly. Inhale and hold the breath. Exhale slowly producing a long continuous buzzing sound, either in the higher or lower pitch. Absorb all the sensations and vibrations produced by these sound waves.

Contraindication: Do not perform this while lying down or if suffering from ear infection.

Benefits:
- Promotes a clear voice with clarity of speech.
- Clears any obstruction in the nose.
- Removes the heavy feeling in the head or forehead.
- Improves lung power, stamina and respiratory system.
- Calms the mind and promotes tranquillity and contentment of the mind.
- Helps singers, swimmers and athletes through improved stamina.
- Relieves tension, stress and reduces high blood pressure.
- Eliminates anger, aggression, anxiety and insomnia.
- Eliminates throat ailments.
- Relieves stress and cerebral tension.
- Speeds up the healing of body tissues.

- Improves the immune system.
- Induces a meditative state.
- Harmonises the mind and directs the awareness inward.
- Excellent for women in labour management during pregnancy.

13. *Namaste Breathing*

In this technique, the gesture of Namaste is used to help increase the breathing capacity through three types of hand positions and breathing.

(a) Abdominal Breathing, (b) Mid or Costal Breathing, and (c) High or Clavicular Breathing

(a) The first type of breathing is the Abdominal or Diaphragmatic deep breathing in which the lower part of the lungs is used. It is best done in a lying position. Join your palms in the 'Namaste' position and place your hands on the navel so that the abdominal movements may be felt. If you breathe with your stomach, you will never fall ill.

(b) The second type is the Thoracic or Chest Breathing in which the middle part of the lungs is used. This is best done in a standing position by joining your palms in a 'Namaste' position at the chest.

Inhale gently, expanding the chest or ribcage and exhale completely, contracting the ribs. In this breathing, avoid any movement of the abdomen.

(c) The third type of breathing is High or Clavicular Breathing where only the upper-most part of the chest and lungs is used. This is best done in a sitting position. The Diamond pose is the most suited. Stretch the arms straight overhead, joining the hands in the 'Namaste' position and folding them backwards and downwards, placing both the thumbs on the upper back. Breathing in this position will be shallow but do not use force to breathe hard. The apex of the lungs is often the most neglected part of the lungs. Therefore, most of the trapped, used-up residual air and toxic waste is accumulated in this region which becomes the breeding place of most of the respiratory diseases. It is, therefore, necessary to activate this part of the lungs. This is done in conjunction with the other two above mentioned types of breathing. However, it is not conducive for everyday breathing as it needs the greatest expenditure of energy with the smallest amount of return.

14. *Harmonious Vibrations of 'OM'—Omkars—Udgeet Pranayam*

Sound Vibrations - '3s'

The Meaning and Importance of AUM/OM

Sound vibrations have a specific effect on our conscious and subconscious mind. AUM/OM is an ancient mantra, a primordial sound used for creating effective sound vibrations through continuous chanting. It is a mantra that is traditionally chanted at the beginning or at the end of yoga sessions to welcome or invoke the higher energy which creates a sense of harmony and unity in a powerful way.

In yogic philosophy it is believed that Aum has more than a hundred meanings. AUM can be fractioned in three letters namely A, U, M which signify the Trinity (Brahma, Vishnu and Mahesh). Aum is also considered as the whole universe as it represents total consciousness—A is the wakeful state, U is the sleep state and M is the deep sleep state. Aum also symbolises the past, present and the future. Meditating on Aum is like dialling the cosmic mobile number. Look at the letter '3s.' It resembles the Sanskrit symbol AUM which creates a protective shield of security, serenity and sanctity. It transports one from this material world to the innermost destination and that is one's true inner self. You become aware of your strength and positive energy. You experience peace. This leads you to a higher level of consciousness and that is total consciousness.

There is a special way to chant 'AUM' and one must have complete faith in it to get the maximum benefits. In reality, Aum is specially meant for those who wish to achieve the difficult state of 'Pratyahara'—the fifth limb in the Ashtanga Yoga System. Once the first four limbs (Yama, Niyama, Asanas and Pranayama) are attained, 'Pratyahara' helps the mind to get detached from the vulnerability of the senses.

Technique: Inhale and hold the breath. Slowly releasing the breath, chant A, then U and finally M as per the phonetics. Think of an imaginary graph which goes up and down. You begin with a brief *Ah* and as the graph goes up chant *Au* till you come to the peak of that mental graph. As it starts coming down, chant *M* till you have exhaled completely. This can also be chanted mentally or silently having a tremendous subliminal effect that works wonders on your subconscious mind.

Benefits: It is believed that chanting Aum through our breath has an uplifting, calming and soothing effect. It improves memory, will power and physical coordination. It arouses the Kundalini power which vibrates and awakens all the chakras. AUM chanting promotes introspection. It protects us from negativity. It improves the respiratory system, functioning of the heart and lowers high blood pressure. Aum blesses us with a vibrant mind by purifying and cleansing it. It has therapeutic benefits as it heals the body, mind and spirit.

If learnt to chant or pronounce properly, the 'Aum' sound creeps into and massages the entire nervous system and promotes well-being. It helps to relax the muscles and reduces stress. It also brings good health and happiness and cures diseases or disorders bringing longevity. There is a great change in the thinking patterns thus removing negative impressions, painful memories, unpleasant past experiences, fear, hostility, resentment, jealousy, etc. Aum builds up tremendous psychic energy therefore positive impressions can be programmed in the subconscious. The practice of Aum increases concentration, memory, logical reasoning and creative thinking. The 'Aum' chanting also clears the throat and the voice modulation.

Contraindications: Hernia.

(B) Concentration—Dharana

The practice of concentration is called Dharana.

Different Techniques in Dharana:
- Concentration through breathing—Pran Dharana
- Concentration through the eyes: 1. Drishti—Thumb-Gazing
                                   2. Tratak—Candle Gazing

Concentration through Breathing—Pran Dharana

Technique: Ideally, this is done sitting in Padmasan (The Lotus Pose) but if found difficult, any meditative or comfortable pose is recommended. Rest your right hand on the centre of your lap, palm facing upward. Keep your left palm facing upward on the right palm and breathe gently for 5–10 minutes. This is called 'Pran Dharana'. Soon you become aware of your whole body which becomes sensitive to the surroundings.

Benefits: The regular practice of Pran Dharana breathing develops awareness of your thought process, talents, self-control and self-confidence, brings about a balance between your will and heart. It promotes a positive attitude which reflects on your thoughts, deeds and speech. Above all, it brings contentment with what you already have and acceptance of life with total satisfaction.

Concentration through the Eyes

Imagine someone standing in front of you and wishing you 'Hello.' What happens exactly? Your eyes meet and you see and accept each other visually. Visual contact involves the use of the greater part of your energy and therefore the eyes are considered as one of the most important sense organs of your body. Whenever you talk or listen to people, you would prefer to have eye contact with them to be able to feel their pulse.

For instance, when you meet your friend after a long time, you will know instantly whether your friend is happy or sad, confident or worried only by the expression in your friend's eyes. How do you know this? It is because our eyes have messages stored in them and speak. They are the windows of our soul because they are intimately connected to our mind and body mechanism, reflecting the mental or physical condition. This is amply proven by the fact that the physical condition of a person is ascertained by the doctor by first examining the patient's eyes. Conversely, when you suffer from any visual defects, your health can also be impaired to a certain extent. This means that the health of your eyes and your physical health are interconnected and interdependent. Yoga, therefore, gives prime importance to the eyes and suggests some simple techniques to keep them healthy through the practice of Dharana, using the eyes.

There is also a close connection between your eyes and your mind.

In yoga, it is believed that wherever your eyes go, your mind follows. If your eyes see too many things, your mind also will be flooded with too many thoughts whereas if you look at one thing steadily, your mind gets the time to lodge on that particular thing. This principle is used to train your mind. When your mind is anchored, it becomes still and improves alertness, concentration, retention, attention span and memory. Especially children need to concentrate, absorb and retain whatever they learn at school. They too will benefit from some of the eye-exercises given below.

In these eye-exercises the simple action of gazing or staring at one object is used. The objects can be different like the sky, the rising sun, the bright full moon or the twinkling stars, any picture of your choice, a candle-flame or it can be as simple as the tip of the nose, the centre of the eyebrows or your thumb. Gazing at any object serves like a psychosomatic exercise because although the eyes i.e. physical organs are involved, there are many physical as well as mental benefits. These are: strengthening the optic nerves and muscles, removing minor defects like a squint or dryness of the eyes and improving alertness, the attention span, coordination, concentration, retention and memory.

1. Drishti—The Gaze

Hold your thumb out an inch away in front of your eyes, in between your eyebrows and gaze at your thumb. Breathe gently and normally. Slowly bring the thumb closer to the bridge of your nose and without blinking, take it further away from you till you straighten your elbow. Then bring your thumb back to the original point and then blink. Your eyes will water or become moist which shows that your eyes are indicating their response to the exercise which serves like the best natural moisturizer for your eyes. Repeat three rounds.

The second movement is holding the right thumb approximately 8–10 inches away from your eyes. Keep looking at the thumb and without moving your head, take the thumb gradually to the right side till it is out of sight. Bring the thumb back to the centre. Repeat the same with your left thumb and then take it to the left side. Again bring it back to the centre. Then blink. Repeat this three times on each side.

The third movement is a circular movement. Hold your thumb approximately 10–12 inches away from your eyes and focus. Slowly form a clockwise circle, of approximately 10–12 inches in diameter with your thumb. Repeat three times and blink. Then similarly make three counter-clockwise circles and blink. Then close your eyes and relax for three minutes.

2. *Tratak—Candle Gazing*

This method is also used as a part of concentration.

Steady gazing or looking at an object without blinking is an excellent eye exercise. Use a candle flame as it is the most widely used object to improve concentration and also because it is easy to hold an *after-image* of the bright flame when you close your eyes. Ideally, the candle is placed at eye level about 18 inches away, in a darkened, draught-free room. As your eyes adapt to the flame, your focus will zero in on the candle flame. This practice leads you to concentrate with pinpoint accuracy and anchor your mind on the flame. Remember, wherever the eyes go, the mind follows as the eyes are the doorway to the mind. When the eyes are steady, the mind too becomes steady. When you fix your gaze on the flame, the mind becomes one-pointed.

Technique:

(a) Breathe gently. Your breath should not cause the candle-flame to flicker.
(b) Start gazing at the candle flame without blinking.
(c) *Do not* stare or gaze *vacantly*, instead look steadily without straining.
(d) When your eyes become moist and begin to water, close your eyes.
(e) Keep your inner gaze steady and visualise the candle flame on your mental screen.
(f) When the after-image vanishes, open your eyes and repeat the same.
(g) Repeat three times and then blow out the candle completely (for safety). (Caution: Avoid undue strain and do not be in a hurry to finish the three rounds).

(h) Close your eyes and breathe gently.

(i) Rub the palms together and place them gently on the closed eyes for 2 minutes.

(j) Sit quietly and relax or lie down and perform Shavasan (the Pose of Tranquillity).

Benefits:

- This improves the eyesight and corrects minor eye weaknesses.
- Cures many eye defects such as dryness of the eyes, floaters, burning, inflammation, short-sightedness, styes, astigmatism, etc.
- Develops the power of concentration, improves the memory and attention span.
- Awakens the inner powers and creativity.

(C) Meditation—Dhyana

The prolonged state of concentration or Dharana leads to Dhyana or Meditation

Dhyana and its Importance

Although meditation is a mighty powered word, in reality it means 'nothing'. When the mind is in its normal active state, doing nothing mentally or having no thoughts is meditation. This is different from mental inertia where the mind is devoid of thoughts due to a lack of energy from exhaustion. Not having thoughts *consciously* is the most difficult thing for the mind because the mind is mental energy and the innate nature of any energy is constant activity. Meditation is making the mind still by disassociating it from its usual state of activity which normally involves a constant search of sensual pleasures. The search for pleasure carries on instinctively even when one is sleeping, waking, eating, walking or talking, in order to assess and ensure that the circumstances one is experiencing are conducive for sensual pleasures.

In fact the unconscious state of having no thoughts is one of the most natural human instincts, exercised unwittingly by all of us without realisation. Every one of us has gone through such inactive moments, sometimes several times a day, when we don't think or analyse and just zero in on nothing. This is a short mental break occurring spontaneously.

At times we are engrossed in some activity or action that is intensely close to our heart and mind. Such activity effortlessly settles our mind into the moment and we feel totally immersed and somewhat beyond emotions. This experience, though subtle, deeply satisfying and very close to meditation, is still not considered meditation. This same experience when used *consciously* as a technique to increase awareness is called Meditation where the state of mind is created to last for a longer time. There is a prolonged contentment which is different from the usual momentary sense of pleasure. Meditative state creates a long term utopia which thwarts the usual emotional roller coaster ride. The mind becomes steadily peaceful and blissful in any given situation and that is called equanimity.

Meditation means different things to different people depending upon their level of exposure and maturity. People meditate for different reasons. Most use it simply as a method for relaxation and to release stress. However, some go deeper and further and use it as a tool for enlightenment, inner awakening, awareness and one-pointed concentration to understand their surroundings and situations and finally to understand the purpose of their existence and its source i.e. the Divine Intelligence. Meditation is also a powerful medium in healing. There are groups who even use meditation to support global peace and bliss.

First find out whether you are truly interested in meditation and if so, what the objective is.

The practice of meditation allows the mind to settle down on any one particular thing and that could be our breathing or chanting. Once we make meditation an integral part of our daily life, we are freed from unnecessary anguish that we often face, most of which is just caused by mental clutter.This kind of awareness created by meditation brings peace and contentment, clarity and enlightenment.

Different Meditation Techniques

The true nature of the mind does not allow it to settle down as the mind is energy and like any other energy, it flows constantly like natural water. We direct the flow of water with boundaries and then turn them into reservoirs. We, similarly, direct our energetic mind by framing it with the boundaries of inhalation and exhalation and allow it to accompany the flow of breath.

Many people are turned off by the concept of meditation as they begin a practice that is either too difficult for them or doesn't suit their temperament. There are various techniques for various temperaments. Whichever technique is chosen, a sustained effort is necessary for the best results.

1. *Japa-Meditation through Prayer Beads*

Japa is meditation through the repeated recitation of holy words or phrases (*mantra*), aided by the synchronised movement of prayer beads. It is a resolve to evolve. However, before embarking upon this spiritual practice, there is a cleansing ritual. The mind must become well established in the basic ethics of non-harming, non-stealing, truthfulness, chastity, contentment, control of the senses, internal and external purity. This means that we should not give in to vices like lust, anger, greed, temptation, pride, ego, jealousy, hatred, unkind and hurtful words, harmful thoughts or actions. When we speak the truth without fear, we are ready for meditation. When the primary resolve has been set right, it will allow us to look within and discover our true self to find peace. It is the best medium through which the life flow (prana) boosts our *sankalp* (resolve).

Technique: There is a universal energy field and there is our own energy field. In order to access universal energy, we need to activate our own energy field to help link up each energy cell with the universal particle. This can be done through prayer beads. Almost every religious practice is associated with a string of prayer beads, the japa-mala, rosary or 'misbaha', used while repeating a name, word or phrase by lightly touching and slipping back each bead, one at a time, using the index, middle finger and the thumb. The beads become the medium between the universal energy and our own energy by acting as a channel between the two. It also acts like a stabiliser regulating the flow of energy into the body and preventing it from coming in bursts. With a lot of practice we establish the bond with the universal energy till our mind becomes still and one with that object.

Benefits: The results from the regular practice of Japa are incredible. Memory improves and self-confidence is heightened. Unknown fears or uncertain feelings disappear to a great extent. Gradually, it dawns on you that life is nothing but an intermission between birth and death. In movie theatres, instead of watching a movie, it would be foolish to give too much importance to the intermission activities like eating popcorn or sipping some soft drink. Similarly, it would be foolish to think about life too passionately and forget the main mission of our existence. If our 'sole' purpose is only to thrive on materialistic things, we lose the 'soul' purpose in life which is to become more evolved and do justice to the human species and its environs. When we arrive in this world, we come as a visitor sent by God but soon forget the main purpose of our existence and start taking the earth and our life for granted. We misuse the earth and abuse our life for our own greed and make our life meaningless. We go away from Nature and finally lose contact with reality. We miss to appreciate nature, the mountains, rivers, the sun and the moon, the stars and rainbows. We are engrossed only in the material world, so much so that even when the time arrives to bid adieu to this earth, we uselessly hang on to the rope of life with the help of unnatural means like a life support system. Although each one of us is allocated a specific time on this earth, we try to overstretch it without contributing much. It is as though our soul clings to our body and is not ready to part with it. We have forgotten the concept of 'let go' without realising that the universe is infinite. Mind is the cause of bondage or freedom. If attached to the material world, it becomes enslaved and if freed from it, it leads to liberation.

2. Meditation on Simple Breathing

The simplest way to meditate is to focus on the breathing and to the sensation of the breath as it enters and leaves the nostrils. Assume that the breath is an object and try to dwell on it without any thoughts. When you inhale, only air should go in and when you exhale, only air should go out. Thoughts should not accompany your breath. Like a sentry, you can patrol your mental innerscape and consciously cast away stray thoughts entering your mind. In case the mind is too restless and defiant, train the mind by labelling each breath by its name as 'in' and 'out' and each thought as 'intruder'. Try not to force your mind. Simply note the sensations as you feel them.This way you will succeed in your initial meditation effort which can then be practised for at least 5–10 minutes everyday and soon you will feel the difference in your mindset and moods.

Benefits:

- Releases stress and negativity
- Overcomes fatigue or sleeplessness
- Promotes anti-ageing and rejuvenation at the cellular level
- Supplies oxygenated blood to the entire system
- Helps you feel the overall sense of well-being
- Helps you experience happiness and peace
- Helps you become more efficient and creative
- Accelerates your inner development

Meditation does not stop at mental experiences alone. It has profound physiological effects resulting, for instance, in a decrease in the oxygen consumption, food consumption, heart rate, respiratory rate, blood pressure and an increase in the intensity of alpha, theta and delta brain waves. This is the key to make the mind relaxed yet alert, a condition which is called 'higher awareness'.

3. *Meditation through a Specific Type of Breathing*

Lie down and place your right palm on your abdomen and the left palm on your chest. Breathe gently and rhythmically and check which palm remains relatively still and which palm moves noticeably. If your left palm on the chest is moving more than the right, it indicates that you are breathing with the chest and not with the diaphragm. If your right palm on the abdomen is moving more than the left, it indicates that you are breathing with your diaphragm. The chest breathing gives you one-third oxygen whereas the diaphragmatic breathing gives you 100 per cent oxygen. The deeper you breathe the more relaxed and focussed you become. If you never forget to breathe deeply, you never forget to forget anything.

4. *Meditation through Image-Visualisation*

Visualisation is fixing your eyes on an object to capture the image which after closing the eyes is reproduced as an after-image by the third eye. Before you begin this meditation technique, you have to develop your inner vision through the third eye. The third eye which lies in the peaceful space between the eyebrows has to be activated and trained to visualise. This can be done by gazing with the two physical eyes at a simple object or a picture of a lotus, lily or any geometrical shape like a triangle, circle or a square. Then close your eyes and attempt to hold the image in front of your third eye. Rest your mind there and enjoy the meditative experience.

A sitting or lying down position is the best but if that makes you restless, engage in moving meditation for instance hopping on to your treadmill. Log on to the rhythm of your pace, matching your breath with every step. In this case the movement or pace is used to develop greater awareness. This practice also encourages mindfulness.

5. *Chakra-Meditation through Colour-Visualisation*

Lie down comfortably. Imagine your entire body being immersed in pure white divine light. Feel the cool air surrounding your body. Disregard all thoughts. Close your eyes. Gently inhale and focus your attention on your navel. Inhale and feel the rise of your stomach. Exhale and feel the fall of your stomach. Access the source of your strength from this belly button. Now let your mind slide down to the basic energy centre, The Root Chakra or 'Mooladhar Chakra'. Imagine the base of the spine drenched in red colour. Think that the root of your spine is immersed in deep red colour and spread this colour throughout your body. Inhale this red colour slowly and exhale this red colour completely.

Focus your attention on the Pelvic Plexus or 'Swaadhishthan Chakra' and imagine it is immersed in orange colour. Unload your mental burden and understand your basic goodness. Absorb the deep, orange colour through the Pelvic Plexus chakra and pass it on upward to the top of the head. Let your energy centre be balanced and harmonised. You begin to feel relaxed. A soothing sensation spreads all over the body. You are drenched in orange colour. Breathe gently. Inhale this orange colour and exhale this orange colour fully.

Visualise your Solar Plexus or 'Manipoor Chakra'. This is your *prana shakti* or solar energy and associate it with yellow golden colour. This is the source of your strength and stamina. Immerse yourself in the golden yellow colour and feel safe and secure. Send this golden colour to the entire body. Your Solar Plexus energy centre is comfortable in golden yellow colour and you are blessed with Divine energy and Grace. Inhale this golden, yellow colour and exhale this golden, yellow colour gently.

Think of your Heart Centre or 'Anahata Chakra' and fill it with green colour. Drench the entire body in soft green colour. Unlock your heart and let it flow with emotions. Your Heart Centre is oozing with light green colour and spreading it throughout your entire body. The green colour is soothing you and you are healing from inside. The green colour is extending your emotional boundaries and love and caring start flowing easily between you and others. Your emotional suffering ends here. You are liberated from sadness and suffering. You are strong and steady. Inhale the green colour gently and exhale green colour completely.

Set your eyes on your Throat Centre or 'Vishuddhi' and fill it with blue colour. Think of the blue colour filling your entire body. You become a channel filled with blue colour. Move it through your entire body. You begin to feel light. The cool, blue colour is gently caressing your body. The blue colour is flowing softly in your veins. Inhale blue colour gently, exhale blue colour completely.

Focus your attention between your eyebrows on your Third Eye Centre or 'Ajna or Adnya Chakra'. This is your main sensor. Fill it with indigo colour. Fill the entire face with the light, indigo colour. Spread this indigo to the rest of your body. Here is your mental strength. Your *Mana Shakti* is filled with indigo colour. The indigo colour blasts your depressing thoughts, ends your circular thoughts and sets you free from the bondage of stale thoughts. The indigo colour now initiates new patterns of creative and inspiring thoughts.

Inhale indigo colour gently. Exhale indigo colour completely.

Now concentrate on the top of your head, The Crown Centre or 'Sahasrara Chakra' and imagine a violet lotus with 1000 petals. Visualise the huge violet lotus doused in that colour as though you are taking a shower in violet coloured water. Imagine dripping the violet colour through your body. Rinse your body in violet colour. Wash away all unwanted thoughts. You begin to unlock and open your heart; unburden your body, feel grounded and feel the calmness of your body. You will gain a crystal clear mind and you will begin to understand your mind. You feel restful and peaceful. The Divine Energy is blessing you. You feel safe and secure. You feel strong and steady. You feel happy and content. Inhale violet colour gently. Exhale violet colour completely.

Summary

And Finally What does Meditation Do?

Meditation is not an intellectual exercise but brings clarity to the mind to find out what life is all about, what you want in life and how to go about achieving it.

Having cultivated an alert yet relaxed mind, you replace a reaction with response. A reactive condition is involuntary, incidental and instinctive but a responsive condition is reacting with understanding. You begin to respond assertively and creatively and more in harmony with your surroundings, with the way things are. You equate with them with ease and confidence.

You may meditate to conquer stress and become free from the harmful effects of stress on your mind and body but be prepared for the motivation to change as you grow in self-awareness and inner peace. Meditation not only changes you but transforms your life for the better. Finally what the practice of mindfulness gradually reveals is that ultimately your entire life can be meditation in action.

Om Shanti Shanti Shantihee!

(D) Relaxation

What is Relaxation?

The mind has one foot in the past and the other in the future and is always vascillating between the past and the future. It never remains still to experience the present moment. Relaxation is bringing the mind to the present moment and making it remain there for a certain period of time. This cannot be done by using force but by exercising through certain gentle techniques.

If you examine the landscape of your mind, you will find many emotions which are related to the past experiences or issues or to the future actions or strategies which constantly interfere with your normal thinking process. The past experiences could begin with the childhood scars and repressed anger, recent anxiety or depression, fears, guilt, worry, resentment, etc., on the one hand and your future hopes, interactions, dreams, strategies, ambitions, fantasies and perhaps wishful thinking on the other hand. This is an internal dialogue in the mind which oscillates between the past and the future. This ongoing process in the mind makes it a control freak that enjoys dominating and controlling us. It is the nature of the mind to think. The problem with the mind is not with its thinking per se, but its retention of the stale and stagnant thoughts and its habit of getting obsessed or influenced with any one thought. In order to break this habit of the mind, and to move away from the haunting or nagging thoughts, there are several relaxation techniques.

How Does Relaxation Function?

The idea of relaxation is to bring new and original thoughts and not getting stuck in mediocre thinking. This needs neutralisation of old habits of the mind like getting habitually stressed, confused or blank while dealing with a dilemma or conflict, getting obsessed with a single issue, over-thinking and mental strain. Relaxation is being aware of the fact that there is a persistent negative thought in the mind. All you have to do is to do nothing about it at that moment and at the same time keeping the mind open and inviting fresh thoughts, some of which will also bring happiness or new ideas. In fact it is unlearning old thought patterns and relearning new methods which help in removing fixed, usual thinking and bringing in a new flow of original and creative thoughts. Soon the mind unfolds its potential for an unlimited capacity which enhances the good side of your nature improving and bringing positivity in the existing situation.

Different Relaxation Techniques

1. *Relaxation through Breath-Workout*

Sit quietly in a comfortable upright position. Interlock your fingers and let your palms face upward and lie gently on your lap. Breathe lightly and easily. Let your attention follow your breathing. When you inhale, feel your breath entering your nostrils and flowing down into your lungs. Do not inhale too deeply or hold your breath for too long; just breathe normally. Close your eyes and focus the mind on your easy, natural breathing. When you exhale, let your attention follow the air out of the lungs, softly out through the nostrils. Repeat this gently. In case you feel that your breathing becomes a bit shallower, let it happen. Return to whatever rate of breathing your body feels comfortable with. If stray thoughts enter your mind, do not participate with them but treat them like your children and tell them gently to stay aside for now, as you are busy with an important meeting and you will deal with them soon. Continue this exercise for at least three to five minutes.

Benefits—With this type of relaxation technique you allow your mind to sink deeper and deeper as though to touch the seabed of tranquillity. You have to try it at least for five minutes to experience this 'high' and you will fall in love with this feeling. The results are amazing. Soon your mind awakens to a new quietude. Your thinking pattern is regulated as if a stabiliser is fixed in your mind. Your thoughts become clear and your speech coherent as you experience the clarity of mind. This is your new formula to give you better perspective and perception to solve problems that becomes your new equation with life. It gives you better insight into day-to-day activities, people, problems, situations and your surroundings in general. This helps your inner strength to surface and your creativity to blossom. Your memory becomes photo-static and you will surprise yourself when solutions to your problems just glide through your mind. Your senses get an overhauling effect.

- You not only see but perceive.
- You not only hear but listen.
- You not only smell but sense the change in the atmosphere.
- You can actually smell the wind, sea-spray, seasons, festivals.
- You not only taste but relish and absorb the nutrients.
- You not only touch but heal.

2. *Psychic Sleep-Yoga Nidra*—*(The Wakeful State of Sleep)*

A Voyage to Relaxation for releasing the fears and healing yourself—Read the following instructions and record them. Then play your voice tape.

"This is a voyage to relaxation. For the next 20 minutes I will be talking to you while you are lying down on your back with your eyes closed. You will be lying down with your eyes closed but you are not asleep. You are relaxed but fully aware. Even if you fall off to sleep, you are not going to worry about it or feel embarrassed. You are going to put all your responsibility on me and unburden yourself. This is a journey to make you feel totally relaxed and truly refreshed. This experience will work wonders for your mind and body and will remove tension and expel anxiety and recharge your batteries with renewed energized cells.

Lie down on the floor, on your yoga mat or towel. Close your eyes. Take a comfortable position and settle down in it. When you close your eyes, you will realise that your eyes become sensitive and serve like a magnet. Your closed eyes will attract everything from your surroundings. You will realise this new awareness. When you close your eyes, your other senses will become sharper and you will be aware of touch, sights, smells, sounds and even taste. This happens because your 'Third Eye' is activated. Your 'Third Eye' is located between your two eyes and cannot be seen from the outside like your physical eyes. It is your body's super sensor and can see and perceive everything around you and project all the stimuli received and perceived by your senses, on your mental screen. In this voyage to relaxation you will be aware of this mental projection and higher awareness which can be used to become acutely aware of your mind and body and also your surroundings without actually opening your eyes. This awareness will help maintain a stable focus and make you concentrate better. There is no need for any kind of fear or anxiety now. Put all your faith and trust in me and relax.

Now inhale gently. Take a full deep breath through your nose. Make sure your breath reaches your abdomen. Now exhale slowly and completely. You may exhale through your mouth, if it makes you feel better. Even if you make a sound while exhaling, that's fine! These are your own releasing sounds. You can say Shh, Aahhh or Hummm while exhaling. Let all the tiredness and tension be released through your breath. Imagine sinking into the floor, deeper and deeper.

Inhale .... Exhale ....
Inhale energy .... Exhale tension ....

340

Keep your eyes closed all throughout and become aware of your entire body, your physical self and allow all your weight to sink onto the floor. Feel grounded. Relax completely. Pass all your tension and unwanted thoughts on to the floor. You will feel your tension dissolving into the floor and you will feel light like a feather. Tightness goes away and lightness comes in. Ease up and feel feather-light.

Continue with your gentle breathing.

Be aware of your toes and relax your toes. Let your feet and the heels relax. Loosen up your ankle joints and release all the tension around them. Relax your shin bones, calves and the knees. Ease up on your outer thighs, inner thighs and the back of the thighs and feel relaxed. Focus on your pelvis and hips. Dissolve all the weight into the floor and bond with Mother Earth. Loosen up your abdomen, the navel and the waist. Release all the stiffness from the midriff, torso and the back.

Remove the stiffness from your shoulders, arms, hands and fingers. Relax your neck, lips, mouth, cheeks, nose, eyes, ears and forehead. Relax your facial muscles. Widen the area between the eyebrows and soften your forehead. Unwind. Let go all the tension. Relax from the top of your head down to your toes. Feel light. Your body feels relaxed now. Your mind is calm and quiet. The feeling of relaxation is spreading right from the top of your head all the way down to your toes.

You become lighter and lighter. Your weight is going out of your body into the floor. You are weightless now. Let Mother Earth hold you in her lap and comfort you to make you feel safe and secure. You feel like a little baby in Mother Earth's lap. Your body feels as light as a feather. Breathe softly. Feel completely peaceful and blissful. You are healing your body and mind. Your gentle breath will calm you down. You experience serenity and tranquillity.

Your body is on a voyage to relaxation and your mind is on a journey to meditation."

3. *Relaxation through Visualisation*

Visualisation to develop the inner vision: Read the following instructions and record them. Then play your voice tape.

"Allow yourself to relax completely. Now gently draw your attention to your mind and peep inside. If you scan your mind you will know that there are no thoughts in your mind whatsoever. Now you are on a journey into the blue sky. You are riding on a white cloud. Little drops of rain are cooling your body. The cool spray smells like rose water which is refreshing you. Your mind is bouncing with joy. You are feeling as light as a feather. You are now entering a beautiful valley full of silvery mist. Your eyes are absorbing the silvery mist. Your eyes are soaked in happiness. You are feeling very happy now. You notice a beautiful rainbow in the distance. The rainbow is full of flowers. The red colour in the rainbow is full of red hibiscus flowers. The orange colour in the rainbow is full of orange marigold flowers. The yellow colour in the rainbow is full of yellow bright sun-flowers. The green colour in the rainbow is full of green fern, lush green fern. The blue colour in the rainbow is full of beautiful blue lotuses. The violet colour in the rainbow is full of gorgeous violet tulips. Your eyes soak in all the colours of the rainbow. Your heart is content to see Nature's beauty. You are enjoying yourself. Every cell of your body is absorbing joy and pleasure. You are savouring sweetness and gentleness. You feel you are in paradise, relishing every serene moment. You are experiencing a sense of harmony and balance. Your mood is very light and cheerful. Every part of body is relaxed and contented. You are happy. You are delighted and you are healing."

Wait for Five to Ten Minutes in this State

Coming Out of the Pose: "Now wiggle your toes, move your fingers. Gently roll your head from side to side. Breathe gently. Slowly raise and bend your right knee keeping your right foot on the floor. Raise and bend your left knee keeping your left foot on the floor. Keep your knees together and gently drop your knees on the floor to the left side. Turn your head and torso slowly to the left side. Stretch your left arm up along the floor and rest your head on your left arm. Place your right arm on your right hip. Breathe gently. Now place your right palm on the floor in front of you, near your heart. Feel the floor with your right palm, push the floor and begin to sit up halfway. Bring your left arm in and use your left palm to push the floor to sit in your usual position.

You have created a powerful and protective energy field around you. Rub your palms in this vibrant, auric energy. Your palms will absorb this energy. Cover your eyes with your palms. Breathe gently and as you inhale, your eyes will absorb this energy that will make you feel relaxed and refreshed. Feel renewed, feel revived; Feel light and happy, feel strong and healthy, feel peaceful and blissful. Now slowly take your palms away from your eyes. Join your palms in 'Namaste' position.

Namaste! The light in me salutes the light in you".

A-1: General Instructions

Consult a Medical Expert before commencing this yoga practice.

1. Follow instructions carefully for every posture.
2. There are 9 interesting headings or key elements in each posture which may serve as a template and help you get an overall view of each posture.
3. Begin each posture with a gentle inhalation and exhalation.
4. After coming out of every posture, inhale and exhale to bring your breathing back to normal. Some postures are hard to perform making breathing either hard or fast and it is important to bring the breathing rate back to normal. This way when you begin the next posture, you have sufficient energy to carry on with other postures.
5. If you have any ailment or particular physical/mental condition which you are aware of, please mention it to your yoga teacher.
6. In case you have any ailment which you are unaware of, you may discover it while performing postures so listen to your body.
7. Yoga postures are meant to detect stiffness or blockage of energy in your body.
8. In case you are in doubt about your physical ailment, please consult your physician.
9. In case you have not understood the posture and are unsure about it, please refrain from doing it until you have consulted with your teacher.
10. Yoga is not merely an athletic system but it works deeper at your cellular level. It stimulates the healthy flow of 'chi' or 'prana' energy throughout the body.
11. Your yoga practice is not your teacher's sole responsibility. It is a shared responsibility between you and the teacher and therefore you cannot hold your teacher entirely responsible for anything untoward that you may encounter while practicing yoga.
12. Yoga is not a religion but a spiritual practice and an approach to 'well-being' with a commitment.

13. Yoga is non-competitive and in fact removes tension caused by competition which blocks off the healthy energy flow.

14. Attending a yoga class can put you in touch with a larger group of like-minded individuals who can revitalise your aura. This is a great way to maintain a 'group spirit'. You may also meet some exceptionally warm and friendly people who may spread and share their kindness with you. You will notice yourself becoming more open and confident.

15. Enjoy your practice with an open mind and a clear heart which will help you increase the awareness of your body, mind and your true spirit. Also at times, remember that making mistakes while practicing yoga is normal & feeling awkward is also natural.

A-2: Instructions for Yoga Students

Please read this before you begin the yoga practice:

1. Please try to come to the yoga class a few minutes early.
2. In each yoga session, you will be performing some new yoga postures which include warm-up, standing, sitting and lying down on the floor, postures.
3. You will begin with your right arm/leg/side but you might see your teacher using his or her left side. That is because your teacher will become your mirror image while demonstrating.
4. When in a pose, muscles that are not involved in the posture should be relaxed.
5. You will be practicing deep breathing and meditation.
6. You will also be practicing visualisation, auto-suggestion and total relaxation techniques.
7. Yoga is about being sensitive to your own body and mind. It is about being sensible to your own physical and emotional needs. It is a healing process and not about getting poses picture-perfect.
8. Each session is so exclusive that no two yoga sessions will feel the same.
9. These yoga postures are specifically, scientifically and specially *designed to detect stiffness or inflexibility in your joints/spine*. Yoga postures remove the stiffness/ blockage and regulate your metabolism.
10. A regular yoga practice breaks through areas that are stiff due to being blocked without vital energy (prana) or due to some unresolved emotional issues.
11. Each time you perform a physical posture, you are working with your physical energy system along with your mental power.
12. Your breath is the main entity that unites your body and mind. You will learn to synchronise each movement with your gentle breathing.
13. Your *easy* pace of breathing will inject life energy in your stiff joints/spine. This energy will flow freely throughout the body to rejuvenate every cell of your body.
14. If you experience pain or discomfort while performing postures, stop and breathe gently. However, you need to continue yoga more than anyone else because pain indicates energy blockage and you need to unblock prana/ energy.
15. Each posture is done with ease and grace and not by force. Please relax and focus your attention on your breathing.

345

16. Each movement will indicate whether it involves inhaling or exhaling.
17. Each inhalation equalises exhalation. After each inhalation and exhalation take a brief pause of 1 second. Focus your attention on this pause. Please be attentive and just follow the instructions on breathing. For some reason, if you cannot keep this pace, please resume your normal breathing pace. (It is not as hard as it may seem or sound.)
18. After each posture, gently inhale and exhale to recharge your breath.
19. Postures are performed in the beginning, followed by deep breathing techniques.
20. Do not force yourself to perform any posture. Stick to your natural limit of flexibility. Eventually, you will overcome all the physical limitations to performing the postures correctly.
21. You will learn some preparatory poses and techniques prior to the postures.
22. You will practice specific postures to stimulate your problem areas/ weak energy spots.
23. You will also learn some balancing postures which help in balancing the cerebral hemispheres.
24. You will also learn some techniques to boost your creativity, memory and ESP.
25. You will not be aware of the time or your surroundings while practising yoga.
26. You will end the yoga practice by performing the Pose of Tranquillity— Shavasan.

    (Coming out of this pose correctly is very important. Avoid any sudden jerks and follow the instructions carefully.)
27. You should feel relaxed, refreshed, renewed and revived after your yoga session. You may take a hot shower soon after the yoga session to avoid muscle soreness.

A-3: Breathing Instructions in Yoga

1. Breathing is the bridge between the body and mind. When you begin a posture, you synchronise breathing with each movement.
2. Each posture begins with an inhalation and ends with an exhalation.
3. Each inhalation lasts for 4 seconds.
4. Each exhalation lasts for 4 seconds.
5. There is a short pause of 1 second in between your inhalation and exhalation.
6. There is also a short pause of 1 second in between your exhalation and inhalation.
7. One inhalation and one exhalation becomes one set of Breath of 10 seconds.
8. You use 2 sets of breaths to go into the pose.
9. You use 4 sets of breaths to remain in the pose. This extended static period in the posture allows the body, mind and spirit to absorb all the benefits of the posture. The first set of breath is to become steady and settle down in the posture, the second set of breath allows you to sink into the dynamics of the posture, the third set of breath is for your mind to reflect on the posture and the fourth set of breath is for your memory to register the posture.
10. You use 2 sets of breaths to come out of the pose. This breathing creates an increased awareness at the physical level. You begin to notice all the sensations in your body (physical sensations). This is known as the increased awareness. With regular practice, the increased awareness turns into the higher awareness (mental sensations). The higher awareness comes directly from an understanding of your mind. When you are aware of your mental sensations, you are no longer uncomfortable in any posture.
11. Totally you breathe 8 times for each posture.
12. Postures give Sthiram (steadiness of the body) and Sukham (comfort of the mind).
13. If you feel pain or discomfort, stop at that level and resume your normal breathing.
14. If you experience pleasure, try not to react to it. Keep breathing gently.
15. If you have any questions, feel free to ask. Thinking aloud is allowed here.

A-4: Salient Features of Yoga Practice

1. This yoga practice adheres to the Traditional Hatha (physical) Techniques.
2. This practice includes fluid and graceful sequences to balance the energy levels.
3. This practice emphasises on precision and form.
4. This practice is perfect for beginners to know themselves better as it serves like a re-introduction to oneself.
5. You learn new techniques and a fresh approach to yoga.
6. You perform all the postures correctly and then improve upon them.
7. This practice can awaken your sense of humour, creativity and psychic powers such as ESP.
8. It is not as physically demanding as Power Yoga.
9. It is not mentally challenging like Kundalini Meditation.
10. It is not Time-Intensive like Kriya Yoga and the cleansing rituals.
11. The practice keeps a comfortable pace from start to finish. A comfortable pace prevents headaches and body aches after the practice.
12. It makes you aware of your limits of flexibility or physical boundaries.
13. It increases your flexibility limits gradually with regular practice.
14. Verbal Instructions on each inhalation and exhalation prepare you for Meditation in the form of 'Meditation in Motion' or 'Moving Meditation'.
15. When you remain focused on a flowing sequence of postures, stray thoughts do not enter your mind.
16. You do not get distracted as you remain connected with the rest of the class.
17. Your yoga practice fosters Self-Empowerment, Self-Improvement, Self-Discipline and Self-Discovery.
18. The choice of postures is designed to accommodate any special need of a practitioner. A customised sheet of postures can be given to you on your request.
19. Your Spiritual Awareness about yourself sets a new record by bringing new dimensions to your perception and perspective.
20. You transform into a 'New and Improved' version of yourself.

348

A-5: Evaluation of Your Yoga Trainer

There are times teachers need to evaluate their own performance and the best way to know is through your students. The following evaluation form filled in by the students not only helps improve the teacher's performance but also helps in bonding with their students and that eventually helps in increasing students' performance as well.

Name: …………………........................   Tel. #…………………………..

1. Does your Yoga session begin on time?
   Yes   No

2. Is the Yoga teacher punctual?
   Yes   No

3. Do you get sufficient practice to your satisfaction?
   Yes   No

4. Are the Yoga timings convenient?
   Yes   No

5. Should the Yoga timings be changed?
   Yes   No

6. Do you feel relaxed after the session?
   Yes   No

7. Do you feel energised after the session?
   Yes   No

8. Have you learned the postures correctly?
   Yes   No

9. Have you learned the preparatory postures and techniques?
   Yes   No

10. Do you have a better control on breathing now?
    Yes   No

11. Have you acquired better control of your postures since you started this practice?
    Yes   No

12. Do you always learn something new in the class?
    Yes   No

13. Do you feel free to ask questions in the class?
    Yes   No

14. Do you get satisfactory explanations in the class?
    Yes   No

15. Do you feel free to express yourself in the class?
    Yes   No

16. Are the instructions clear in terms of:
    English language   Yes   No
    Voice modulation   Yes   No
    Clarity of speech   Yes   No

17. Regular yoga practice in the class:
    (a) has given you a better physical flexibility
    (b) has given you better mental/emotional stability
    (c) has made you 'feel good' physically/mentally

18. Is your yoga trainer professional?
    Yes   No

19. Is your Yoga trainer qualified/certified?
    Yes   No

20. Is your Yoga trainer:
    A performer   A transformer

21. Your Yoga trainer:
    Inspires you   Depresses you

22. Does your Yoga trainer understand your needs?
    Yes   No

23. Does the Yoga session give you good value for money?
    Yes   No

24. Is the Yoga session:
    Boring   Interesting

25. Does the Yoga practice bring out your best potential?
    Yes   No

26. This yoga class is:
    Average   Different from the rest

Any other comments....

A-6: Additional Questions about Your Trainer

Here are some additional questions you could include in your evaluation:

1. Are you satisfied with your Yoga Trainer?
2. Is your yoga trainer trained in exercise physiology?
3. Is he/she certified by a recognised organisation/institute?
4. Is he/she trained in Safety and First Aid including CPR, in case of an emergency?
5. Does he/she explain the importance and benefits of yoga postures?
6. Does he/she create a non-competitive atmosphere?
7. Does he/she make the yoga session enjoyable?
8. Does he/she know your fitness/flexibility level?
9. Does he/she assess your mental/psychological/emotional aspect?
10. Does he/she compromise your health for the sake of the yoga session?
11. Does he/she offer an effective yoga practice?
12. Does he/she create a friendly environment?
13. Does he/she practise yoga postures along with you?
14. Does he/she know the difference between the beginners and non-beginners and treats them accordingly?
15. Does he/she supervise and give individual attention?
16. Does he/she correct your postures with a personal touch?
17. Does he/she choose good/soothing yoga music?
18. Does he/she provide enough space to perform postures?
19. Does he/she teach proper techniques to simplify yoga?
20. Is the Yoga trainer polite and friendly?
21. Does he/she instil confidence in you?
22. Is he/she punctual and regular?
23. Does he/she answer your queries after the class?
24. Does he/she seem concerned about your difficulties/problems?
25. Does he/she motivate you to perform challenging poses?
26. Does he/she force you to do difficult postures when you are not ready?
27. Does he/she give attention to breathing and cues accordingly?
28. Are his/her verbal instructions clear and audible?
29. If you have any other expectations about your yoga class and trainer, could you please take the time off to write them down along with any other comments.

A-7: Special Instructions for Yoga Teachers

1. Make sure your yoga students know that you are a YOGA TEACHER WHO IS:

   (a) Professional (b) Qualified (c) Certified and (d) Registered
2. Make sure you begin the yoga session on time.
3. A teacher should always be more punctual and regular than the students.
4. Always give sufficient practice to your students' satisfaction.
5. Ensure that the yoga timings are convenient for both you and your students.
6. Find out the purpose of joining the yoga class from your students.
7. Ask your students how they feel before they begin the yoga practice.
8. Ask your students how they feel after the class.
9. Teach them preparatory poses and preliminary techniques.
10. Teach them complementary poses.
11. Teach them about contraindications.
12. Teach them introductory breathing series.
13. Encourage them to ask questions before or after the class.
14. As far as possible provide them absolutely correct and short explanations to the point.
15. In case you do not know the answer to their question, you should tell them that you will find out and come back with an explanation later.
16. Remember that the students' attention span is not too extended.
17. You should feel free to express yourself and explain in the class.
18. If you feel any pressure from any of your students, you need to have a talk with that student.
19. Your yoga instructions should be clear in terms of

    (a) Language (b) Voice Modulation (c) Clarity of Speech

    (d) Do not worry about your accent as people are used to global accents
20. Do not become a Performer in yoga poses but become a Transformer for your yoga students. Transform them into better human beings.
21. You should be mentally alert and vigilant.
22. You should be emotionally stable and happy while teaching yoga.
23. You should inspire your students with occasional encouraging comments like 'good', 'very good', 'excellent' or 'bravo'.
24. Try to understand your students' needs.

25. Make your session interesting by using certain accessories like incense sticks, candles, soothing yoga music, flowers, lucky bamboo, crystals, gem-stones, Feng Shui arrangements, etc.
26. Make your session motivating by using props like blocks, straps and eye-masks.
27. Bring your students' best potential out through your good inputs in them.
28. Make your yoga class unique by reflecting your own creativity and individuality.
29. Always be open to new ideas from your students.
30. Do not be fazed by any of your students' baseless criticism as they have their own reasons to do so.
31. Do not be flattered by their sycophancy as they have their own ulterior motives.
32. Differentiate between genuine appreciation and flattery.

1. You should be trained in Exercise Physiology.
2. You should be certified from a reputed institute or a qualified yoga guru.
3. You should have safety training in case of an emergency.
4. You should explain the benefits/importance of each yoga posture.
5. You should caution them with the contraindication of each pose.
6. Create a non-competitive atmosphere in the class.
7. Allow the students to get connected with their selves.
8. Discourage the comparison between advanced and beginner students.
9. Make sure they remain within the natural limits of their flexibility.
10. Assess their physical, mental and emotional level.
11. Teach stretchy and challenging poses but keep safety in mind.
12. Do not have too stringent rules about yoga, be flexible at times.
13. Demonstrate yoga postures to the students.
14. Allow them to perform and watch them.
15. Assist them when they need that little extra help.
16. Manipulate their body if required.
17. Find out and know the difference between the beginners and non-beginners. Many students are not aware whether they are beginners or non-beginners.
18. Supervise each student and give individual attention.
19. Choose some good and soothing yoga music.
20. Do not play favourites.
21. Provide them with enough space/place to perform stretchy postures.
22. Teach them conventional/traditional yoga postures and if they cannot perform them, then teach them the simplified version.
23. Arrange beautiful structured sequences using the complementary poses.
24. Always be polite and friendly and do not get hassled by any untoward factor in the class.
25. Take the initiative to change the unwanted factor to suit your requirements.
26. Adapt to the surroundings in a friendly and tactful manner.
27. Answer all the queries and concerns of your students.
28. Motivate some beginners to perform challenging postures once in a while.
29. Do not force them to perform hard and difficult postures if they are not ready.
30. Instruct them with breathing cues—when to inhale and when to exhale in a pose.
31. Your verbal instructions should be clear and audible while breathing cues are given.

www.ingramcontent.com/pod-product-compliance
Lightning Source LLC
Chambersburg PA
CBHW080411270326
41929CB00018B/2979